Fetal Islet Transplantation

Fetal Islet Transplantation

Edited by

Charles M. Peterson,
Lois Jovanovic-Peterson, and
Bent Formby

Sansum Medical Research Foundation
Santa Barbara, California

Springer Science+Business Media, LLC

Library of Congress Cataloging-in-Publication Data

Fetal islet transplantation / edited by Charles M. Peterson, Lois Jovanovic-Peterson, and Bent Formby.
p. cm.
"Proceedings of the Second International Sansum Symposium on Human Fetal Islet Transplantation, held October 27-30, 1994, in Santa Barbara, California"--T.p. verso.
Includes bibliographical references and index.
ISBN 978-1-4613-5816-9 ISBN 978-1-4615-1981-2 (eBook)
DOI 10.1007/978-1-4615-1981-2
1. Islands of Langerhans--Transplantation--Congresses. 2. Fetal tissues--Transplantation--Congresses. 3. Diabetes--Surgery--Congresses. I. Peterson, C. M. II. Jovanovic-Peterson, Lois. III. Formby, Bent. IV. International Sansum Symposium on Human Fetal Islet Transplantation (2nd : 1994 : Santa Barbara, Calif.)
[DNLM: 1. Islets of Langerhans Transplantation--congresses. 2. Fetal Tissue Transplantation--congresses. 3. Islets of Langerhans--embryology--congresses. 4. Diabetes Mellitus--surgery--congresses. WK 800 F419 1995]
RD599.5.I84F48 1995
617.5'570592--dc20
DNLM/DLC
for Library of Congress 95-13980
CIP

Proceedings of the Second International Sansum Symposium on Human Fetal Islet Transplantation, held October 27–30, 1994, in Santa Barbara, California

ISBN 978-1-4613-5816-9

Originally published by Plenum Press in 1995
Softcover reprint of the hardcover 1st edition 1995

10 9 8 7 6 5 4 3 2 1

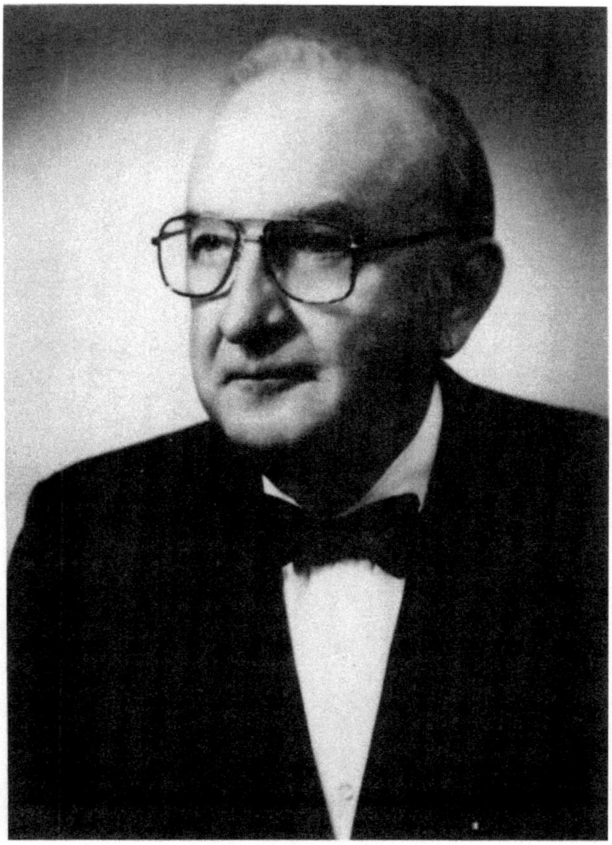

This book contains selected proceedings from a Symposium on Fetal Islet Transplantation held at Sansum Medical Research Foundation in Santa Barbara, California October 27-30, 1994. On October 28, 1994, Paul E. Lacy, M.D., Ph.D. received the W.D. Sansum Award in Science. The W.D. Sansum Award commemorates Dr. William D. Sansum, the first to isolate and give insulin to patients with insulin-dependent-diabetes in the United States in May of 1922. The award is given to scientists whose achievements in medical research have had an impact on the community and the world and who by example and effort have fostered the careers of younger investigators. The W.D. Sansum Award symbolizes the context in which this volume is dedicated to Dr. Lacy. Since completion at Ohio State University of his Masters Thesis in 1948 entitled Studies in Whole Organ Culture, Dr. Lacy had maintained an interest in isolation and preservation of tissue. Luckily for those in the field of endocrine pancreatic studies he soon turned his attention to the islets of the pancreas. Following his doctoral studies at the Mayo Foundation of the Graduate School of the University of Minnesota he made his intellectual home at Washington University School of Medicine in St. Louis, Missouri. At that institution he served as Chairman of the Department of Pathology and Edward Mallinckrodt Professor for over 20 years. He became the Robert L. Kroc Professor of Diabetes and Endocrine Diseases to concentrate full time on research.

Dr. Lacy created a laboratory and environment where a person could become more than even he or she expected. He also communicated a sense of optimism and humor that spread far beyond his own laboratory. His studies of the endocrine pancreas and transplantation have in many ways defined the field. On behalf of those of us who have learned from him, physicians in practice, and above all persons with diabetes everywhere, this book is dedicated to Paul E. Lacy.

PREFACE

Despite the advent of insulin for clinical use in 1922, our ability to control hyperglycemia and prevent the long term sequelae of the disease remains limited. Thus normalization of the *milieu interieur* with physiologic responses of insulin and metabolites remains an elusive but critically important goal. The developing endocrine pancreas provides a model system that speaks to many challenges of the transplantation biologist. Thus the attempt to recapitulate the ontogeny of vascularization, growth and development, immunologic tolerance, and glucose responsive insulin secretory capacity of fetal islet tissue provides a tantalizing possibility to replace insulin secreting tissue in persons with diabetes. Studies of this tissue are also important because of the implications such investigations have for genetic and molecular biological approaches to restoring insulin secretion as well as for providing clues to enhancing the growth and repair of islets that have been the target of autoimmune disease.

Investigators in the area of fetal islet transplantation comprise a small group scattered throughout the world scientific community. Therefore it seemed important to provide a forum where these scientists could gather, share ideas, and achieve consensus such that progress in this rapidly evolving area could be facilitated. The conference would have remained a dream if the support of the Okla Basil Meade, Jr. family had not made it manifest. With this generous core support, other sources were able to contribute to assure success of the Symposium on Fetal Islet Transplantation held at Sansum Medical Research Foundation, October 27–30, 1994. Neither the Symposium nor the resulting volume would have been possible without the support of the American Diabetes Association of Santa Barbara and its Support Group for Parents of Children with Diabetes, Cure Diabetes Now, the Diabetes Treatment Centers of America, Miles, Inc., Mini-Med, Inc., Ross Laboratories, Schaub Design Group, Upjohn, and every member of the Sansum Medical Research Foundation.

The present volume provides the foundation for anyone interested in the areas of fetal islet growth, differentiation, and immunology, as well as transplantation. The ultimate success of the book will be the stimulation of clinical protocols that provide non-toxic achievement of insulin independence as defined in the Consensus Statement at the end of this volume. We feel honored for the opportunity to be able to help foster that goal and work with this group of scholars.

Charles M. Peterson, M.D.
Lois Jovanovic-Peterson, M.D.
Bent Formby, Ph.D., D.Sc.
Santa Barbara

PREFACE

CONTENTS

PROTOCOLS FOR ENHANCING FUNCTION OF FETAL ISLETS IN VITRO AND FOLLOWING TRANSPLANTATION

Alberto Hayek* and Gillian M. Beattie

The Islet Research Laboratory at The Whittier Institute
Department of Pediatrics
The University of California, San Diego—School of Medicine
9894 Genesee Avenue
La Jolla, CA 92037

INTRODUCTION

The significant differences in the in vitro and in vivo behavior of fetal islet cells from different animal species are important considerations in the interpretation of experimental data, specially as they are made to apply to the study of growth and differentiation of human fetal pancreatic cells. For example, methods that work very efficiently in rats for fetal islet isolation (24) prove considerably less efficient in mice despite good matches of gestational age, enzymatic and media conditions. Thus, if methods to isolate fetal endocrine cells produce different results, not surprisingly similar methods to enrich and enhance function of purified endocrine cell populations in different species, are also bound to produce distinct results as already shown in reports dealing with responses to growth factors (6,40), pharmacologic agents and more conventional peptide hormones such as insulin, growth hormone and prolactin (9). Of importance also in the interpretation of functional effects on islets is the consideration of whether homologous hormones are used to induce specific effects (10).

Because of the above considerations and of the main interest which attaches to human fetal pancreatic islets and in view of their potential role in therapy, and because these facts have guided our efforts, this review will focus primarily on the biology of human fetal islets.

TISSUE PROCUREMENT, PROCESSING AND CHARACTERIZATION

It seems evident by now that fetal tissue obtained from spontaneous abortions or ectopic pregnancies will be neither suitable nor adequate for biological studies and much

* Correspondence: Alberto Hayek, M.D., The Whittier Institute, 9894 Genesee Avenue, La Jolla, CA 92037. Telephone: (619) 450-4257; FAX: (619) 558-3495.

Fetal Islet Transplantation
Edited by C. M. Peterson, L. Jovanovic-Peterson, and B. Formby, Plenum Press, New York, 1995

less for transplantation in insulin-dependent diabetes (8). Thus, tissues from elective abortions constitute the most significant source of cells for developmental, clonal expansion and future gene therapy studies. It is anticipated, however, that the future introduction of RU486 will substantially decrease the availability of fetal tissues for basic and clinical research, an important issue where significant amounts of cells may be needed if cell-based insulin replacement in type I, or even type II diabetes using fetal tissue reaches the stage for clinical trials.

The human pancreatic tissue is obtained at one of several procurement centers after termination of pregnancy by dilatation and extraction between 12 and 24 weeks gestation. The tissue arrives at our laboratory after periods of 5 min and 24 h of warm and cold ischemia, respectively. For the last 3 years, viability of tissues under these conditions has exceeded 98%, a fact that facilitates the transport of tissues across the country without the worry of tissue necrosis. After arrival, the tissue is minced into l-mm pieces in cold Hanks' Balanced Salt Solution and digested with 5.5 mg/mL collagenase while shaking vigorously for about l5' in a water bath at 37°C. Contrary to the situation with the adult pancreas where the type and lot number of collagenase is crucial to successful islet isolation, most commercially available collagenases appear equally suitable for digestion of human fetal tissue. After several washes with the same salt solution, the digest is placed into 60-mm petri dishes that discourage cell attachment in RPMI-1640 containing l0% pool human serum, obtained from discarded umbilical cords, and antibiotics (l00 U/mL penicillin, 0.1 mg/mL streptomycin and l mg/mL Amphotericin-B). Medium is changed every other day.

Generation of Islet-Like Cell Clusters (ICCs)

After 3-5 days in culture, following tissue digestion with collagenase, islet-like cell clusters are easily identified and recovered using a stereomicroscope and positive displacement micropipeters. This digestion-culture method, originally described for the fetal rat pancreas (24), leads to the isolation of large number of rat islets but, in the case of the human fetal pancreas, the end results are ICCs as originally termed by Sandler et al (48). Most of the studies reviewed here from our laboratory have used ICCs rather than fresh or uncultured tissue as discussed in the Chapter by Dr. Bernard Tuch. A simple procedural difference that may be important in the generation and eventual in vitro and in vivo behavior of ICCs is that the Swedish investigators (29,46,48) used culture dishes that allow cell attachment while we used exclusively petri dishes that discourage attachment and incubation times of 5 to 7 days. Under direct vision with a stereomicroscope, we pick ICCs with diameters ranging from 50 to 150 μm (Fig. 1). The average number of ICCs collected after 7 days in culture is 13.4 per mg of starting tissue and the yield is not affected by gestational age between 17 and 24 weeks (38).

Cellular Content of ICCs

The cellular composition of ICCs is very heterogeneous comprising epithelial cells, stromal cells, primarily fibroblasts and endothelial cells. ICCs with high epithelial content (~ 75% of the total surface area) are smaller and more translucent. Because we recently reported on the differential integrin expression in epithelial cells in the human fetal pancreas (30), we took advantage of the high affinity binding between the invasin protein of *Yersinia pseudotuberculosis* and many βl integrins to isolate highly enriched populations of fetal pancreatic epithelial cells in ICCs. In the epithelial rich ICCs, the total surface area of the combined hormone-containing endocrine cells is about 13% with insulin-positive cells usually occupying only ~ 3%. Thus, most of the epithelial cells within ICCs we believe are the precursors of the endocrine cells that eventually will form the adult pancreatic islet.

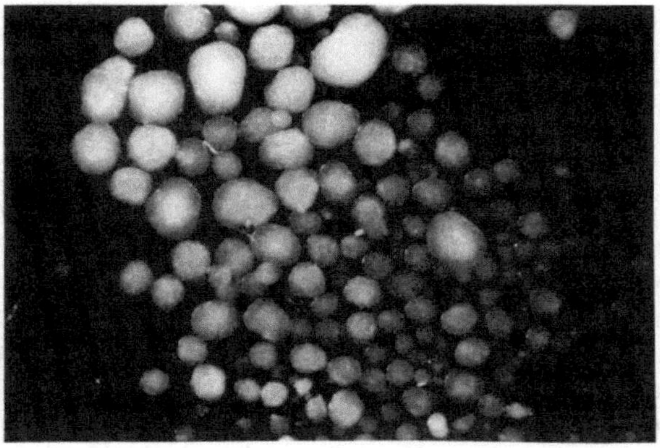

Figure 1. Photomicrograph of ICCs from collagenase digested fetal pancreas showing the typical heterogeneity of preparation; original magnification 35x, reduced 66%.

The Search for Cellular Markers of Endocrine Cell Precursors

Evidence from several sources indicates that the ductal epithelium in the embryonic pancreas is the source of the endocrine tissue that as the pancreas matures, localizes in the islets of Langerhans (4). Expression of catecholaminergic enzymes such as tyrosine hydroxylase was first suggested by Teitelman et al (53) in the rodent pancreas to represent cells with the potential for transformation into endocrine cells. Further observations by the same authors showed the transient co-expression of the enzyme in glucagon positive cells during development in vitro and during regeneration following removal of the dorsal pancreas at 11 days of gestation in the mouse (54). In transgenic mice models of islet regeneration, Gu et al (19) have found transitional cells in regenerating pancreas as duct epithelial cells co-expressing carbonic anhydrase II and amylase, an exocrine enzyme. As the cells progress through their differentiating pathways and begin their migration from the duct, the dual expression of exocrine and endocrine products is also observed in the progression to fully functional and strictly differentiated endocrine cells.

Beattie et al (4), in our laboratory, recently showed that acid β-galactosidase (β-gal) could be used as a developmentally regulated marker of endocrine cell precursors in the human fetal pancreas. In these studies, ICCs rich in the enzyme, after transplantation into nude mice showed a high rate of endocrine cell differentiation which coincided with a significant decrease in β-gal content in the graft 12 weeks after transplantation. In the fresh pancreas, the enzyme localized to discrete areas within ductal epithelium and sorting analysis of β-gal rich cell populations demonstrated that the enzyme was found mainly in epithelial cells and that tyrosine hydroxylase in the fetal pancreatic cells colocalized strictly to high β–gal containing cells. We have been unable in our laboratory to demonstrate the exocrine enzyme amylase in the fetal pancreas. In fact, using sensitive ribonuclease protection assays, amylase transcripts were not detected in any of the fetal pancreases studied, but it was present postnatally (32). Thus, the expression of this enzyme as a marker of transitional cells in the fetal pancreas is probably restricted to the experimental model in mice induced by the transgene state. The only other exocrine protein that we have looked for expression of the gene is the reg gene in the human fetal pancreas. Its expression, quite low before 16 weeks gestation shows a sudden increase in the mRNA levels through 24 wk gestation, at which point it reaches levels comparable to those seen in the adult pancreas (32). Localized by in situ hybridization to the exocrine pancreas in our human fetal preparations, the reg gene may be an important regulatory element in processes involving differentiation and/or replication of fetal β-cells (41).

FUNCTIONAL ASPECTS IN VITRO

Fetal vs Adult Human Islets

Inasmuch as there are species differences in islet cell development and function, significant differences are also present in the in vivo and in vitro function of human fetal as compared to adult islets. The human fetal islet cell is virtually glucose unresponsive in terms of insulin release, and only around 20 weeks of gestation is a low-magnitude monophasic insulin response elicited; a biphasic type of response, characteristic of mature β-cell is clearly a postnatal event (42). The nature of the glucose unresponsiveness is not known but it does not appear to be related to the lack of expression of the glucose sensor apparatus, constituted by the enzyme glucokinase and the glucose transporter 2, since the gene transcripts for these proteins have been detected as early as in the 13-wk fetal pancreas (32). Also, the unresponsiveness is selective to glucose since other secretagogues which increase cyclic AMP in the β-cell elicit brisk insulin responses (36).

Significant differences are also present when adult and fetal cells are kept in culture and put in conditions that facilitate attachment, migration and in the case of fetal cells, proliferation. Isolated adult islets kept free floating, for 7 days, in culture medium containing glucose in concentrations exceeding 11 mM glucose, show significant impairment in insulin release in response to higher concentrations of glucose (16). If, on the other hand, human adult islets are placed in culture conditions that facilitate attachment, such as culture dishes coated with the matrix produced by bovine corneal endothelial cells, insulin release in response to glucose is, if anything, very much enhanced (3). More surprisingly, insulin release under these conditions is further enhanced when the attached islets are kept in medium containing 22.2 mM glucose or insulin in concentrations as high as 10 μg/ml and, if fibroblastic cells are eliminated from the culture (3).

In contrast to the above information, free floating ICCs at 20 weeks gestation release more insulin into medium than clusters attached to substrates similar to those used in the culture of adult islets (Fig. 2). No difference was observed in ICCs obtained at 18 or 20 wk gestation, and both showed the same decrease in insulin release over the 7 day culture period (Fig. 3). If the cultures are continued for as long as 18 days, insulin release ceases after 2 weeks in the monolayer cultures, but it is still measurable in the free-floating ICCs (Fig. 4). Not unexpectedly, preliminary evidence obtained in our laboratory shows a negative correlation between cell replication and function in cultured fetal pancreatic cells.

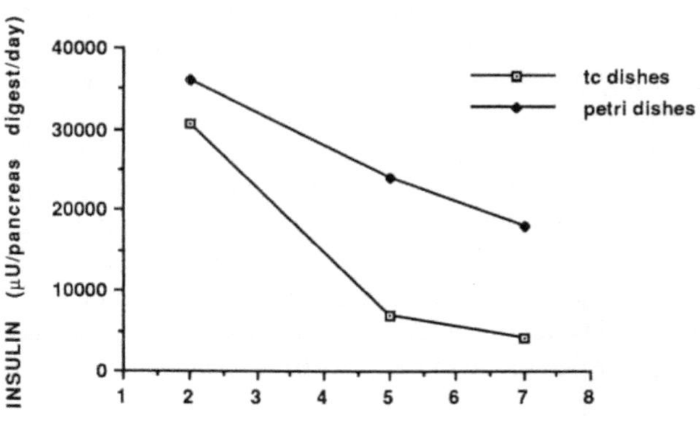

Figure 2. Difference in insulin release from cell clusters (50-150 μM) kept free floating vs. cell clusters attached in tissue culture dishes.

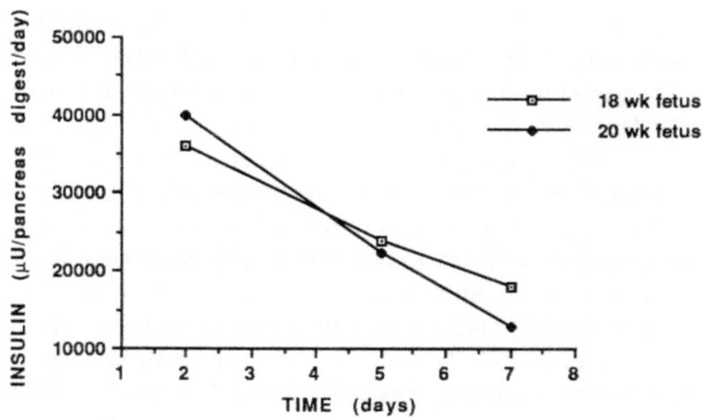

Figure 3. Decrease in insulin release into medium from cell clusters in the first week of incubation.

Effects of Growth Factors

The importance of growth factors in human fetal islets is described in detail in the Chapter by Dr. Debra Hullett. Here we would like to summarize some of our studies of selected growth factors for their morphogenic, mitogenic and insulinotropic activity in primary organ cultures of midgestation human fetal pancreases. As detailed below, of all the growth factors tested in our system, hepatocyte growth factor/scatter factor (HGF/SF) gave the most interesting results.

HGF/SF, first recognized as a growth factor involved in hepatic regeneration, exerts a wide variety of biological effects on many cell types, particularly of epithelial and endothelial origin (18,51). These activities include mitogenic activity for hepatocytes and several other epithelial cells, potent mitogenic (motility-inducing) effects on many epithelial cell lines in vitro (cell scattering (62)), a morphogenic effect on kidney tubular cells (tubule formation (35) and breast carcinoma cells (lumen formation (55)), and an angiogenic effect, which is due to mitogenic and motogenic stimulation of vascular endothelial cells (11,17). It appears that the HGF/SF gene is only expressed in cells of mesenchymal origin (50), although the immunoreactive protein may be detected also in epithelial cells (63). However, mesenchymal cells in general do not express the HGF-receptor, which is the product of the c-met proto-oncogene (7). In contrast, the receptor is highly expressed in many epithelial tissues (13,31,43,50), including pancreas (43,50). Based on this pattern of expression it has been proposed that HGF/SF could act as an important mediator of signal exchange between mesenchyme and epithelium during development (50). HGF/SF has been detected in tissue

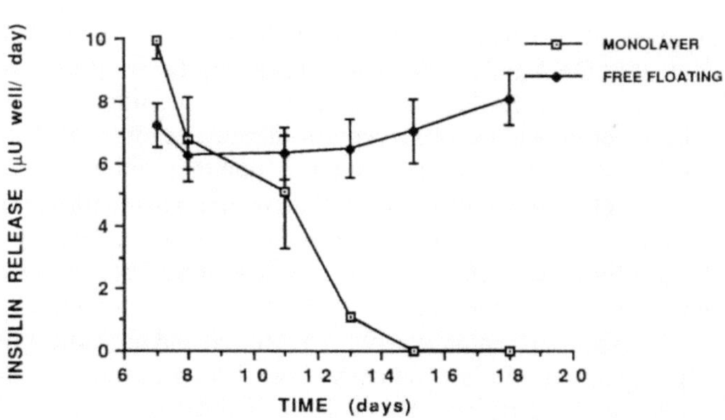

Figure 4. Insulin release from free floating clusters into medium compared to cells in monolayer formation.

extracts of rabbit pancreas, and localized by immunohistochemical analysis in the exocrine portion (63). In a subsequent report, high HGF/SF immunocrossreactivity was found in glucagon-containing islet cells in both man and rat (56) indicating a possible role for HGF/SF in islets.

Previous studies have suggested a role for the insulin-like growth factors in fetal islet development. In the rat, IGF-I is produced by islet cells, which also express IGF-I receptors, and the peptide is mitogenic for endocrine cells (reviewed in (25,52)). In the regenerating rat pancreas, IGF-I expression is focally increased in areas of ductal proliferation (34,49). However, in the human fetal pancreas, while IGF-II is highly expressed, IGF-I is barely detectable (34). TGF-α is structurally related to EGF, and both peptides bind to the same receptor (EGF-R). TGF-α has traditionally been considered as a fetal form of EGF, but is now known to be expressed also in adult tissues (12). A high level of TGF-α expression has been detected in the human fetal pancreas, involving both the acinar and islet cells (33). EGF-R is also expressed in the fetal pancreas (33) and in the ICCs (34).

The induction of endocrine development in the fetal islet is mediated by fetal mesenchyme (14) and several of the growth factors and other mediators of mesenchymal-epithelial interaction have been identified. These include the epithelial-cell specific FGF-7 (17), HGF/SF (51) and TGF-α and -β.

Identification of HGF/SF as Mitogen for Human Pancreatic β-Cells

There have been relatively few studies exploring the role of growth factors in islet cell growth and development. Most of the work was performed with isolated fetal or neonatal rodent islets, and generally the effects of a single, or a few growth factors were tested (reviewed in (25,52)). Because the experimental conditions in these studies often involved the use of highly purified endocrine cells, the assays may not have been suitable for the detection of important developmental effects, such as the proliferation and differentiation of endocrine precursor cells. For this reason, we used primary organ cultures, ICCs, of midgestational human fetal pancreases to examine the potential role of selected growth factors. Although only a small minority of the cells in the ICCs express islet hormones, significant β-cell differentiation can be induced in vitro, and especially after transplantation into nude mice as previously indicated (5,39,48).

We examined the morphogenic, mitogenic and insulinotropic activities of several growth factors, including those that are thought to be important in epithelial growth and morphogenesis, such as keratinocyte growth factor (FGF-7) and HGF/SF, but that had not previously been studied in the context of pancreatic islet development.

In our laboratory, out of all the different growth factors tested, HGF/SF was the only one that clearly induced in vitro development of epithelial cell clusters containing increased numbers of β-cells (40). Our data indicate an increase in the number of ICCs, in the total content of DNA and insulin, and in the proportion of β-cells within the HGF/SF-treated ICCs (Figs. 5 and 6). HGF/SF increased the total number of β-cells 3- to 6-fold during a 6-day culture period and the observed 3-fold higher number of BrdU-labeled insulin-positive cells confirmed that this was at least partly due to a mitogenic effect of HGF/SF on β-cells.

FGF-2 induced a nearly 3-fold increase in the formation of ICCs from digested human fetal pancreatic tissue. However, the total insulin content was increased only 1.9-fold, and the insulin content per DNA was decreased by 30%, implicating that the expansion of cell mass was mainly due to the growth of non-insulin-containing cells.

As described previously (15) Hullett and her colleagues have described enhancement of β-cell activity in fetal pancreatic pro-islet preparations cultured with IGF-I. In our model system, under different experimental conditions, exogenously added IGFs had little effect.

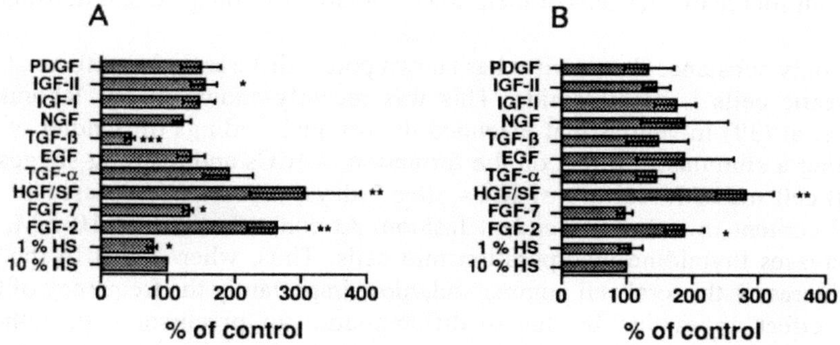

Figure 5. Effects of growth factors on the formation of ICCs (A) and their total insulin content (B) after 5 days in culture. *;**;***; p<0.05; 0.01; 0.001.

This might be due to a high endogenous level of the IGFs and their binding proteins, either present in the human serum used or produced by cells in culture. However, when we used a monoclonal antibody to block the IGF-I receptor, utilized by both IGF-I and IGF-II, the marked inhibition of ICC formation suggested that the IGFs played a limited role in this process. The same is true for PDGF, which has been shown to be mitogenic for fetal rat islet cells (31). We were also unable to detect any effect of PDGF or NGF.

The highest level of insulin content per DNA was obtained when TGF-β was added to the culture medium. This was, however, entirely due to the decrease in DNA content, a reflection of the dramatic decrease in the number of epithelial cells. These results were not surprising since TGF-β is known to be a potent inhibitor of the proliferation of many epithelial cell types (23,44). We also showed that blocking TGF-β with a neutralizing antibody results in effects opposite to those of the peptide, indicating that TGF-β exerts an inhibitory action on epithelial cell proliferation. However, the increase in total insulin content after culture with the TGF-β antibody suggests that TGF-β also plays a role in the regulation of β-cell growth and/or differentiation. These data are summarized in Figures 5 and 6.

Thus, according to this information, HGF/SF is the most potent stimulus for ICC formation, and most importantly, HGF/SF is the only factor that increases the epithelial and β-cell content of cultured fetal pancreatic tissue (40). Our studies have provided the first evidence for a significant role of certain mesenchyme-derived heparin-binding growth factors in human islet development. Particularly, HGF/SF may prove useful in generating a

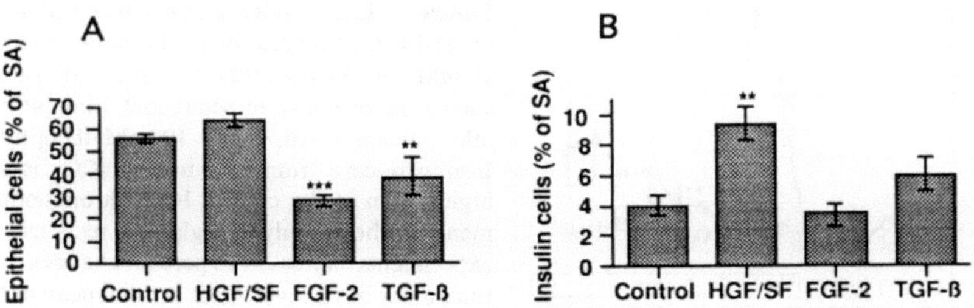

Figure 6. Effect of selected growth factors on the proportion of epithelial cells (A) and β-cells (B) within the ICCs. S.A., surface area. **;***; p<0.01;0.001.

more abundant source of islet cells or their precursors for physiological and transplantation studies.

The only substance that in vitro has shown potent differentiating effects of human fetal pancreatic cells is nicotinamide. This was recently shown in our laboratory by Otonkoski et al (39) in studies that extended the original findings of Sandler et al (47) demonstrating a stimulatory effect on the formation of ICCs and a strong suggestion of increased β-cell mass. In culture of ICCs after 7 days, nicotinamide increases insulin release and content in a dose-dependent fashion. At concentrations of 10 mM, nicotinamide increases thymidine incorporation into cells. Thus, when added to the culture medium it increases the total cell number and, more importantly the frequency of β-cells. This latter effect appears to be due to differentiation of precursor cells rather than replication of existing β-cells, a conclusion based mainly on morphological observations. Nicotinamide also increases the transcription of islet hormone specific genes which correlates nicely with induced maturation of glucose-induced insulin secretion. When ICCs previously exposed to nicotinamide were perifused, insulin release exhibited a 4-fold first-phase insulin release and, although attenuated, a second phase was also evident (Fig. 7). All of these findings support the view of nicotinamide as a true enhancer of endocrine differentiation in the human fetal pancreas.

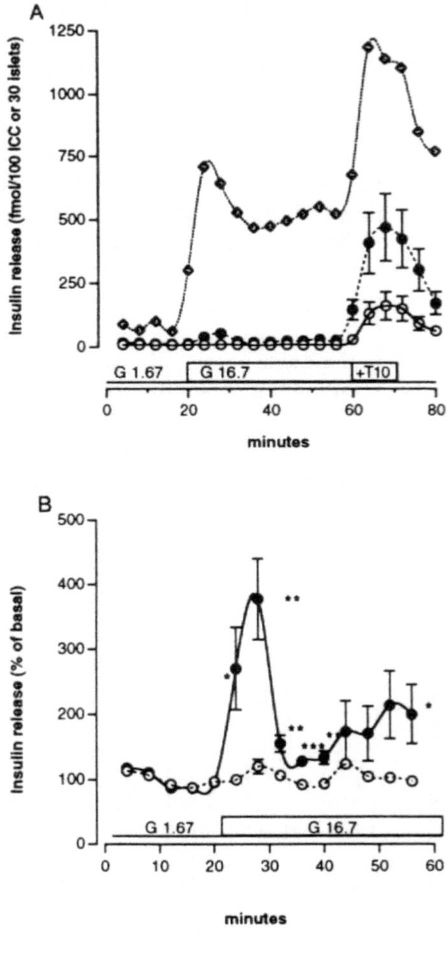

Figure 7. Insulin release in perfusion of adult islets (–) or fetal ICCs cultured for 7 d in standard medium (○) or 10 mM NIC medium (●). A, expressed in absolute units, shows the response to sequential stimulation with 16.7 mM glucose (G16.7) and 10 mM theophylline (T10). Insulin release from NIC-treated ICCs is significantly higher than in the control ICCs throughout the experiment. B shows only the glucose response of the fetal experiments expressed as percent changes from the prestimulatory basal level. Data are the mean of two separate experiments with adult islets and the mean +SEM of six fetal experiments; very small error bars are not shown. *;**;***; $p<0.05$; 0.01; 0.001***.

FUNCTIONAL ASPECTS IN VIVO

ICCs After Transplantation

Korsgren et al (28) have shown that pretreatment of fetal porcine pancreatic cells in culture with nicotinamide accelerates reversal of diabetes after transplantation to nude mice (28). In contrast, we have not been able to enhance function of transplanted human fetal pancreatic cells into nude mice. Thus, while nicotinamide in vitro causes the remarkable effects described above, pretreatment of human fetal pancreatic cells with nicotinamide causes no discernible effects (39). Our results however do not exclude the possibility that the same treatment protocol in vitro of human fetal cells, followed, for example, by nicotinamide supplementation of the drinking water during the period of engraftment, might either enhance function or accelerate differentiation of fetal endocrine cells decreasing in this way the mandatory 12 wk period necessary to obtain full function (4). We have recently demonstrated that grafts of ICCs treated in vitro with HGF/SF are morphologically and functionally similar to grafts of untreated ICCs (37).

Short- and Long-Term Effects on Morphology and Function

In a longitudinal study undertaken to study the growth and differentiation of β-cells in human fetal ICCs implanted under the kidney capsule in normoglycemic mice over a 12 month period, we showed that grafted tissue, predominantly ductal in appearance, was unresponsive to glucose 2-4 weeks after grafting, and only a few sporadic cells were insulin positive. Circulating serum human C-peptide was first detectable 2 months post implantation in 40% of animals. At that time transplanted tissue seemed more abundant, consisting of both endocrine and exocrine elements with 10% of the surface area immunostaining for insulin. The grafted endocrine tissue had assumed the trabecular column-like architecture of adult islets by 3 months (Fig. 8) with a concomitant 3-4 fold increase in serum human-C peptide concentration after glucose stimulation in all animals. This finding indicated functional maturation of fetal β-cells, now comprising 55% of the surface area of the graft, which represents ~20 fold increase over the starting material (4). It is important to note that after 5 days of tissue culture and 3 months engraftment, the "absolute age" of cells from 18-24 week fetuses would be 32-37 weeks, close to term, when normal physiological maturation is expected. Transplanted tissue was capable of releasing C-peptide for at least 12 months (see Table 1) and the proportion of insulin containing cells in the graft was comparable to that of the grafts at 3 and 4 months (Fig. 9), showing that human ICCs after transplantation

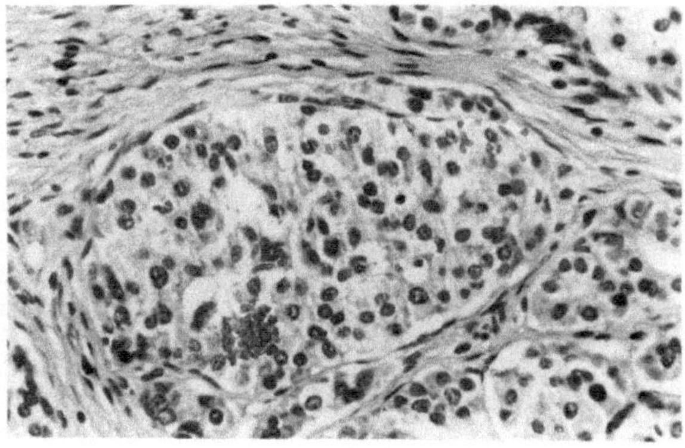

Figure 8. Photomicrograph of grafted human fetal ICCs 3 mo after transplantation under the kidney capsule of a nude mouse demonstrating the morphological appearance of adult islets; original magnification 800x, reduced by 66%.

Table 1. Basal and Glucose Stimulated Serum Human C-peptide Levels in Grafted Athymic Nude mice.

Time since engraftment	C-peptide (pmols/L) Basal (0 min)	Stimulated (30 min)	Stimulation index
2 weeks	0,0,0,0,0	0,0,0,0,0	
1 month	0,0,0,0,0	0,0,0,0,0	
2 months	0,0,0,101,133	0,0,0,118,232	
3 months (n=6)	255 ±32	924 ±165	3.6±0.4
4 months (n=5)	261± 48	1120 ±216	4.3±0.5
12 months (n=3)	265 ±71	540 ±75	2.2±0.4*

Data are expressed as pmols /L ± s.e.m. serum human C-peptide measured before and 30 min after stimulation with 3 g/kg glucose i.p.
* p>0.02 compared to 4 month stimulation index. Reproduced with permission from Cell Transplantation ( ).

under the kidney capsule remain functionally viable for virtually the life span of immunocompromised rodents (1).

Implantation Site

Not taking into account the issue of rejection, it is likely that factors such as the site of implantation will place a critical role in differentiation, replication and adequacy of response to physiologic stimulation. After transplantation of fragments of human fetal pancreas to athymic nude mice, Tuch et al compared the subcutaneous site to the kidney capsule, spleen and liver and found the subcutaneous space inferior (58,59). In most studies of transplantation of human fetal pancreas to nude mice, the kidney capsule has been the preferred site (4,26,27,39,48,57,60,61). In our laboratory, using a syngeneic rat model, the transplantation of neonatal islets into diabetic rats produced equally good results in the metabolic response when the grafts were placed into the spleen or kidney, both sites being preferable to the omentum (22). Extending these studies in inbred rats we have shown that pancreas (21) and lung (20) have proven also to be efficacious sites for islet transplantation. Currently clinical transplantation of adult islets uses the portal vein for islet embolization to the liver (45). Based on the results of these previous studies, we undertook a pilot study to evaluate the spleen, liver, lung and pancreas and the kidney as potential recipient sites to study the growth and differentiation of human fetal endocrine cells, cultured as ICCs, in

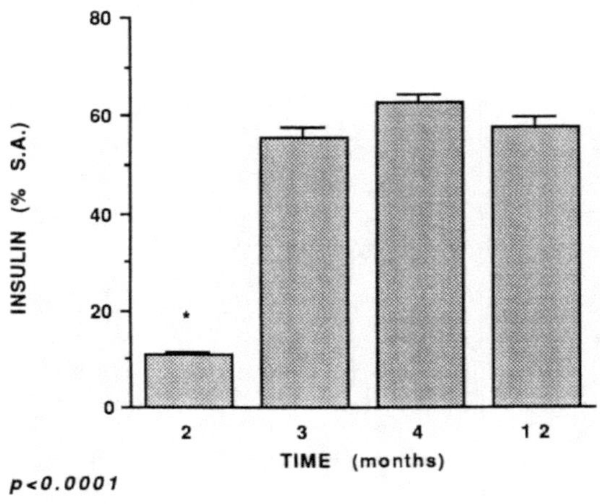

Figure 9. Comparison of immunostaining of grafted human fetal ICCs 3, 4 and 12 months after transplantation under the kidney capsule of nude mice. Percentage of surface area of graft immunoreactive with insulin antibody was quantitated using a computerized image analysis system. + Adapted with permission from the *American Diabetes Association, Inc.* (41). ++ Reproduced with the permission from *Cell Transplantation* (1). +++ Reproduced with permission from the *Journal of Clinical Investigation* (40)

athymic nude mice. Preliminary results of this study, based on serum human C-peptide responses following glucose stimulation and immunohistochemical analyses of the tissue at the site of implantation, indicate that pancreas and kidney are optimal sites to allow for growth and maturation of human fetal ICCs. Surprisingly, the results of transplantation of ICCs into the liver, lung and spleen were not too encouraging, possibly due to lack of differentiation and maturation factors at the site of implantation (2).

The information reviewed in this chapter indicates that fetal pancreatic cells have all the potential for careful scrutiny in well planned clinical transplantation studies where adequate immunosuppression is already required.

REFERENCES

1. Beattie, G.M.; Butler, C.; Hayek, A. Morphology and function of cultured human fetal pancreatic cells transplanted into athymic mice: a longitudinal study. Cell Transplantation 3:421-425, 1994.
2. Beattie, G.M.; Hayek, A. Outcome of Human Fetal Pancreatic Transplants According to Implantation Site. Transplantation Proceedings 26:3299; 1994.
3. Beattie, G.M.; Lappi, D.A.; Baird, A.; Hayek, A. Functional impact of attachment and purification in the short term culture of human pancreatic islets. J.Clin.Endocr.Metab. 73:93-98; 1991.
4. Beattie, G.M.; Levine, F.; Mally, M.I.;et al,. Acid β-galactosidase: A developmentally regulated marker of endocrine cell precursors in the human fetal pancreas. J.Clin.Endocrinol.Metab 78:1232-1240, 1994.
5. Beattie, G.M.; Otonkoski, T.; Lopez, A.D.; Hayek, A. Maturation and function of human fetal pancreatic cells after cryopreservation. Transplantation 56:1340-1343; 1993.
6. Bonner-Weir, S.; Smith, F.E. Islet cell growth and the growth factors involved. Trends Endocrin.Metab. 5(2):60-64; 1994.
7. Bottaro, D.P.; Rubin, J.S.; Faletto, D.L.; et al. Identification of the hepatocyte growth factor receptor as the c-met proto-oncogene product. Science 251:802-804; 1991.
8. Branch, D.W.,et.al. Human Fetal Tissue Working Group. Suitablility of fetal tissues from spontaneous abortions and from actopic pregnancies for transplantation. Journal of American Medical Association 1994.
9. Brelje, T.C.; Allaire, P.; Hegre, O.; Sorenson, R.L. Effect of prolactin versus growth hormone on islet function and the importance of using homologous mammosomatotropic hormones. Endocrinology 125:2392-2399; 1989.
10. Brelje, T.C.; Scharp, D.W.; Lacy, P.E.; et al. Effect of Homologous Placental Lactogens, Prolactins, and Growth Hormones on Islet β-Cell Division and Insulin Secretion in Rat, Mouse, and Human Islets: Implication for Placental Lactogen Regulation of Islet Function During Pregnancy. Endocrinology 132(2):879-887; 1993.
11. Bussolini, F.; Di Renzo, M.F.; Ziche, M.; et al. Hepatocyte growth factor is a potent angiogenic factor which stimulates endothelial cell motility and growth. J.Cell Biol. 119:629-641; 1992.
12. Derynck, R. The physiology of transforming growth factor-α. Adv. Cancer Res. 58:27-52; 1992.
13. Di Renzo, M.F.; Narsimhan, R.P.; Olivero, M.; et al. Expression of the Met/HGF receptor in normal and neoplastic human tissues. Oncogene 6:1997-2003; 1991.
14. Dudek, R.W.; Lawrence, I.E.; Hill, R.S.; Johnson, R.C. Induction of islet cytodifferentiation by fetal mesenchyme in adult pancreatic ductal epithelium . Diabetes 40:1041-1048; 1991.
15. Eckhoff, D.E.; Soillinger, H.W.; Hullett, D.A. Selective enhancement of β-cell activity by preparation of fetal pancreatic proislets and culture with insulin growth factor 1. Transplantation 51(6):1161-1165; 1991.
16. Eizirik, D.L.; Korbutt, G.S. ; Hellerstrom, C. Prolonged exposure of human pancreatic islets to high glucose concentrations in vitro impairs the β-cell function. JCI 90:1263-1268, 1992.
17. Finch, P.W.; Rubin, J.S.; Miki, T.; Ron, D.; Aaronson, S.A. Human KGF is FGF-related with properties of a paracrine effector of epithelial cell growth. Science 245:752-755; 1989.
18. Furlong, R.A. The biology of hepatocyte growth factor/scatter factor. Bioessays 14:613-617; 1992.
19. Gu, D.; Lee, M-S.; Krahl, T.; Sarvetnick, N. Transitional cells in the regenerating pancreas. Development 120:1873-1881; 1994.
20. Hayek, A.; Beattie, G.M. Reversal of experimental diabetes by injection of syngeneic islets into perpheral veins. Cell Transplantation 1:83-85; 1992.
21. Hayek, A.; Beattie, G.M. Intrapancreatic islet transplantation in experimental diabetes in the rat. Metabolism 41:1367-1369; 1992.

22. Hayek, A.; Lopez, A.D.; Beattie, G.M. Factors influencing islet transplantation - number, location , and metabolic control. Transplantation 49:224-225; 1990.
23. Heine, U.I.; Munoz, E.F.; Flanders, K.C.; et al. Role of transforming growth factor-β in the development of the mouse embryo. Journal Cell Biology 105:2861-2876; 1987.
24. Hellerstrom, C.; Lewis, N.J.; Borg, H.; Johnson, R.; Freinkel, N. Method for large-scale isolation of pancreatic islets by tissue-culture of fetal rat pancreas. Diabetes 28:766-769; 1979.
25. Hellerstrom, C.; Swenne, I. Functional maturation and proliferation of fetal pancreatic β-cells. Diabetes 40:89-93; 1991.
26. Hullett, D.A.; Bethke, K.P.; Landry, A.S.; Leonard, D.K.; Sollinger, H.W. Successful long-term cryopreservation and transplantation of human fetal pancreas. Diabetes 38:448-453; 1989.
27. Hullett, D.A.; Falany, J.L.; Love, R.B.; Butler, J.A.; Sollinger, H.W. Human fetal pancreas: Potential for transplantation. Transplantation Proceedings XIX, No.1:909-910; 1987.
28. Korsgren, O.; Andersson, A.; Sandler, S. Pretreatment of fetal porcine pancreas in culture with nicotinamide accelerates reversal of diabetes after transplantation to nude mice. Surgery 113:205-214; 1993.
29. Korsgren, O.; Sandler, S.; Landstrom, A.S.; Jansson, L.; Andersson, A. Large-scale production of fetal porcine pancreatic isletlike cell clusters. Transplantation 45:509-514; 1988.
30. Levine, F.; Beattie, G.M.; Hayek, A. Differential integrin expression facilitates isolation of human fetal pancreatic epithelial cells. Cell Transplantation 3:307-313, 1994.
31. Lyer, A.; Kmiecik, T.E.; Park, M.; et al. Structure, tissue-specific expression, and transforming activity of the mouse met protooncogene. Cell Growth Diff. 1:87-95; 1990.
32. Mally, M.I.; Otonkoski, T.; Lopez, A.D.; Hayek, A. Developmental gene expression in the human fetal pancreas. Pediatric Research 36:537-544, 1994.
33. Miettinen, P.J.; Heikinheimo, K. Transforming growth factor-alpha (TGF-α) and insulin gene expression in human fetal pancreas. Development 114:833-840; 1992.
34. Miettinen, P.J.; Otonkoski, T.; Voutilainen, R. Insulin-like growth factor-II and transforming growth factor-α in the developing human fetal pancreatic islets. J. Endocr. 138:127-136; 1993.
35. Montesano, R.; Matsumoto, K.; Nakamura, T. Identification of a fibroblast-derived epithelial morphogen as hepatocyte growth factor. Cell 67:901-908; 1991.
36. Otonkoski, T. Insulin and glucagon secretory responses to arginine, glucagon and theophylline during perifusion of human fetal islet-like cell clusters RUNNING TITLE: Secretory responses of human fetal islets. J.Clin. Endocrinol. Metab 67:734-740; 1988.
37. Otonkoski, T.; Beattie, G.M.;Lopez, A.D.; Hayek, A. Use of Hepatocyte Growth Factor/Scatter Factor to Increase Transplantable Human Fetal Islet Cell Mass. Transplantation Proceedings 26:3334; 1994.
38. Otonkoski, T.; Beattie, G.M.; Mally, M.I.; Hayek, A. Assessment of human fetal islet cell preparations. Methods in Cellular Transplantation, IN PRESS 1994.
39. Otonkoski, T.; Beattie, G.M.; Mally, M.I.; Ricordi, C.; Hayek, A. Nicotinamide is a potent inducer of endocrine differentiation in cultured human fetal pancreatic cells. J. Clin. Invest. 92:1459-1466; 1993.
40. Otonkoski, T.; Beattie, G.M.; Rubin, J.S.; Lopez, A.D.; Baird, A.; Hayek, A. Hepatocyte growth factor/scatter factor induced growth of human fetal pancreatic β-cells in vitro. Diabetes 43:947-953, 1994.
41. Otonkoski, T.; Mally, M.I.; Hayek, A. Opposite effects of β-cell differentiation and growth on reg expression in human fetal pancreatic cells. Diabetes 43:1164-1166, 1994.
42. Otonskoski, T.; Andersson, S.; Knip, M.; Simell, O. Maturation of insulin response to glucose during human fetal and neonatal development. Diabetes 37:286-291; 1988.
43. Prat, M.; Narsimhan, R.P.; Crepaldi, T.; Nicotra, M.R.; Natali, P.G.; Comoglio, P.M. The receptor encoded by the human c-met oncogene is expressed in hepatocytes, epithelial cells and solid tumors. Int. J. Cancer 49:323-328; 1991.
44. Rizzino, A. Transforming growth factor-β: multiple effects on cell differentiation and extracellular matrices. Dev. Biol. 130:411-422; 1988.
45. Robertson, R.P. Seminars in Medicine of the Beth Israel Hospital, Boston. Pancreatic and islet transplantation for diabetes - cures or curiosities? New England Journal of Medicine 327 (26):1861-1868; 1992.
46. Sandler, S.; Andersson, A.; Korsgren, O.; et al. Tissue culture of human fetal pancreas: Growth hormone stimulates the formation and insulin production of islet-cell like clusters. J.Clin.Endocr.Metab. 65:1154-1158; 1987.
47. Sandler, S.; Andersson, A.; Korsgren, O.; et al. Tissue culture of human fetal pancreas. Effects of nicotinamide on insulin production and formation of islet-like cell clusters. Diabetes 38 (Suppl. 1):168-171; 1989.
48. Sandler, S.; Andersson, A.; Schnell, A.; et al. Tissue culture of human fetal pancreas. Development and function of β-cells in vitro and transplantation of explants to nude mice. Diabetes 34:1113-1119; 1985.

49. Smith, F.E.; Rosen, K.M.; Villa-Komaroff, L.; Weir, G.C.; Bonner-Weir, S. Enhanced insulin-like growth factor I gene expression in regenerating rat pancreas. Proc.Natl.Acad.Sci.USA 88:6152-6156; 1991.
50. Sonnenberg, E.; Meyer, D.; Weidner, K.M.; Birchmeier, C. Scatter Factor/Hepatocyte growth factor and its receptor, the c-met tyrosine kinase, can mediate a signal exchange between mesenchyme and epithelia during mouse development. J. Cell Biol. 123(1):223-235; 1993.
51. Strain, A.J. Hepatocyte growth factor: Another ubiquitous cytokine. J. Endocr. 137:1-5; 1993.
52. Swenne, I. Pancreatic beta-cell growth and diabetes mellitus. Diabetologia 35:193-201; 1992.
53. Teitelman, G.; Joh, T.H.; Reis, D.J. Transformatin of catecholaminergic precursors into glucagon (A) cells in mouse embryonic pancreas. Proc.Natl.Acad.Sci.USA 78:5225-5229; 1981.
54. Teitelman, G.; Lee, J.; Reis, D.J. Differentiation of prospective mouse pancreatic islet cells during development in vitro and during regeneration. Dev.Biol 120:425-433; 1987.
55. Tsarfaty, I.; Resau, J.H.; Rulong, S.; Keydar, I.; Faletto, D.L.; Vande Woude, G.F. The met Proto-Oncogene Receptor and Lumen Formation. Science 257:1258-1261; 1992.
56. Tsuda, H.; Iwase, T.; Matsumoto, K.; et al. Immunohistochemical localization of hepatocyte growth factor protein in pancreas islet A-cells of man and rats. Jpn.J.Cancer Res. 83:1262-1266; 1992.
57. Tuch, B.E. Reversal of diabetes by human fetal pancreas. Transplantation 51:557-562; 1991.
58. Tuch, B.E.; Grigoriou, S.; Turtle, J.R. Growth and hormonal content of human fetal pancreas passaged in athymic mice. Diabetes 35:464-469; 1986.
59. Tuch, B.E.; Grigoriou, S.; Turtle, J.R. Comparison of liver, spleen, and kidney as sites for xenografting human fetal pancreas in the nude mouse. Transplantation Proceedings 19(2):2907-2909; 1987.
60. Tuch, B.E.; Ng, A.B.P.; Jones, A.; Turtle, J.R. Histologic differentiation of human fetal pancreatic explants transplanted into nude mice. Diabetes 33:1180-1187; 1984.
61. Tuch, B.E.; Ogersby, K.J. Maturation of insulinogenic response to glucose in human fetal pancreas with retinoic acid. Horm.Met.Res. 25 (Supplement):233-238; 1990.
62. Weidner, K.M.; Arakaki, N.; Hartmann, G.; et al. Evidence for the identity of human scatter factor and human hepatocyte growth factor. Proc.Natl.Acad.Sci.USA 88:7001-7005; 1991.
63. Zarnegar, D.P.; Muga, S.; Rahija, R.; Michalopoulos, G. Tissue distribution of hepatopoietin-A: a heparin-binding polypeptide growth factor for hepatocytes. Proc.Natl.Acad.Sci.USA 87:1252-1256; 1990.

2

EXPRESSION OF TWO NON-ALLELIC REG GENES IN THE DEVELOPING HUMAN PANCREAS: EFFECTS IN VITRO OF NICOTINAMIDE AND MATERNAL GROWTH FACTORS

Bent Formby, Jean Falzone and Sheng Loh

Sansum Medical Research Foundation
Santa Barbara, California, USA

INTRODUCTION

Several characteristics make fetal tissue superior to adult tissue for transplantation (1). Thus, fetal cells can often differentiate in response to environmental signals or according to an intrinsic program. This plasticity means that such cells may migrate, grow and establish functional connections with other cells. Additionally, fetal cells may proliferate more rapidly and more often than mature, fully differentiated cells. They may produce high levels of angiogenic factors, which enhance their ability to grow once they are grafted and may also facilitate regeneration of surrounding host tissues (2). Major histocompatibility antigens (HLA's) are expressed at lower levels in some fetal tissues than in corresponding adult tissues, which makes the fetal tissue less susceptible to rejection by the recipients immune system. Fetal tissue is more resistant to ischemic damage during in vitro manipulation or after transplantation (3), and therefore can survive at lower oxygen tensions than adult tissue, which probably explains why fetal tissues and cells better survive refrigeration or cryopreservation than those of adults (4).

Standard insulin-replacement therapy often does not prevent complications, including nephropathy, cardiovascular disease and retinopathy, which as already suggested by Banting and Best (5) could be prevented by the more precise regulation of plasma glucose levels resulting from a successful transplantation of pancreatic islet cells. Because the fetal pancreas has a high ratio of endocrine to exocrine tissue and lack of mature antigenic passenger leucocytes it is considered preferable to adult pancreas tissue, which convincingly has been documented in nude mice with experimentally induced diabetes: human fetal pancreatic islets were able to survive, develop and restore normal blood glucose levels (6-10). On the basis on these observations more than 1500 fetal pancreas allografts reported in the literature have been attempted in patients with insulin-dependent diabetes (11-14). Unfortunetely, many of the reports lack the details needed for critical evaluation, but the overall picture shows 18-25% of recipients having measurable C-peptide levels up to 45 months after transplantation. Thus several fundamental problems may have contributed to this relatively poor success rate, e.g. HLA-mismatched, culture conditions of fetal pancreatic tissue prior to transplantation, lack of immunosuppression of recipients.

It is therefore conceivable that a detailed characterization of the physiological and molecular mechanisms involved in the development of the human fetal pancreatic islet cells can contribute to design of improved cultivation procedures that will optimize fetal islet insulin secretory capacity and increase the number of β-cells prior to their transplantation into insulin-dependent diabetic recipients.

We specifically investigated in vitro a possible association of insulin secretory capacity with growth of β-cell mass induced by maternal growth factors and nicotinamide as well as the relevance of two non-allelic Reg genes in the adaptive growth response of fetal islets to maternal growth factors and nicotinamide.

ADAPTATION OF PANCREATIC ISLETS TO PREGNANCY: CORRELATION BETWEEN THE ONSET OF PLACENTAL LACTOGEN SECRETION AND INCEASED MATERNAL ISLET CELL PROLIFERATION AND INSULIN SECRETION

Parsons et al. (15) studied islet cell proliferation and insulin secretion during gestation in the rat. Their results demonstrated a marked increase of maternal β-cell BrdU-labeled nuclei which correlated with a similar pattern of changes in insulin secretory profiles observed with perfused pancreata of pregnant rats. These changes in islet β-cell proliferation and insulin secretion correlated with increased serum levels of placental lactogen (PL), hence providng support for the hypothesis that PL is involved in pancreatic adaptation to pregnancy. Of note is the observation that the secretory capacity of rat islets that have adapted to pregnancy is such that they can secrete up to 10-fold more insulin in the presence of normal blood glucose levels in part explained by the observed islet cell proliferation. A consequence of the increased insulin secretion observed during pregnancy is a dramatic lowering of the threshold of glucose-stimulated insulin secretion. With a reduction of the threshold from 5.5-6.0 to 3.5-5.0 mM glucose, several-fold increase in insulin release occurs at normal serum glucose levels.The importance of this increased sensitivity of β-cells to glucose is critical because if the threshold were to remain unchanged, then the enhanced above threshold secretion would only result in a small increase in circulating insulin. Also, the sustained hyperglycemia necessary to meet the increased demands for insulin if increased sensitivity of β-cells to glucose did not occur could have detrimental effects on the developing fetus. Collectively, this adaptation allows maternal islets to maintain elevated insulin secretion without the need for sustained hyperglycemia. As mentioned above the temporal changes of threshold and secretion were similar to that observed for islet cell proliferation, and again correlate with the profile of PL serum levels. In the pregnant rat peak secretion and minimal threshold occurred on day 15 and then returned to normal levels by day 20. These results suggest that counterregulatory influences are competing with lactogenic effects on islets during the later stages of pregnancy. A possibility to explain return toward normalcy is that there is down-regulation of β-cell lactogen receptors in the presence of sustained high concentrations of PL. That this actually accurs is indicated by the elevated PL levels maintained until term. An alternative mechanism to account for the return of islet β-cell proliferation and insulin secretion to normal levels in the face of high concentrations of PL is the presence of high levels of steroids during the later states of pregnancy (16).

In humans PL secretion is first detected in maternal plasma at 6 weeks gestation and increases until about 30th week of gestation, when peak concentrations of 5-10 μg/ml are observed (17). Although a similar increase in prolactin occurs during gestation, with peak concentrations of 130-200 ng/ml (18), pituitary growth hormone expression is suppressed with plasma levels relatively unchanged at 4-6 ng/ml (19). Also in humans the onset of PL secretion temporally coincides with the increased glucose-stimulated insulin secretion, thus further suggesting that PL regulates islet function during pregnancy.

ROLE OF PL AND NICOTINAMIDE IN DEVELOPMENT OF HUMAN FETAL PANCREATIC CELLS

High-affinity PL receptors are abundant in animal and fetal tissues, indicating a role for PL in fetal development. PL can attain concentrations of 10 nM in the human fetal circulation (20, 21), approximately 1/14th its concentration in maternal serum. In vitro data strongly suggest anabolic and mitogenic actions for PL on fetal tissues, including amino acid transport, hepatic glycogenesis, protein synthesis, and stimulation of IGF-1 and insulin release (20). Despite these findings, definitive evidence is lacking that PL contributes to maturation of human fetal pancreatic islet cells. Therefore we investigated in tissue culture experiments the ability of PL and maternal serum to alter insulin secretory capacity as well as transcript levels of insulin and Reg proteins from cultured human fetal pancreatic fragments.

Insulin secretory capacity was assessed by insulin responses to two successive 1 hr static batch incubations and calculated as the amount of insulin secreted per hour as percent of total insulin. The first incubation (F1) was in low glucose (2 mM) medium while the second incubation (F2) included 25 mM glucose and 10 mM theophylline as potentiator (22). The fractional stimulatory ratio (FSR defined as F2/F1) was used as an index of insulin secretory capacity of a given fetal pancreatic preparation to secrete insulin at a steady state in response to various stimuli. An FSR value of one theoretically represents no stimulation.

We investigated the effect of PL, maternal serum, FBS and nicotinamide (NA) on the insulin secretory capacity of 18-24-week old fetal pancreata, and observed, as shown in Table 1, a rather strong increase in FSR-values after cultivation for 4 days in the presence of either15% maternal serum or 15% maternal serum plus 10 mM NA. The significant 3-fold increase in FSR-value reached in the presence of maternal serum was reduced by a polyclonal antibody against PL to a FSR-value close to one indicating an almost completely block of stimulation. Although not conclusive because the polyclonal antibody against PL might

Table 1. FSR-Values* Calculated from Radioimmunoassays of Secreted and Non-secreted Insulin in Two Successive One-Hour Static Batch Incubations of Human Fetal Pancreatic Fragments after Cultivation under Various Conditions for Four Days

Culture conditions**	FSR-value (mean±1SD (n))
+ 15% FBS	1.28±0.20 (6)
+15% FBS plus 1μg hPL/ml	2.18±0.42 (4)
+ 15% FBS plus 10 mM NA	2.38±0.22 (8)
+15% maternal serum	4.22±1.07 (15)
+15% maternal serum plus 75μg polyclonal anti-hPL antibody/ml	1.09±0.11 (6)
+15% maternal serum plus 10 mM NA	5.08±0.71 (5)

*For calculation of FSR-value see text. ** complete RPMI 1640 medium.

crossreact with other maternal growth factors (e.g. growth hormone which in humans is structurally similar to PL) our data confirm data obtained with rat neonatal islets after cultivation for 4 days in the presence of 1 μg/ml rPL-1 which demonstrated a 2-fold increase in insulin secretion (23). Interestingly and shown in Table 1 we also found a 2-fold increase in FSR-value when human fetal pancreatic fragments were cultured in the presence of 1 μg/ml PL, suggesting other growth factors exist in maternal serum and have a stimulatory effect on fetal insulin secretion e.g. prolactin and growth hormone (23,24). Otonkoski et al. (25) recently reported that NA is a potent inducer of endocrine differentiation in cultured human fetal pancreatic cells. These investigators found treatment of human fetal pancreatic cells with 10 mM NA resulted in a 2-fold increase in DNA content, a 3-fold increase in insulin content and a 2-fold increase in insulin release. As shown in Table 1 we also found a 2-fold increase in FSR-value after cultivation of fetal pancreatic fragment in the presence of 10 mM NA, hence confirming the data reported by Otonkoski et al (25). Four days cultivation of fetal pancreatic fragments in the presence of 15% maternal serum plus 10 mM NA resulted in a 4-fold increase in FSR-value (Table 1). Collectively, our data together with results reported by others indicate that maternal growth factors, in particular PL, and NA potentiate the insulin secretory machinery of human fetal pancreatic cells. These observations promoted our study of possible molecular mechanisms involved in the response of human fetal pancreatic islet cells to maternal growth factors and/or NA.

THE REG GENES

Reg (regenerating gene) was first isolated from a rat regenerating islet-derived cDNA library (26). Watanabe et al (27) isolated the human Reg cDNA and gene encoding a 166-amino acid protein which exhibited 70% homology with rat Reg protein. Recently, several Reg-related genes and proteins have been isolated (28) and demonstrated to be derived from a multigene family, the Reg/PSP gene family (29). Based on the primary structure, the proteins have been grouped into three subclasses. Activation of type I Reg gene participates in rat pancreatic β-cell regeneration. Recently, Moriizumi et al (30) isolated a novel human gene and cDNA encoding a member of the Reg proteins, Reg1β. The gene encodes a 166-amino acid protein which has 22 amino acid substitutions in comparison with the previously isolated human Reg1α protein. Reg1β was only expressed in the pancreas, whereas Reg1α was expressed in the kidney and stomach as well as in the pancreas.

FUNCTION OF REG PROTEINS

Yonomura, Y. et al (31) reported that the administration of DNA repair enzyme inhibitors cuch as NA to 90% depancreatized rats induced islet regeneration, and let to an improvement in the surgical diabetes. Screening of the regenerating islet-derived cDNA library from the rats revealed a novel single copy gene which encodes a 165 amino acid secreted protein. Further studies identified the Reg-protein in the insulin-containing secretory granules of rat β-cells (32). Subsequent studies in both in animal models of islet regeneration and in tumor cell lines have confirmed enhanced Reg gene transcription, hence linking expression to normal and transformed cell proliferation (33). Although these studies implied a tropic role for the Reg gene in rat β-cells, a recent report described the existence of a clear parallel association between increases in rat islet cell replication and Reg mRNA expression (34). In the light of additional reports (35) emphasizing the close association between Reg gene expression and regeneration or growth of rat islet β-cells in vitro and in vivo, Reg protein would appear to act on panceatic β-cells as an autocrine growth factor. This issue was also addressed in experiments performed by Miyaura et al. (29) where Reg gene expression was measured in rats after implantation and resection of a solid insulinoma tumor, which is a maneuver known, respectively, to reduce and reexpand the volume of β-cells. Thus, animals with an implanted insulinoma tumor became profoundly hypoglycemic. Islet β-cells declined from normal 75% of total islet volume to less than 30%, in conset with a marked reduction in the Reg mRNA level. Removal of the tumor resulted in a sharp increase in β-cell replication, as measured by ^{3}H-thymidine incorporation and a return to normal β-cell volume within 4 days of tumor resection. This was associated with a transient induction in Reg gene expression compared to that of tumor-bearing animals, effectively returning the amount of Reg mRNA to the levels found in normal animals within 48 hours; at later time points after tumor removal (3-7 days) Reg gene expression declined, but then rose toward normal. In situ hybridization analysis localized the initial induction in Reg mRNA expression to the exocrine pancreas. Continous infusion of insulin into normal rats for 4 days, a maneuver that does not significantly reduce β-cell mass, resulted in dramatically reduced insulin mRNA in islets, but no change in the levels of Reg mRNA. These observations clearly suggest that the diminution in pancreatic β-cell mass caused by subcutaneous implantation of an insulinoma is associated with reduced Reg gene expression and that the increase in β-cell replication after resection of the tumor is preceded by return of Reg gene expression toward normal.

Although it was thought that there was only a single locus for Reg protein in the mammalian genome, Unno et al (28) in a recent study isolated from mice two distinct cDNAs and genes, one of which was a mouse homologue to rat and human Reg gene, the other another type of Reg gene. These two mouse genes were designated Regl and Reg2, respectively. The two proteins encoded by these genes share 76% amino acid sequence identity with each other. Both genes span about 3 kb pairs, and the genomic organization of six exons and five introns is conserved between them. Chromosomal mapping studies indicated that the Regl gene was localized on mouse chromosome 12, whereas the Reg2 gene was localized on chromosome 3. By northern blot analysis, both Regl and Reg2 mRNAs were detected in the normal pancreas and hyperplastic islets of aurothioglucose-treated male NON mice, but not in the normal islets. By slot blot analysis, the amounts of Regl mRNA and Reg2 mRNA in the hyperplastic islets, which consist predominantly of β-cells, were estimated as 1.57 and 1.17 ng/μg RNA, respectively. By the same analysis, the amounts of Regl mRNA and Reg2 mRNA in normal islets were determined to be less than 0.06 ng/μg RNA. Regl mRNA and Reg2 mRNA in normal pancreas were 1.30 and 0.41 ng/μg RNA, respectively. These results suggest that expression of members of the Reg gene family are importent in β-cell proliferation and/or differentiation. The physiological reasons for the maintenance of two functional non-allelic reg genes encoding proteins of different amino acid sequence in the mice are still unclear. Recently Moriizumi et al (30) reported the isolation of a novel human gene and cDNA encoding a member of the Regl proteins, Reg 1β. The novel gene is composed of the Goldberg-Hogness promotor sequence (tataaa) and six exons encoding a 166-amino acid protein. The comparison of the novel gene with the human Reg gene revealed that the coding regions of the Reg gene and the corresponding regions of the novel gene exhibited 91% homology. Reglβ mRNA of 0.9 kbp was only expressed in the pancreas and was not detected in any other tissues. Interestingly, the 5'-flanking regions of both Reg genes carry several E-box core motifs, NNCANNTGNN, that are protein-binding sites in gene enhancers and are present in the regulatory regions of pancreas-specific genes such as insulin, amylase, chymotrypsin and trypsin 1 genes (36). Thus, data published recently in the literature combined with the observation made by us and Otonkoski et al (25) that the human fetal pancreas expresses Reglα mRNA provide the rationale for studying the molecular mechanisms by which the two non-allelic Reg genes and their products may be involved in replication of human fetal pancreatic islet cells, and how these genes may be regulated by lactogenic hormones and NA.

EXPRESSION OF NON-ALLELIC REG GENES IN HUMAN FETAL PANCREATA

Human fetal pancreata used in our research are obtained through a nonprofit organ procurement center (Advanced Biosciences Resources, Oakland, CA). Patient consent for tissue donation is obtained by the procurement center. The tissue is obtained by dilation and extraction, and shipped on ice in RPMI 1640 containing 10% FBS and antibiotics (100 U/ml penicillin, 0.1 mg/ml streptomycin and 1 μg/ml amphotericin). The tissue is received in the laboratory within 18-24 hours, cut into fragments and cultured under various conditions described in following the text.

EXTRACTION OF mRNA AND SYNTHESIS OF cDNA

Poly(A^+)mRNA was isolated from cultured human fetal pancreatic fragments by absorption on oligo(dT) cellulose using Micro-FastTrack mRNA isolation kit(Invitrogen, San Diego, CA). The mRNA was used directly as template for first strand synthesis of cDNA in a reaction mixture containing 1000 U Moloney murine leukemia reverse transcriptase, 40 U rRNasin, 50 μM random hexamer, 50 mM Tris-HCl (pH 8.3); 75 mM KCl; 10 mM dithiothreitol; 3 mM MgC12; 0.5 mM each of dGTP, dTTP, dATP, dCTP all brought to a total volume of 60 μl with DEPC (diethyl pyrocarbonate)-treated water. cDNA used for comparison between groups was simultaneously prepared using identical RT reaction mixes.

AMPLIFICATION OF cDNA

A PCR method was used that estimates the relative abundance target transcripts normalized to GADPH (glyceraldehyde-3-phosphate dehydrogenase) mRNA. GADPH is amplified along with target sequences from the same cDNA in the same (multiplex) or separate reaction tubes. Normalization to GAPDH controls for variation in the efficiency of mRNA extraction and cDNA synhesis. GAPDH was judged a suitable housekeeping gene because processed pseudogenes were not detected in genomic DNA of any of the fetal pancreatic specimens tested. Also, GAPDH levels did not vary between the goups compared.

For PCR, 4 μl of cDNA was used in a modified hot start method as described previously (37). Briefly, cDNA was added to 30 μl of a master mix containing 0.8 μmol of each primer, 17 mM Tris-HCl (pH 8.3), and 80mM KCl. Water was added to the cDNA reactions to a final volume of 40 μl. All reactions were overlaid with light mineral oil and heated to 99°C. After 10 min, the reactions were cooled to 94°C, and a 10 μl volume containing 7 mM MgC12, 1 mM each of dATP, dTTP, dGTP and dCTP, and 1.2 U Taq polymerase was added directly through the oil overlay. Reactions were then temperature modulated for 28 to 32 cycles as follows: 95°C for 60 sec; 58°C for 30 sec; 72°C for 30 sec, with the extension segment automatically increased 3 sec/cycle. PCR products were electrophoretically separated on agarose gels containing ethidium bromide at 0.5 μg/ml. Following electrophoresis, gels were photographed (Polaroid 667 film) and scanned at 600 dpi in 8-bit (256 levels) gray scale. A gray scale value (GSV) was defined as the mean gray scale level (0-255) multiplied by the total number of prixels in the scanned PCR band, and used to indicate DNA content. These measurements were performed using commercially available software and a Macintosh IIci personal computer. Upon PCR amplification of serial dilutions of sample cDNA, a concomittant decrease in the PCR product was observed. For semiquantitative comparisons template dilutions were chosen to fall within the range in which input tempate concentration correlated with the intensity of amplification product. Similarly, varying the number of PCR cycles did not change the relative differences between samples. These basic studies indicated that our PCR conditions never were within the plateau phase of amplification. Plateau occurs at higher cycles during PCR when band intensity no longer increases or even decreases due to build up of higher molecular weights products. Comparison of gene upregulation following stimulation during cultivation and the relative abundance of mRNA between samples was given by comparing the GSV ratios of Reg1α or Reg1β to GADPH at any template dilution subplateau. All comparisons are expressed as means of this ratio ± 1 SD, averaged from a minimum of 3 separate mRNA extractions. Our RT-PCR method is sensitive to at least 25% differences in cellular mRNA transcripts.

PCR PRIMERS AND ENDONUCLEASE DIGESTS

Oligonucleotide primers were synthesized commercially and reconstituted to 40 μM in DEPC-treated water. Primer sequences were: Reg1α sense, GAC-CAGCTCATACCTCATGCT, antisense, CCCAGGTCTGCG-GTCTTC; Reg1β sense, AACTCGTTCCATGCTATC, antisense, GACACC-AGGTTGCCTGAATTC; Insulin sense, GAGGGGAGCACATGCTGGT, antisense, CCACCCATGGCAAATTCCATGGCA; GADPH sense CCACCCATG-GCAAATTCCATGGCA, antisense, TCTA-GACGGCAGGTCAGGTCCACC; phosphorothiorate Reg1α antisense AUG deoxynucleotide, CTGAGCCATGCTGAGCTG. All PCR primer pairs used to assess the relative levels of gene expression span introns, as none amplified bands from genomic DNA. PCR product intensities, therefore, reflect the amplification of cDNA only and not co-extracted genomic DNA. For restriction endonuclease digestion, 5-20 μl of PCR product was incubated with 2 U of enzyme for 60 min directly in PCR buffer at 37°C.

EFFECT OF MATERNAL SERUM AND NA ON LEVELS OF EXPRESSED REG1α AND REG1β mRNA IN HUMAN FETAL PANCREATA AFTER CULTIVATION FOR 4 DAYS

Human fetal pancreatic fragments (~1 mm^3) of gestational age from 18 to 23 weeks were cultured 4 days in RPMI 1640 supplemented with either (1), 15% FBS with or without 10 mM NA or (2), matched 15% maternal serum with or without 10 mM NA. Total cellular mRNA from each culture experiment was used for first strand cDNA synthesis. PCR amplification was carried out separately for Reg1α, Reg1β, insulin and GADPH using oligonucleotides amplimers which targeted known cDNA sequences spanning at least one intron. Fig.1 shows representative PCR products from four human fetal pancreata of gestational ages ranging from 18 to 23 weeks cultured for 4 days in media containing 15% maternal serum plus 10 mM NA. Reg1α mRNA produced by pancreatic fragments was generally more abundant than Reg1β mRNA when visualized by ethidium bromide staining. For Reg1β, stronger ethidium bromide staining was detected in pancreatic fragments isolated from embryos older than 18 gestational weeks, which probably coincide with rapid expansion of islet cell mass between 18 and 24 gestational weeks (24). We found marked expression of the Reg1α gene, but not the Reg1β gene, in two 15 gestational weeks pancreata (data not shown), suggesting the Reg1α gene is

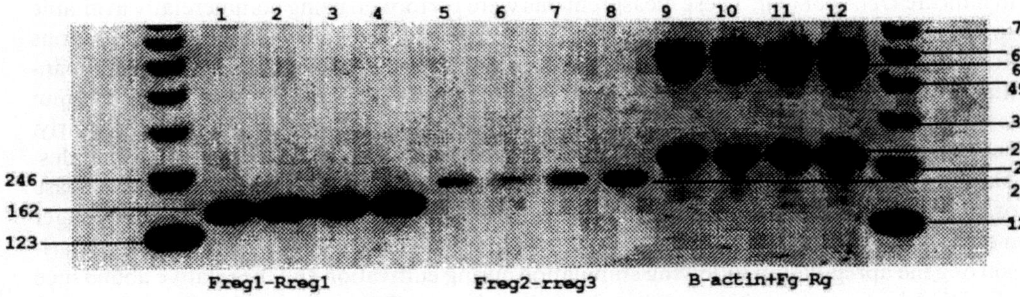

Figure 1. RT-PCR analysis of Reg1α (lanes1-4) and Reg1β (lanes8-8) gene expressions in four human fetal pancreata after cultivation for 4 days in RPMI 1640 culture media supplemented with 15% matched maternal serum plus 10 mM nicotinamide. The products of PCR amplificatrion of cDNA were separated by agarose gel electrophoresis, visualized by ethedium bromide, photographed (Polaroid 667 film) and scanned at 600 dpi in 8-bit (256 levels) gray scale, which is shown in the figure. **Lanes 1,5 & 9,** 20 week human fetal pancreas. cDNA amplified with primers FRegl and RRegl produced a product of 162 bp (lane 1, Reg1α gene expression). cDNA amplified with primers Freg2 and rreg2 produced a product of 240 bp (lane 5, Reg1β gene expression). GADPH (618 bp, primers FG/RG) and β-actin (252 bp) transcripts in lane 9 are controls and corfirm equal amounts of RNA were reversed transcribed and loaded on gel. **Lanes 2,6 & 10,** 18 week human fetal pancreas. cDNA amplified with the same primers as in lanes 1,5 & 9. **Lanes 3,7 & 11,** 21 week human fetal pancreas.cDNA amplified with the same primers as in lanes 1,5 & 9. **Lanes 4,8 & 12,** 23 week human fetal pancreas. cDNA amplified with the same primers as in lanes 1,5 & 9.

the only Reg gene functioning in the early stages of pancreatic development. cDNA levels of the two housekeeping genes, GAPDH and β-actin, visualized by ethidium were almost identical (fig.1). The specificity of the amplification bands was confirmed by analysis of restriction fragment sizes obtained from the PCR products after cleavage with enzymes, that cut at positions between the PCR primers. Thus, HpaII produced fragments of the predicted sizes: 93 and 69 bp (Reg1α amplified product is 162 bp), and Alu produced fragments of predicted sizes: 117 and 123 bp (Reg1β amplified product is 240 bp). Serial 2-fold dilutions (1/4, 1/8 and 1/16) of input cDNA template in each culture experiments were used in order to make semiquantitative comparisons. Scanning area density of each band digitized at 400 dpi in 8-bit gray scale was normalized to the scanning area density in the control GADPH band. Mean relative densitometric values of cDNA template dilutions are shown in Table 2. Maximal increased expression of both Reg genes in pancreatic fragments was found after cultivation for 4 days in the presence of 15% maternal serum plus 10 mM NA. Lower Reg1α and Reg1β mRNA levels were observed after cultivation for 4 days in the presence of 10 mM NA. The following should be noted from Table 2; (i) Reg1β mRNA was not found after cultivation for 4 days in the presence of 15% maternal serum or 15% FBS; (ii) cultivation of pancreatic fragments in the presence of 10 mM NA, but not 15% maternal serum significantly enhanced the levels of Reg1α transcripts in comparison with cultivation of pancreatic fragments in 15% FBS; (iii) levels of insulin mRNA was significantly ($p=0.028$, $n=4$) increased after cultivation for 4 days in the presence of 10 mM NA, but not 15% maternal serum. As demonstrated in Table 1, 10 mM NA only weakly potentiated the stimulatory effect of 15% maternal serum on insulin secretory capacity (FSR, $p=0.2$). It is relevant to note that cultivation of fetal pancreatic fragments for 24 hours in the presence of 16 μM phosphorothioate Reg1α antisense AUG deoxynucleotide did not affect levels of insulin mRNA, suggesting the Reg1α gene product does not regulate the transcription of the insulin gene. We did not fing Reg1α, Reg1β and insulin genes expressed in control human fetal spleens or adult human peripheral blood lymphocytes.

Table 2. Relative Densitometric Values of Serial Dilutions of Template cDNA (mean±SD (n))

STIMULI:	15% maternal serum, 10 mM NA	10 mM NA	15% maternal serum	15%FBS
Reg1α/GADPH[a]	1.16±0.08 (5)	0.75±0.31(3)[b]	0.54±0.17(5)[c]	0.35±0.10(5)[d]
Reg1β/GADPH	0.44±0.06 (3)e	0.26±0.06(3)[f]	0	0
Insulin/GADPH	ND	0.80±0.26 (3)[g]	0.25±0.21 (3)[h]	0.31±0.26(3)[i]

Students T-test: a) vs b), p=0.028; b) vs c) NS; b) vs d), p=0.034; c) vs d), NS; e) vs f), p=0.025; g) vs h), p=0.045; h) vs i), NS.
18 to 23 weeks old human fetal pancreata were cut into small fragments as described in the text and cultured for 4 days at 37C in complete RPMI 1640 medium supplemented with various stimuli mentioned above. mRNA was isolated as described in the text. PCR products are from serial dilutions (1/2, 1/4, 1/8) of template cDNA. Ratios of relative amount of target gene to constitutively expressed GAPDH gene were calculated after scanning of PCR products in the linear phase of amplification (see also text).

Our studies on midgestational human fetal pancreata show in addition to insulin, the transcriptional levels of two non-allelic Reg genes are enhanced after cultivation for 4 days in the presence of maternal serum plus NA. The demonstration of increased Reg gene expression when cells are stimulated with maternal serum suggest an association between Reg gene expression and growth factors, which provides a basis for further clarification of which growth factors in the maternal serum (e.g. placental lactogen, prolactin, growth hormone) alone or in concert regulate growth and differentiation of the fetal endocrine pancreas. The precise fetal pancreatic responder cells involved remain elusive although the marked NA induced improvement in the glucose sensivity of insulin release combined with the increased transcriptional level of the insulin gene suggests existing β-cells or undifferentiated endocrine cells could be the site of action. Recent evidence in isolated rat islets of a close association between expression of Reg1α protein in β-cell secretory granules and growth of islet β–cells induced by various growth factors, links Reg1α gene at least in rodents intimately with β-cell proliferation.

Mally et al.(38) recently reported the Reg1α gene localizes to the human fetal pancreatic acinar cells. Currently we are therefore studying a possible role of the non-allelic Reg1β gene in the development and differentiation of the human fetal endocrine pancreas as well as to whether Reg1β transcripts are localized to fetal exocrine or endocrine cells. If most of the Reg mRNA expression, as suggested by Mally et al (38), occur in the exocrine fetal pancreas, it raises the possibility of a symbiotic relationship between the fetal exocrine and endocrine pancreas, a concept which is fundamentally attractive, because it may explain why the islets are developed in an otherwise seemingly irrelevant digestive organ.

REFERENCES

1. Edwards, R.G., 1992, in Fetal Tissue Transplants in Medicine, Cambridge University, Cambridge, England.
2. Bjorklund, A., Lindvall, O., and Isacson, O., 1987, Michanisms of action of intracerebral neural implants: studies on nigral and striatal grafts to the lesioned striatum. Trands Neurosci. 10:509-516.
3. Lacy, P., and Davie, J., 1984. Transplantation of pancreatic islets. Ann. Rev. Immunol. 2:183-199.
4. Sandler, S., Andersson, A., and Schnell, A., 1985. Tissue culture of human fetal pancreas. Diabetes 34:1113-1119.
5. Bliss, M., 1982. The discovery of insulin. University of Chicago Press, Chicago, 28-29.
6. Tuch, B., Ng, A., and Jones, A., 1984, Transplantation of human fetal pancreatic tissue into diabetic nude mice. Transplant. Proc. 16:1059-1061.

7. Hullett, D., Falany, J.L., and Love, R.B., 1987. Human fetal pancreas - a potential source for transplantation. Transplantation 43:18-22
8. Bethke, K., Hullett, D., Falany, J., and Love R.B.,1988. Cultured human pancreatic tissue reverses experimentally induced diabetes in nude mice. Curr Surg. 45:123-126.
9. Elias K., Noonan, R., and Zayas, J., 1990. Development of human fetal xenograft transplants in diabetic nude mice. Transplant. Proc. 22:806-807.
10. Tuch, B., Monk, R.S., Beretov, J., 1991. Reversal of diabetes in athymic rats by transplantation of human fetal pancreas. Transplantation 52:172-174
11. Groth, C.G., Andersson, A., and Bjorken, C. 1980. Transplantation of fetal pancreatic microfragments via the portal vein to a diabetic patient. Diabetes 29 (suppl 1):80-83.
12. Hu, Y-F., 1985. Clinical studies on islet transplantation in 39 patients with insulin-deprendent (type 1) diabetes mellitus. in Wuhan international symposium on organ transplantation. Wuhan, China, 39-40.
13. Benikova, E.A., Turchin, I.S., and Beliakova, L.S., 1987. Experience with the treatment of children with diabetes mellitus using allo- and xenografts of cultures of pancreatic islets. Probl. Endokrinol. (Moskwa), 33:19-22.
14. Farkas, G., Karacsonyi, S., Szabo, M., and Voros, P. 1990. Alteration in diabetic retinopsathy and nephropathy following islet transplantation. Transplant.Proc. 22:765-766.
15. Parsons, J.A., Brelje, T.C., and Sorenson, R.L., 1992., Adaptation of islet of Langerhans to pregnancy: increased islet cell proliferation and insulin secretion correlates with the onset of placental lactogen secretion. Endocrinology 130:1459-1466.
16. Bartholomeusz, R.K., Bruce, N.W., Martin, C.E., Hartman, P.E., (1976). Serial measurement of arterial plasma progesterone levels throughout gestation and parturition in individual rats. Acta Endocrinol (Kbh) 82:436-443.
17. Ogren, L., and Talamantes, F., 1988. Prolactins of pregnancy and their cellular source. Int. Rev.Cytol. 112:1-65.
18. Tyson,P., Hwang, P., Guyda, H., Friesen, H.G., 1972. Studies of prolactin in human pregnancy. Am.J.Obstet. Gynecol. 113:14-20.
19. Handwerger, S., Freemark, M., 1987. Role of placental lactogen and prolactin in human pregnancy. Adv.Exp.Med.Biol.219:399-420.
20. Hill, D.J., 1992. What is the role of growth hormone and related peptides in implantation and the development of the embryo and fetus. Hormone Research 38 (suppl 1):28-34.
21. Freemark, M., Kirk, K., Pihoker, C., Robertson, M.C., Shiu, R.P., Driscoll, P., 1993. Pregnancy lactogens in the rat conceptus and fetus:circulating levels, distribution of binding, and expression of receptor messenger ribonucleic acid. Endocrinology 133:1830-1842.
22. Formby, B., Walker, L., Peterson, C.M., 1987. Effects of duration of cold storage and gestational age on the insulin secretory capacity of human fetal pancreatic islets. Diabetes Research 4:113-116.
23. Brelje, T., Scharp, D., Lacy, P., Ogren, L., Talamantes, F., Robertson, M., Friesen, H., Sorensen, R., 1993. Effect of homologous placental lactogens, prolactins, and growth hormones on islet B-cell division and insulin secretion in rat, mouse and human islets: implication for placental lactogen regulation of islet function during pregnancy. Endocrinology 132:879-887.
24. Formby, B., Ullrich, A., Coussens, L., Walker, L., Peterson, C.M. 1988. Growth hormone stimulates insulin gene expression in cultured human fetal pancreatic islets. J. Clin.Endocrinol.Metab. 66:1075-1079.
25. Otonkoski, T., Beattie, G.M., Mally, M.I., Ricordi, C., Hayek, A., 1993. Nicotinamide is a potent inducer of endocrine differentiation in cultured human fetal pancreatic cells. J.Clin.Invest. 92:1459-1466.
26. Terazono, K., Yamamoto, H., Takasawa, S., 1988. A novel gene activated in regenerating islets. J.Biol.Chem. 263:2111-2114.
27. Watanebe, T., Yonekura, H., Terazono, K., 1990. Complete nucleotide sequence of Human Reg gene and its expression in normal and tumoral tissues. J.Biol.Chem. 265:7432-7439.
28. Unno, M., Yonekura. H., Nakagawara, K., 1993, Structure, chromosomal localization, and expression of mouse reg genes, regI and regII. J.Biol.Chem. 268:15974-15982.
29. Miyaura, C., Chen, L., Appel, M., 1991. Expression of reg/PSP, a pancreatic exocrine gene: relationship to changes in islet beta-cell mass. Mol.Endocxrinol. 5:226-234.
30. Moriizumi, S., Watanabe, T., Unno, M., 1994. Isolation, structural determination and expression of a novel reg gene, human reg1β. Biochim.Biophys. Acta 1217:199-202.
31. Yonomura, Y., Takashima, T., Miwa, K. (1984). Amelioration of diabetes mellitus in partially depancreatized rats by poly(ADP-ribose) synthetase inhibitors: evidence of islet β-cell regeneration. Diabetes 33:401-404.

32. Terazano, K., Uchiyama, Y., Yde, M. 1990. Expression of reg protein in rat regenerating islets and its co-location with insulin in the beta cell secretory granules. Diabetologia 33:250-252.
33. Unno, M., Itoh, T, Watanabe, T. 1992. Islet beta-cell regeneration and reg genes. Adv. Expl. Med.Biol. 321:61-66.
34. Francis, P.J., Southgate, J.L., Wilkin, T.J. 1992. Expression of an islet regenerating (reg) gene in isolated rat islets: effects of nutrient and non-nutrient growth factors. Diabetologia 35:238-242.
35. Watanabe, T., Yonemura, Y., Yonekera, H. 1994. Pancreatic beta-cell replication and amnilioration of surgical diabetes by Reg protein. Proc.Natl.Acad.Sci. (USA) 91:3589-3592.
36. German, M.S., Moss, L.G., Wang, J.,Rutter, W.J. 1991. The insulin and islet amyloid polypeptide genes contain similar cell-specific promotor elements that bind identical beta-cell nuclear complexes. Mol. Cell. Biol. 12:1777-1788.
37. Pearce, R.B., Trigler, L., Svaasand, E.K., Peterson, C.M. 1993, Polymorphism in the mouse Tap-1 gene. Association with abnormal CD8 T cell development in the nonobese nondiabetic mouse. J.Immunol. 151:5338-5347.
38. Mally, M.I., Otonkoski, T., Lopez, A.D., Hayek, A. 1994. Developmental gene expression in the human fetal pancreas. Pediatr. Res. 36:537-544.

3

PREPARATION OF FETAL ISLETS FOR TRANSPLANTATION: IMPORTANCE OF GROWTH FACTORS

Debra A. Hullett,* Debra A. MacKenzie, Tausif Alam, and Hans W. Sollinger

Department of Surgery
University of Wisconsin-Madison
Madison WI 53792

1. INTRODUCTION

It is estimated that approximately 1.4 million people in the United States suffer from insulin dependent diabetes mellitus (IDDM). Daily insulin therapy and whole organ pancreas transplantation are the only treatments currently available. Results of the diabetes complications and control trial have indicated that while tight control of circulating glucose levels significantly reduced the complications associated with IDDM, it does not prevent them. Insulin replacement therapy is not sufficient to prevent the macrovascular and microvascular complications that make IDDM the third leading cause of death. Pancreas transplant suffers from a shortage of donor organs and requires that the recipient be placed on lifelong immunosuppressive therapy. Adult islet transplantation has met with little success and also suffers from a shortage of donor organs and the need for potent immunosuppression. In contrast, human fetal pancreas (HFP) is readily available, has the potential for further growth and differentiation following transplantation and can be cultured *in vitro*. This gives HFP the potential for immunologic manipulation such that immunosuppressive therapy may be significantly reduced or eliminated. The growth and differentiation of HFP may be accelerated with short-term culture in growth factors.

2. THE POTENTIAL OF HFP FOR TRANSPLANTATION

The potential of HFP transplantation for the treatment of IDDM has been shown in experimental animal model systems (1,2). Human fetal pancreas is readily available, has the potential for further growth and differentiation, and is easily transplanted. In our experience

* Address Correspondence to: Debra A. Hullett, Department of Surgery, University of Wisconsin, H4/749 CSC, 600 Highland Ave., Madison, WI 53792

Fetal Islet Transplantation
Edited by C. M. Peterson, L. Jovanovic-Peterson, and B. Formby, Plenum Press, New York, 1995

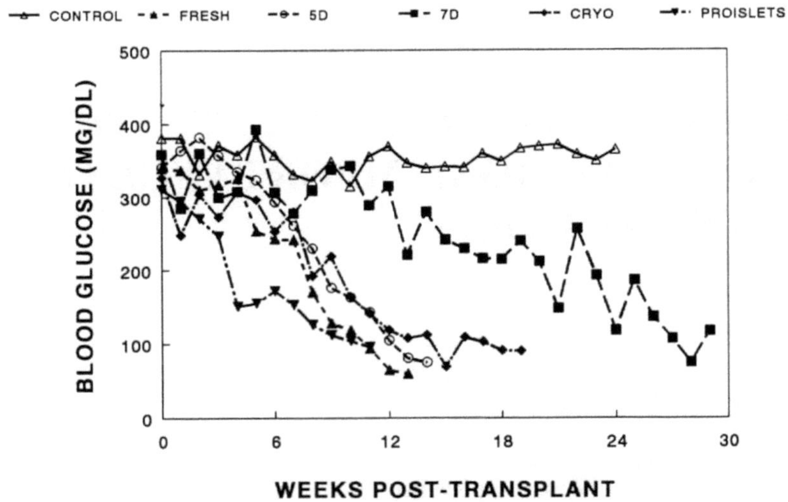

Figure 1. Reversal of hyperglycemia in streptozotocin-induced diabetic nude mice following transplantation of HFP. Nude mice were transplanted with 4-5 mg of HFP tissue and blood glucose levels determined on a weekly basis.

with over 1000 HFP tissues, we have shown that HFP explants, either cyropreserved, cultured or prepared as proislets reliably reverse experimentally-induced diabetes in immunoincompetent nude mouse recipients (Figure 1). Normal glucose control is restored following transplantation (1, 3-6). Grafted HFP responds normally to glucose challenge, while fresh HFP is not responsive to glucose indicating that further growth and differentiation occurs following transplantation.

To date, there has been limited success in the clinical transplantation of HFP; no recipient has been successfully removed from insulin therapy. However, in a limited study carried out by Lafferty and colleagues, 9 of 15 recipients demonstrated reduced insulin requirements following HFP transplantation (7). The reduction in insulin requirement was dependent on the amount of HFP transplanted. In addition, intact islets staining positively for insulin, glucagon, and somatostatin were detected in biopsy specimens. These results demonstrate the potential of HFP for clinical transplantation.

A. Problems Facing HFP Transplantation

There are two major problems facing the successful clinical transplantation of HFP. First HFP is extremely immunogenic. Fetal pancreatic tissue is more immunogenic that adult islets, requiring significantly longer culture periods to achieve prolonged allograft survival (8-10). Simeonovic, et al. have shown that murine proislets preparations (prepared by limited collagenase digestion) are less immunogenic and contain significantly fewer donor antigen presenting cells (APC), endothelial cells and less exocrine tissue (9,10). We have obtained similar results with HFP proislets in that proislets are less efficient stimulators of proliferation in a one way mixed lymphocyte culture. Other methods to decrease the immunogenicity of HFP and improve the allograft survival of endocrine tissues include, hyperbaric oxygen culture (HOC [11,12]), high oxygen culture (13,14), UVB irradiation (15) and low temperature culture (16). The primary focus of these techniques has been donor APC removal. However, results with HOC and UVB irradiation have suggested that other mechanisms may be involved in mediating graft prolongation (17-19). We have shown that HOC of murine thyroid tissue results in the down-regulation of MHC class I surface expression, prolongation of graft survival, and induction of recipient tolerance to a non-treated second allograft (11,19). We have observed recipient unresponsiveness to simultaneously transplanted HOC- and non-treated thyroid allografts in which fully functional donor APC are present in the non-treated graft. Our results suggest that clonal deletion is not the mechanism, rather the evidence now suggests that presentation of donor alloantigen by naive splenic B cells may be responsible for the induction of T cell anergy. Recent results suggest that HOC can be successfully applied to HFP. Thus, it may be possible to transplant HFP without the use of immunosuppressive therapy.

The second major problem facing successful HFP transplantation is the time required for the development of glucose responsiveness following transplantation. Fresh HFP is non-responsive to glucose challenge. Approximately 3 months is required for beta cells to differentiate, mature and restore normoglycemia in streptozotocin-induced diabetic nude mice (1). Most acute rejection episodes occur within the first 3 months post-transplant. Since HFP is not responsive to glucose, there is no effective way of monitoring for either transplant rejection episodes or early function during the HFP maturation period. Work from several laboratories has suggested that the differentiation and maturation of HFP can be accelerated with the use of short-term culture in growth factors (6, 20-22).

3. NORMAL DIFFERENTIATION OF HFP

The pancreas is derived from an epithelial evagination of the foregut endoderm into the splanchnic mesoderm from which both acinar and islet cell differentiation occurs(20). It is generally believed that beta cells are derived from cells which bud from embryonic duct-like cells. The processes which drive the differentiation of budding cells to glucose responsive beta cells remain unclear. Sarvetnick and colleagues have describe the presence of transitional cells which stain positively for multiple exocrine and endocrine hormones. They have proposed a differentiation pathway which proceeds from ductal epithelium to ductal acinar phenotype to ductal endocrine phenotype to cells with either a acinar or endocrine phenotype (23).

A. Genetic Markers of Beta Cell Differentiation

A number of genes have been identified as markers of beta cell differentiation including adenine nucleotide translocator (ANT), acid β-galactosidase, and reg (24-27). ANT is a mitochondrial protein which forms a membrane pore allowing the transport of ATP and ADP. Welsh and colleagues have characterized the expression of ANT (24). The level of ANT increased with increasing degree of islet functional response, i.e. fetal islets contain less ANT whereas adult islets responding to a high glucose challenge contain the most. Interestingly, the authors suggest that defects in the expression of this gene are associated with decreased glucose sensitivity. This may result from the lower energy level within the cell.

A second gene associated with HFP differentiation is acid β-galactosidase. Beattie, et al. noted that following collagenase digestion and culture of HFP, free floating islet-like cell clusters were obtained that contained a high number of undifferentiated cells (25). Histochemical analysis revealed that greater than 70% of these cells stained positively for acid beta-galactosidase. The expression of acid-β galactosidase was developmentally regulated; expression peaked at 18-24 weeks gestational age and was greatly diminished following transplant into nude mice when mature differentiated islets were present. In comparison to ANT, which appears to be a marker of functionally differentiated beta cells, acid-β galactosidase appears to be a marker of the immature beta cell.

A third gene associated with beta cell replication is the reg gene. Watanabe, et al. have shown that reg is expressed in regenerating islets but not in normal adult islets (26). In a second series of experiments using a 90% pancreatectomy model, rats receiving recombinant reg protein reversed their diabetes and significantly increased their beta cell mass (27). *In vitro* studies with isolated islets showed that addition of reg protein significantly increased ^{3}H-thymidine incorporation. In studies designed to distinguish between fetal growth and differentiation, Hayek and colleagues examined the level of reg gene expression during HFP culture in the presence of nicotinamide (promotes HFP differentiation) or hepatocyte growth factor/scatter factor (mitogenic for HFP (HGF/SF)[27]). Reg expression was elevated 3-fold in cultures containing HGF/SF and only marginally in nicotinamide culture. It is likely that the reg gene plays a role in beta cell replication and may have little to do with beta cell differentiation.

In summary, little is known about which gene products influence the development of a glucose responsive beta cell from a budding ductal cell. It is likely that genes active during fetal development will be different than those active during adult beta cell regeneration.

B. Growth Factors Influencing Beta Cell Differentiation

Soluble peptide growth hormones have also been implicated in the differentiation of beta cells. The growth factors TGF-α, TGF-β, gastrin, and insulin-like growth factor-1 (IGF-1) have been shown to influence the growth and differentiation of beta cells (6, 21, 28,29). Recent experiments by Bonner-Wier and colleagues using transgenic mice expressing TGF-α and gastrin under the control of the insulin promoter suggest that islet growth may be stimulated by both gastrin and TGF-α since expression of neither transgene alone was sufficient to promote islet growth (29). Several groups have demonstrated that gastrin is expressed in fetal beta cells but not in adult islets. In addition, gastrin has been described as a pancreatic growth factor. In fact, neoplastic transformation of adult beta cells results in the re-expression of gastrin. Positive regulatory sequences located in the gastrin promoter region resemble the islet-specific enhancer elements of the insulin gene (30). This suggests that a coordinate or regulated expression of gastrin and insulin may occur in fetal beta cells. Thus, gastrin in either a paracrine or autocrine fashion could promote the differentiation of beta cells to a glucose responsive state. Rorsman, et al. have suggested that rat fetal pancreatic beta cells are unresponsive to glucose due to an insensitivity of ATP-regulated K+ channels (31). It is possible that gastrin may be involved in regulating the sensitivity of K+ channels.

In the Bonner-Wier transgenic mouse studies expression of TGF-α alone resulted in the development of metaplastic ductules which contained numerous insulin positive cells. Bonner-Wier has suggested that TGF-α is induced during the early ductal expansion phase and that other factors such gastrin and IGF-I are induced later when islets begin to differentiate. Other experiments using immunoperoxidase staining techniques have shown a differential expression of TGF-β2 and TGF-β3 in the endocrine pancreas, suggesting a role for these factors in both insulin secretion and in the differentiation of beta cells (32). Finally, TGF-β1 has been shown to inhibit the growth of acinar tissue (33). The role of TGF-β in the growth and differentiation of beta cells may be multifactorial. TGF-β is an inhibitor of cell proliferation at higher concentrations (nanomolar range), and is a potent stimulator of extracellular matrix deposition at lower concentrations (femtamolar concentrations) (34-36). The composition and extent of extracellular matrix may influence the differentiation state of the beta cell. Sjoholm and Hellerstrom have recently demonstrated that TGF-β1 was effective in blocking the mitogenic effect of glucose on rat fetal islets but also stimulated insulin secretion (28). Thus, while TGF-α may influence the early beta cell replication and the early development of the beta cell, TGF-β1 may influence terminal beta cell differentiation.

Another growth factor recently identified as potentially important for the growth and differentiation of HFP is hepatocyte growth factor/scatter factor. Otonkoski, et al. compared the ability of HGF/SF, basic fibroblast growth factor-2, keratinocyte growth factor, and IGF-II to promote the formation of islet-like cell clusters (proislets) during *in vitro* culture (37). Both HGF/SF and keratinocyte growth factor stimulated proislet formation by 2-3 fold. Only culture in HGF/SF increased insulin content per DNA and increased the number of replicating cells (by 3-fold).

The somatomedins, of which IGF-1 is a member, have been shown to influence the growth and maturation of fetal pancreas. Fetal islet cell cultures have been shown to produce and accumulate IGF-1 and IGF-2 in the culture media (38). Both growth factors have mitogenic effects on fetal islet beta cells. Exogenous IGF-1 addition to human fetal islet-like cell clusters induced a 2-fold increase in DNA content (39).

In a model employing 90% pancreatectomy, Smith et al. have shown that IGF-1 expression is localized in focal areas of regeneration near proliferating ductules (21). We have used culture in IGF-1 to accelerate the maturation of HFP (6). HFP explants or proislets were placed in culture in the presence of IGF-1, IGF-2 or both IGF-1 and IGF-2 (72h 100ng/ml) and the amount of insulin released in response to high glucose and theophylline challenge determined. As shown in Figure 2, insulin release was greatest in the IGF-2 culture. Explants or proislets were then placed beneath the kidney capsule of streptozotocin-induced diabetic nude mice. Culture in the presence of IGF-1 significantly decreased the time required for return to normoglycemia. IGF-2 or IGF-1 + IGF-2 cultured HFP did not significantly decrease the time required for reversal. Hematoxylin and eosin staining of IGF cultured HFP explants revealed a more organized appearance, with less exocrine tissue and with an overall structure more analogous to mature islets than present in explants cultured in medium alone. Immunocytochemical analysis showed an increased number of insulin-positive cells in IGF-treated cultures. Additionally, the positive cells were located in organized clusters near ductal elements. These results suggest that IGF-I culture may enhance the differentiation of HFP explants and proislets.

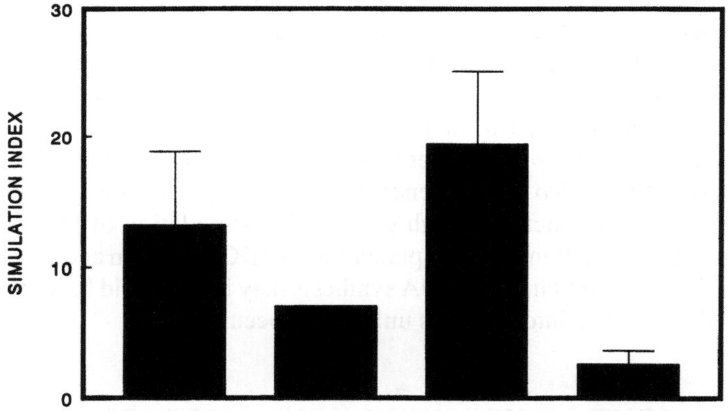

Figure 2. Regulatory control of IGF-1 or IGF-2 cultured HFP. A stimulation index (ng insulin released in response to low glucose/ng insulin released in response to high glucose and theophylline) was used to quantify regulatory control.

4. ENHANCEMENT OF FUNCTION WITH CHEMICAL AGENTS

Nicotinamide is an inhibitor of the enzyme poly(ADP-ribose) synthetase which is a nuclear protein whose function is unclear. However, it is postulated that poly(ADP-ribose) synthetase may function to ribosylate nuclear proteins effecting modifications in chromatin structure and the transcription of previously inactive genes. Nicotinamide has been shown in *in vitro* studies to stimulate adult islet and human fetal pancreatic cell DNA replication and to increase the insulin content by 3-fold (40). Initial studies have suggested that nicotinamide also promotes beta cell differentiation (22). Otonkoski, et al. report the development of beta cell outgrowths for epithelial cell clusters (41). These clusters showed an increase in the expression of insulin, glucagon and somatostatin. An *in vivo* study performed by Korsgren, et al. demonstrated that addition of nicotinamide to the drinking water (2.5 mM) significantly decreased the time required for reversal of diabetes in alloxan-induced diabetic nude mice by fetal porcine islet-like cell clusters from 8 weeks to 3-4 weeks (22). Assessment of graft function demonstrated normal insulin release in low glucose and enhanced insulin release in response to 16.7 mM at 4 weeks post-transplant. However, insulin release in response to high glucose was decreased at 8 weeks despite a significant increase in the insulin content of the graft. Thus, long-term effects of nicotinamide may not be advantageous to stable graft function. Perfusion of graft bearing kidneys from mice that had received nicotinamide treated islet-like cell clusters rather than nicotinamide in the drinking water, showed nearly a 3-fold increase in the amount of insulin released in response to glucose challenge 18 weeks post-transplant. Therefore, *in vitro* exposure to nicotinamide prior to transplant may activate unknown gene products leading to the differentiation of beta cells.

5. ENHANCEMENT OF HFP FUNCTION WITH GENETIC MANIPULATION

A novel approach for enhancing the rate of replication in fetal beta cells has been to introduce selected oncogenes into pancreatic cells under the control of the insulin promoter localizing the growth to the beta cell (42-45). Welsh and colleagues transfected fetal rat islets with v-*src*, c-*myc* and c-Ha-*ras* and measured the rate of replication by ^{3}H-thymidine incorporation. Transfection with v-*src* and c-*myc* significantly enhanced the replication rate (43). In a second series of experiments, the platelet derived growth factor (PDGF) B chain was co-transfected with the PDGF-β-receptor into a beta cell enriched cell suspension (44). Co-transfection with the PDGF-B chain or addition of 10% fetal calf serum resulted in a significant stimulation of DNA synthesis. Finally, purified islets transfected in vitro with the oncogene v-src and transplanted to diabetic recipients showed a small increase in DNA synthesis in contrast to *in vitro* experiments where maximum stimulation was achieved in 16.7 mM glucose (45). *In vivo* the influence of other regulatory factors may dominate the action of the oncogene products and high glucose. No stimulation of DNA synthesis was observed following transfection and transplantation of PDGF B-chain and PDGF β-receptor. One reason for the low stimulation of DNA synthesis may be the rapid loss of plasmid DNA from transfected cells since integration is unlikely to occur.

6. ENHANCEMENT OF HFP WITH GENE THERAPY TECHNIQUES

Until recently, genetic alteration of mammalian cells was primarily accomplished by stable transformation or retroviral-mediated transfection. Gene transfer by stable transformation is inefficient, requiring a time consuming analysis of the stable clones and is not suited for use in the whole organ or animal. Although the vectors used in retroviral-mediated gene transfer have improved in safety, they are dependent on the integration of reverse transcribed viral DNA into the genomic DNA of the host (46). This event requires active host cell division and carries the risk of undesirable transformation because of insertional mutations or by activation of certain oncogenes. In one instance, retroviral gene transfer resulted in the generation of lymphomas in nonhuman primates (47).

The use of replication-defective adenoviruses as vectors for delivery and expression of genes of interest has emerged as an attractive alternative to conventional methods because they efficiently infect non-dividing cells. A number of serologically distinct adenoviruses from various species have been identified, including over 50 subtypes from humans, of which two (Ad2 and Ad5) are the most studied. Adenoviruses contain a double stranded DNA genome of 36Kb in a 70 nm icosahedron particle. Adenoviruses infect the host via an unknown ubiquitous cell surface receptor, replicate episomally and propagate through a lytic cycle (46). The wild type Ad5 genome has been rendered replication-defective by deletion of the E1 genes (48). In the last four years replication-defective adenovirus systems have been used to efficiently deliver genes of interest to mammalian cells in primary culture as well as to various tissues *in vivo* (49-52). Because adenovirus replicates episomally, gene expression is transient (53). As a consequence, it is an ideal vector for the delivery of genes whose products are needed and desired only for a limited period of time, such as growth factors. It is likely that adenovirus-mediated expression of growth factors in HFP explants or proislets will accelerate the development of glucose responsiveness such that graft function can be monitored soon after transplantation and that appropriate therapy can be used to prevent acute graft rejection.

It has recently been shown in isolated primary rat hepatocytes cultures that replication-defective adenovirus was able to transfect at least 85% of all cells and was able to direct the synthesis of high levels of a functionally active muscle glycogen phosphorylase (50). It has also been shown that the β-galactosidase containing adenovirus (AdCMV.β-gal) can successfully transfect isolated adult rat islets, resulting in a high level of enzyme expression without impairing insulin response to glucose challenge (Alam et al. unpublished observations).

We have begun initial studies using adenovirus to transfect HFP with the growth factor IGF-I. To determine whether adenovirus would transfect HFP as well as it does fully differentiated mature issues, HFP proislets were prepared by limited collagenase digestion. After overnight culture in supplemented RPMI 1640 medium, proislets were transfected with the replication-defective adenovirus AdCMV.β-gal and cultured for four additional days. Transfected proislets showed intense blue staining following X-gal staining. To determine if AdCMV.β-gal transfection was specific for beta cells insulin positive cells were identified by immunofluorescence. Results showed some cells positively stained for both β-gal and insulin; no preferential transfection of the beta cells was observed. There was no discernible difference in the insulin release of β-gal transfected proislets and control cultured non-transfected proislets in response to high glucose (16.7 mM) and theophylline (10 mM). These results provide a starting point for HFP transfection studies with adenovirus constructs containing growth factors as a means to enhance or accelerate HFP function following transplantation.

Unfortunately, several studies have suggested that deletion of the E1 genes is not sufficient to prevent development of an immune response to adenoviral proteins expressed on the cell surface (51). A cytotoxic T cell response has been described following the in vivo transfection of rat hepatocytes with E1a- and E1b-deleted recombinant adenovirus containing the human gene for LDL receptor (51). Similar results have been described in mice transfected with E1a-deleted recombinant Adenovirus containing the CF transmembrane conductance regulator (52). When a second generation virus—not only deleted of E1a and E1b, but also crippled by a temperature-sensitive mutation in the E2a gene— was used to transfect mice, substantially longer gene expression and less inflammation was observed (54).

7. SUMMARY

The process of beta cell differentiation and maturation to a glucose responsive cell remains largely undefined. It is clear that gene products involved in fetal development are different from those that are involved in the replication and regeneration of adult islets. Defining which growth and differentiation factors mediate beta cell development remains a goal of future research efforts.

Human fetal pancreas transplantation is a viable alternative to whole organ or adult islet transplantation. Significant progress has been made in overcoming the problems of HFP immunogenicity and lack of glucose responsiveness. The use of short-term culture or gene therapy techniques to increase the expression of certain growth factors, particularly IGF-1 and TGF-β, will enhance HFP function and allow for the monitoring of acute rejection by graft function in the early period following transplantation. Many of the currently available immunosuppressive agents affect beta cell function. Thus, the development of techniques, such as HOC, which allow transplantation in the absence immunosuppressive therapy will further enhance the potential for successful HFP transplantation.

ACKNOWLEDGEMENT

This work was supported National Institutes of Health grants DK-35446 and HD-32137.

REFERENCES

1. Hullett, D. A., Falany, J.L., Love, R.B., Burlingham, W.J., Pan, M., and Sollinger, H.W. Human fetal pancreas - a potential source for transplantation. Transplantation 1987;43:18.
2. Tuch, B.E., and Simpson, A.M. Experimental fetal islet transplantation. In: Pancreatic Islet Cell Transplantation. Ricordi, C. ed. R.C. Landers, Co., Austin, TX. 1992. p294.
3. Bethke, K.P., Hullett, D.A., Falany, J.L., Love, R.B., and Sollinger, H.W. Cultured human fetal pancreatic tissue reverses experimentally induced diabetes in nude mice. Curr. Surg. 1988;45(2):123.
4. Hullett, D.A., Landry, A.S., Leonard, D.K., and Sollinger, H.W. Improved human fetal pancreatic tissue survival following hyperbaric oxygen culture. Transplan. Proc. 1989;21(1):2659.
5. Hullett, D.A., Bethke, K.P., Landry, A.S., Leonard, D.K., and Sollinger, H.W. Successful long-term cryopreservation and transplantation of human fetal pancreas. Diabetes 1989;38(4):448.
6. Eckhoff, D.E., Sollinger, H.W., and Hullett, D.A. Selective enhancement of B cell activity by preparation of fetal pancreatic proislets and culture with insulin growth factor 1 (IGF-1). Transplantation 1991;51(6):1161.
7. Lafferty, K.J., and Hao, L. Fetal pancreas transplantation for treatment of IDDM patients. Diabets Care 1993;16:383.
8. Mandel, T.E., and Koulmanda, M. Effect of culture conditions on fetal mouse pancreas in vitro and after transplantation in syngeneic and allogeneic recipients. Diabetes 1985;34:1082.
9. Simeonovic, C.J., Hodden, M.J., and Hume, D.A. Role of Ia- positive leukocytes and F4/80 positive macrophages in the immunogeneity of fetal mouse proislets and fetal pancreas. Transplant. Proc. 1988;20:68.
10. Simeonovic, C.J., and Lafferty, K.J. Immunogeniety of isolated fetal mouse pancreas. Aust. J. Exp. Biol. Med. Sci. 1982;60:391.

11. Hullett, D.A., Landry, A.S., Leonard, D.K., and Sollinger, H.W. Enhancement of thryoid allograft survival following organ culture: alteration of tissue immunogenicity. Transplantation 1989;47(1):24.
12. LaRosa, F.B., and Talmage, D.W. The failure of major histocompatibility antigen to stimulate a thyroid allograft reaction after culture in oxygen. J. Exp. Med. 1983;157:898.
13. Talmage, D.W., and Dart, G.A. Effect of oxygen pressure during culture on survival of mouse thyroid allografts. Science 1978;200:1066.
14. Lafferty, K.J., Bootes, A., Kilby, A.A., and Barch, W. Mechanism of thyroid allograft rejection. Aust. J. Exp. Biol. Sci. 1976;54:573.
15. Hardy, M.A. Reemtsma, K. Lau, H.T. Induction of indefinite rat islet allograft survival with direct ultraviolet irradiation and peri-transplant cyclosporine. Transplant. Proc. 1985;17:423.
16. Markmann, J.F., Tomaszewski, J., Posselt, A.N., Levy, A.R., Woehrle, M., Barker, C.F., and Naji, A. The effect of islet cell culture *in vitro* at 24^{0}C on graft survival and MHC antigen expression. Transplantation 1990;49:272.
17. LaRosa, F.G., Smilek, D., Talmage, D.W., Lafferty, K.J., Bauling, P., and Ammons, T.J. Evidence that tolerance to cultured thyroid allografts is an active immunological process. Protection of third party grafts bearing new antigens when associated with tolerogenic antigens. Transplantation 1992;53:903.
18. Simon, J.C., Tigelaar, R.E., Bergstresser, P.R., Edelbaum, D., Cruz, P.D.Jr., Ultaviolet B radiation converts langerhans cells from immunogenic to tolerogenic antigen- presenting cells. J. Immunol. 1991;145(2):485.
19. Everlith, K.M., Landry, A.S., Sollinger, H.W., and Hullett, D.A. Induction of recipient tolerance by hyperbaric oxygen culture may be mediated by anergic CD8+ T cells. Transplant. Sci. 1993;3:20.
20. Rosenberg, L., Vinik, A.I., and Duguid, W.P. Islet neogenesis. In: Pancreatic Islet Cell Transplantation. Ricordi, C., ed. R.C. Landers, Co. Austin, TX, 1992; p.58.
21. Smith, F.E., Rosen, K.M., Villa-Komaroff, L. Wier, G.C., and Bonner-Wier, S. Enhanced insulin-like growth factor I gene expression in regenerating rat pancreas. Proc. Nat'l. Acad. Sci. USA 1991;88:6152.
22. Korsgren, O., Andersson, A., and Sandler, S. Pretreatment of fetal porcine pancreas in culture with nicotinamide accelerates reversal of diabetes after transplantation to nude mice. Surgery 1993;113:205.
23. Gu, D., and Sarvetnick, N. Epithelial cell proliferation and islet neogenesis in IFN-γ transgenic mice. Development 1993;118:33
24. Welsh, N., Svensson, C., and Welsh, M. Content of adenine nucleotide translocator mRNA in insulin-producing cells of different functional states. Diabetes 1989;38:1377.
25. Beattie, G.M., Levine, F., Mally, M.I., Otonkoski, T., O'Brien, J.S., Salomon, D.R., and Hayek, A. Acid β- galactosidase: a developmentally regulated marker of endocrine cell precursors in the human fetal pancreas. J. Clin. Endocrinol. and Metab. 1994;78:1232.
26. Watanabe, T., Yonemura, Y., Yonekura, H., Suzuki, Y., Miyashita, H., Sugiyama, K., Moriizumi, S., Unno, M., Tanaka, O., Kondo, H., Bone, A.J., Takasawa, S., and Okamoto, H. Pancreatic beta-cell replication and amelioration of surgical diabetes by Reg protein. Proc. Nat'l. Acad. Sci. USA 1994;91:3589.
27. Otonkoski, T., Mally, M.I., and Hayek, A. Opposite effects of β-cell differentiation and growth on reg expression in human fetal pancreatic cells. Diabetes 1994;43:1164.
28. Sjoholm, A., and Hellerstrom, C. TGF-β stimulates insulin secretion and blocks mitogenic response of pancreatic β- cells to glucose. Am. J. Physiol. 1991;363:C1046.
29. Wang, T.C., Bonner-Wier, S., Oates, P.S., Chulak, M. Simon, B., Merlino, G.T., Schmidt, E.V., and Brand, S.J. Pancreatic gastrin stimulates islet differentiation of transforming growth factor α-induced ductular presursor cells. J. Clin. Invest. 1993;92:1349.
30. Wang, T.C., and Brand, S.J. Islet cell-specific regulatory domain in the gastrin promoter contains adjacent positive and negative DNA elements. J. Biol. Chem. 1990;265:8908.
31. Rorsmam, P., Arkhammer, P., Bokvist, K., Hellerstrom, C., Nilsson, T., Welsh, M., Welsh, N., and Berggren, P. Failure of glucose to elicit a normal secretory response in fetal pancreatic beta cells results from glucose insensitivity of the ATP-regulated K+ channels. Proc. Nat'l. Acad. Sci. USA 1989;86:4505.
32. Yamanaka, Y., Friess, H., Buchler, M., Beger, H.G., Gold, L.I., and Korc, M. Synthesis and expression of transforming growth factor β-1, β-2, and β-3 in the endocrine and exocrine pancreas. Diabetes 1993;42:746.
33. Logsdon, C.D., Keyes, L., and Beauchamp, R.D. Transforming growth factor-β (TGF-β1) inhibits pancreatic acinar cell growth. Am. J. Physiol. 1992;262:G364.
34. Mii, S., Ware, A., and Kent, K.C. Transforming growth factor-beta inhibits human vascular smooth muscle cell growth and migration. Surgery 1993;1145:464.
35. Majack, P.A. Beta-type transfroming growth factor specifies organizational behavior in vascular smooth cell cultures. J. Cell Biol. 1987;105:965.

36. Parekh, T., Saxena, B., Reibman, J., Cronstein, B.N., and Gold, L.I. Neutrophil chemotaxis in response to TGF-β isoforms (TGF-β1, TGF-β2, TGF-β3) is mediated by fibronectin. J. Immunol. 1993;151:1147.
37. Otonkoski, T., Beattie, G.M., Rubin, J.S., Lopez, A.D., Baird, A., and Hayek, A. Hepatocyte growth factor/scatter factor has insulinotropic activity in human fetal pancreatic dells. Diabetes 1994;43:947.
38. Swenne, I., Hill, D.J., Strain, A.J., and Milner, R.D.G. Growth hormone regulation of somatomedin C/insulin-like growth factor I production and DNA replication in fetal rat islets in tissue culture. Diabetes '1987;36:288.
39. Otonkoski, T., Knip, M., Wong, I., and Simell, O. Effects of growth hormone and insulin-like growth factor I on endocrine function of human fetal-like cell clusters during long-term tissue culture. Diabetes 1988;37:1678.
40. Sandler, S., Anderson, A., Korsgren, O. et al. Tissue culture of human fetal pancreas: effects of nicotinamide on insulin production and formation of isletlike cell clusters. Diabetes 1989;38(suppl 1):168.
41. Otonkoski, T., Beattie, G.M., Mally, M.I., Ricordi, C., and Hayek, A. Nicotinamide is a potent inducer of endocrine differentiation in cultured human fetal pancreatic cells. J. Clin. Invest. 1993;92:1459.
42. Welsh, M., Mares, J., Oberg, C., and Karlsson, T. Genetic factors of importance for β-cell proliferation. Diabetes/Metab Rev. 1993;9(1):25.
43. Welsh, M., Welsh, N., Nilsson, T., Arkhammar, P., Pepinsky, R.B., Steiner, D.F., and Berggren, P. Stimulation of pancreatic islet beta-cell replication by oncogenes. Proc. Nat'l. Acad. Sci. USA 1988;85:116.
44. Welsh M., Claesson-Welsh, L., Hallberg, A., Welsh, N., Betsholtz, C., Arkhammar, P., Nilsson, T., Heldin, C., and Berggren, P. Coexpression of the platelet-derived growth factor (PDGF) B chain and the PDGF β receptor in isolated pancreatic islet cells stimulates DNA synthesis. Proc. Nat'l. Acad. Sci. USA 1990;87:5807.
45. Welsh, M., and Andersson, A. Transplantation of transfected pancreatic islets: stimulation of β cell DNA synthesis by the src oncogene. Transplantation 1994;57:297.
46. Varmus, H. Retroviruses. Science 1988;240:1427.
47. Donahue, R.E., Kessler, S.W., Bodine, D., McDonagh, K., Dunbar, C., Goodman, S., Agricola, B., Byrne, E., Raffeld, M., Moen, R., Bocher, J., Zsebo, K.M., and Neinhaus, A.W. Helper virus induced T cell lymphoma in nonhuman primates after retroviral mediated gene transfer. J. Exp. Med. 1992;176:1125.
48. Graham, F.L., and Prevec, L. Manipulations of adenovirus. In: methods in Molecular Biology, Murray, E.J. ed. The Humanna Press, Inc., Clifton, NJ. 1991;7:109.
49. Statfor-Perricaudet, L.D., Levrero, M., Chasse, J.F., Perricaudet, M., and Briaud, P. Evaluation of the transfer and expression in mice of an enzyme-encoding gene using a human adenovirus vector. Human Gene Therapy 1990;1:241.
50. Gomez-Foix, A.M., Coats, W.S., Baque, S., Alam, T., Gerard, R.D., and Newgard, C.B. Adenovirus mediated transfer of the muscle glycogen phosphorylase gene in hepatocytes confers altered regulation of glycogen metabolism. J. Biol. Chem. 1992;267:25129.
51. Yang, Y., Ertl, H.C.J., and Wilson, J.M. MHC class I restricted cytotoxic T lymphocytes to viral antigens destroy hepatocytes in mice infected with E1-deleted recombinant adenovirus. Immunity. 1994;1:433.
52. Simon, R.H., Engelhardt, J.F., Yang, Y., Zepeda, N., Weber- Pendleton, s., Grossman, M., and Wilson, J.M. Adenovirus- mediated transfer of the CFTR gene to lung of nonhuman primates: toxicity study. Hum. Gene. Ther. 1993;4:771.
53. Herz, J., and Gerard, R.D. Adenovirus-mediated transfer of low density lipoprotein receptor gene acutely accelerates cholesterol clearance in normal mice. Proc. Nat'l. Acad. Sci. USA 1993;90:2812.
54. Engelhardt, J.F., Ye, X., Doranz, B., and Wilson, J.M. Ablation of E2a in recombinant adenoviruses improves transgene persistence and decreases imflammatory response in mouse liver. Proc. Nat'l. Acad. Sci. USA 1994;91:6196.

4

STUDIES OF FETAL PORCINE ISLET-LIKE CELL CLUSTERS—A TISSUE SOURCE FOR XENOTRANSPLANTATION IN INSULIN-DEPENDENT DIABETES MELLITUS?

S. Sandler,* L. Jansson, J.-O. Sandberg, N. Salari-Lak, A. Andersson, and C. Hellerström

Department of Medical Cell Biology, Uppsala University
Biomedicum, P. O. Box 571
S-751 23 Uppsala, Sweden

INTRODUCTION

Insulin-dependent diabetes mellitus (IDDM) is an autoimmune disease characterized by the selective destruction of the insulin-producing β-cells from the pancreatic islets (Gepts, 1965; Eisenbarth, 1986). The disease is insidious, and does not become manifest until approximately 90% of the β-cells are lost. The disease can be treated with insulin which, despite its prolongation of life of the patients, cannot succesfully prevent long-term complications of the disease, such as blindness, nephropathy, neuropathy and cardiovascular disease. To obtain a strictly physiological minute-to-minute regulation of the glucose metabolism, the only possible treatment today is replacement of the lost pancreatic β-cells. This can be accomplished by transplantation of the whole pancreas, meaning that only 1% of the transplanted organ, i.e. the islets, are really necessary. This treatment is hampered by technical complications (Robertson, 1992), and to transplant only the needed endocrine component of the pancreas would therefore be preferable. The isolation and purification of islets from adult cadaveric human donors has now become sufficiently successful to warrant clinical trials (Gray et al., 1984, Ricordi et al., 1988), and a few patients have been, at least temporarily, cured of their disease (Scharp et al., 1991; Warnock et al., 1991). These results are encouraging since they demonstrate that this surgically simple procedure may offer a new treatment modality for IDDM. One major drawback with transplantations in IDDM is the immunogenicity of the implanted islets, which may result both in graft rejection and disease recurrence with the development of the underlying disease also in the graft (Gill and

* Telephone: +46 (0)18 174430; FAX: +46 (0)18 556401.

Fetal Islet Transplantation
Edited by C. M. Peterson, L. Jovanovic-Peterson, and B. Formby, Plenum Press, New York, 1995

Lafferty, 1989). However, the development of new and more specific immunosuppressive drugs, in combination with advances in immunoalterations and immunoisolation would obviate the present day problems with immunosuppression. Despite the promising results obtained so far several other, non-immunological drawbacks to islet transplantations exist. The major problem is to obtain sufficient quantities of viable and functionally intact endocrine cells for subsequent implantations. With the presently available isolation techniques several donors are normally required for each successful human allogeneic islet transplantation. This would therefore lead to an even greater demand on donor organ supply than the present whole organ transplantations.

In view of this consideration other sources of endocrine pancreatic tissue for transplantations must be sought for. In this context the use of xenogeneic tissues is of great interest provided that the immunological problems can be solved. Even though the islets from sub-human primates cannot be used, due both to ethical and practical (possible transmission of contagious diseases) constraints, other animals such as pigs would provide an almost unlimited number of possible donors. However, the practical difficulties to isolate islets from adult pig pancreata are considerable. The interest has therefore also been focused on the possibilty to use fetal porcine pancreases for this purpose. The possibilty to use fetal pancreatic tissue in curing diabetic rodents was first demonstrated 20 years ago (Brown et al., 1974), and has later been repeatedly confirmed in small laboratory animals and miniature pig animal models of diabetes; for a review see (Andersson and Sandler., 1992). The fetal endocrine pancreas is not only easily available (if a xenogeneic source is used), but the hormone prodoucing cells have also a great potential for growth and differentiation, all of which makes it a prime candidate as a future source for pancreatic islets intended for transplantation in IDDM. Moreover, porcine insulin has proven its efficacy for more than 70 years in the treatment of human IDDM.

In this chapter we will describe our experimental and clinical findings from the use of the fetal porcine pancreas in an attempt to treat patients with IDDM. For this purpose, we took advantage from our previous experience in preparing explants for in vitro tissue cultures from the fetal rat (Hellerström et al., 1979) and the fetal human pancreas (Sandler et al., 1985). Thus, we worked out a method for preparation of so called islet-like cell clusters (ICC) from the fetal porcine pancreas (Korsgren et al., 1988). These explants, which show a marked potential for further differentiation in vivo into mature pancreatic islets after transplantation, can easily be produced in large quantities from the fetal porcine pancreas by a simple culture technique.

METHODOLOGY USED

Preparation and Culture of Fetal Porcine Pancreas

Pregnant sows belonging to a local stock were killed by means of a slaughtering mask. The length of gestation was 70-75 days (full-term $\approx$ 115 days). The fetuses (10-15 per litter) were immediately collected from the uterus and placed on ice during transport to the laboratory.

After aseptic removal the pancreatic glands were put in cold Hanks' solution containing benzylpenicillin and streptomycin, minced to fragments with a size of 1-2 mm^3 and treated with approximately 10 mg/ml of collagenase (Collagenase A from Clostridium histolyticum, Boehringer Mannheim, Mannheim, Germany) as described elsewhere (Korsgren et al., 1988). After washing, the digested tissue was explanted into culture dishes allowing cellular attachment (Nunclon, Nunc, Kamstrup, Denmark). During the initial 2-3 days there was a outgrowth of a monolayer of fibroblasts. On top of this layer, there is a gradual appearance of spherical cell aggregates, with a diameter of 200-400 μm, that are loosely attached to the fibroblastoid cells. The cell aggregates could easily be detatched by flushing culture medium with a syringe, and then harvested by a pipette. In the stereomicroscope the cell aggregates resembled isolated pancreatic islets in shape and size, but since only a minority of the cells at this stage stained positively for islet hormone content we have designated them as ICC.

The culture medium was RPMI 1640 (11.1 mM glucose; HyClone, Cramlington, UK) and the cultures were supplemented with either 1% or 10% (v/v) pooled human serum (1% HS or 10% HS; The Blood Center, Huddinge Hospital, Huddinge, Sweden). In some culture dishes 10 mM nicotinamide (Sigma Chemicals, St Louis, MO, USA), 200 ng/ml dexamethasone (Sigma) or 2 mM sodium butyrate (Sigma) was added. In the cultures to which the factors were added, the serum supplement was 1% HS.

The culture medium was exchanged after two days and after four days ICC were harvested and examined as descibed below. In some experiments the culture medium was then changed in all groups to RPMI 1640 + 10% HS, without any further addition and the ICC were cultured for another four days, when their function was examined.

Transplantation of ICC to Mice

Male, inbred athymic nude C57BL/6 mice (Bomholdtgaard, Ry, Denmark) and normal male inbred C57BL/6 mice, belonging to a locally bred stock originally obtained from the Jackson Laboratory, Bar Harbor, ME, USA, were used as recipients of ICC. In some animals diabetes was induced by an intravenous injection of alloxan (90 mg/kg body weight; Sigma) four days prior to transplantation.

Transplantation of ICC was performed, under anaesthesia using tribromoethanol, after 4-5 days of culture (Korsgren et al., 1991). The ICC were deposited under the left renal capsule after a small incision using a braking pipette. Depending on the type of experiment about 100-600 ICC, corresponding to a volume of approximately 1-6 μl of ICC, were implanted. All animals had free access to pelleted chow (Type R34; AnalyCen, Lidköping, Sweden) and tap water, throughout the experiments.

Immunosuppressive Treatment of Mice Grafted with ICC

C57BL/6 mice animals transplanted with ICC were treated for two weeks by subcutaneous daily injections with 100 μl of either saline, cyclosporine A (CsA; 12.5 mg/kg body weight, Sandoz Pharma, Basel, Switzerland), 15-deoxyspergualin (DSG; 5.0 mg/kg body weight, Behringwerke AG, Marburg, Germany) or RS-61443 (70 mg/kg body weight, Syntex, Palo Alto, CA, USA) . Mice treated with cyclophosphamide (CYP; 70 mg/kg body weight, Orion-Farmos Corporation, Turku, Finland) were given subcutaneous injections every second day.

Morphological Examinations of Grafted ICC

The effect of the different immunosuppressive protocols on the graft survival was evaluated by light microscopical examinations. The graft-bearing kidneys were removed 14 days after transplantation, fixed in formalin, embedded in paraffin, sectioned (7 μm thick) and stained with hematoxylin-eosin. Morphological scoring of the grafts was performed with the examiner unaware of the origin of the sections. The morphology of the grafts was ranked according to an arbitrary four grade scale: Grade 1, rejected graft with absence of endocrine and epithelial cells and a fulminant mononuclear cell infiltration; grade 2, only a few remaining endocrine and epithelial cells and a heavy infiltration of mononuclear cells; grade

3, almost intact graft, but with some mononuclear cells present; grade 4, intact graft without any visible mononuclear infiltration (Sandberg et al.,1993).

DNA and Insulin Content of ICC and in Grafted ICC

ICC in groups of 50 were homogenized by ultrasonic disruption in 200 µl redistilled water. An aliquot of 50 µl was mixed with 125 µl acid ethanol (0.18 M HCl in 95% [v/v] ethanol) and extracted overnight at 4°C. The insulin concentration of the extract was measured by radioimmunoassay (Heding, 1972). Two 50 µl aliquots of the homogenate were analyzed by fluorophotometry for their DNA content (Kissane and Robins, 1958; Hinegardner, 1971).

After killing by cervical dislocation and removal of the kidney from the transplanted animals, the grafts were localized under a stereomicroscope, and carefully dissected free from the renal parenchyma and renal capsule. The grafts were subsequently immersed in 1.0 ml of acid ethanol (95%) and homogenized by ultrasonic disruption, after which insulin was extracted and measured as described above.

Insulin Release from ICC in vitro

Triplicate groups of 50 ICC were incubated for 3 consecutive hours at 37°C (CO_2:O_2; 5:95) in glass vials with Krebs-Ringer bicarbonate buffer (Krebs and Henseleit, 1932) containing 10 mM Hepes (Sigma) and 2 mg/ml of bovine serum albumin (BSA; Fraction V, Miles Laboratories, Slough, UK). The medium was supplemented with 1.7 mM glucose during the first hour of incubation, with 16.7 mM glucose during the second hour and with 16.7 mM glucose + 5 mM theophylline during the last hour. The incubation media were kept frozen at -20°C until analysis for insulin by radioimmunoassay (Heding, 1972).

Measurement of Poly(ADP-Ribose) Polymerase (PARP) Activity

This assay has been modified from a previously described procedure (Benjamin and Gill, 1980). Groups of 100 ICC were transferred to test tubes containing medium RPMI 1640 and centrifuged at 1500 rpm for 1 min. The supernatant was removed and 0.5 ml of a lysis buffer (10 mM Tris-HCl, 1 mM EDTA, 4 mM $MgCl_2$ x 6 H_2O, 30 mM 2-mercaptoethanol, 0.05% Triton X-100; pH 7.8) was added to the tubes. Then the ICC were disrupted by sonication for 3 sec. After a 30 min incubation at +4°C, 0.5 ml of a reaction buffer (30 mM Tris-HCl, 1 mM EDTA, 40 mM $MgCl_2$ x 6 H_2O, 20 mM 2-mercaptoethanol, 0.05% Triton X-100, 200 µM NAD and 0.05 µCi/ml nicotinamide[U-^{14}C]adenine dinucleotide (purchased from Amersham International, Amersham, UK); pH 7.8) was added. The samples were subsequently incubated for 60 min at 37°C, whereupon 2 ml of 10% (w/v) trichloroacetic acid (TCA) was added to precipitate proteins. The TCA precipitate was filtered through glass microfiber filters (GF/A; Whatman International, Maidstone, UK). After drying overnight at +60°C, the radioactivity of the filters was determined by liquid scintillation counting. Two blank samples, not containing any ICC, were run in parallel in each assay, and the radioactivity in these samples was substracted from the ICC-containing samples. The PARP activity was subsequently calculated as dpm/100 ICC.

Perfusion of ICC Graft-Bearing Kidneys

Experiments were performed on kidneys from both normoglycemic control mice and alloxan-treated mice 2, 4 or 6 months after transplantation, according to previously developed methodology (Korsgren et al., 1988; Korsgren et al., 1989). Thus, the graft-bearing kidney was removed under pentobarbital anaesthesia (60 mg/kg body weight intraperitoneally; Mebumal Vet, Nordvacc, Solna, Sweden), together with the abdominal aorta and vena cava. Aorta was cannulated with a polythene cathether for infusion of the perfusion medium, which was Krebs-Ringer bicarbonate buffer (Krebs and Henseleit, 1932) supplemented with 10 mM Hepes, 2.0% (w/v) BSA and 2.0% Dextran T 70 (Pharmacia Fine Chemicals, Uppsala, Sweden). The medium was gassed (95% O_2 and 5% CO_2) continuously and the flow rate was adjusted to 1 ml/min without recycling. An incision was made in the renal vein and the ureter in order to allow a free flow of the perfusate. The experiments started with a 30-min perfusion with medium supplemented with 2.8 mM glucose, followed by a 45-min interval with 16.7 mM glucose, 15 min at 2.8 mM glucose, 20 min at 16.7 mM glucose + 10 mM theophylline, and finally 15 min at 2.8 mM glucose. Samples for measurement of the insulin concentration were collected with either 1, 3 or 5 min intervals.

EXPERIMENTAL FINDINGS WITH PORCINE PANCREAS

Ontogeny of the Fetal Porcine Endocrine Pancreas

Cells containing islet hormones have been demonstrated by immunocytochemical examination of the fetal porcine pancreas at four weeks of gestation (Alumets et al., 1983). While the ventral bud contained PP cells, insulin, glucagon and somatostatin containing cells were present in the dorsal bud. At midgestation (8-10 weeks) the endocrine cells were arranged into strands and nests, whereas islets of an adult type could not be observed until at a very late gestational stage, and sometimes not until several weeks after birth. Even in the adult pig the islets are often very irregular in shape, which might contribute to the difficulties most investigators have experienced when attempting to isolate islets by collagenase digestion from these animals.

An interesting feature of developing endocrine islet cells is the co-localization of the different islet hormones to the same cell and even to the same secretory granule. This probaby reflects that early progenitor cells to the pancreatic islets are multipotential and that several islet-specific genes are active, but when fetal development proceeds the expression of specific genes are becoming restricted to individual cells (Teitelman and Lee, 1987; Teitelman 1993). However, during certain stresses on islet cells, this fetal trait might reappear in adult islet cells (Teitelman, 1993). Using a double immunogold labeling technique it was demonstrated that in the fetal porcine pancreas (gestational days 50-90) several cells showed co-localization of the islet hormones (Lukinius et al., 1992). At 70 days of gestation monohormonal cells started to appear, but polyhormonal cells were still found in the pancreas of newborn pigs. In the human fetal pancreas a similar phenomenon has been demonstrated up to week 22 of gestation, but not at any later stage (DeKrijger et al., 1992; Lukinius et al., 1992).

Development of Porcine ICC after Transplantation into Nude Mice

Porcine ICC grafted under the kidney capsule of normal nude mice, could easily be distinguished as a whitish spot by visual inspection four weeks after implantation. In paraffin-embedded sections of graft-bearing kidneys, immunocytochemically stained for glucagon and insulin, there was a large number of islet-like structures containing a majority of endocrine cells (Korsgren et. al., 1988). The insulin-positive cells were frequently organized into duct-like structures, a pattern resembling that previously observed when human fetal ICC were transplanted into nude mice (Sandler et al., 1985).

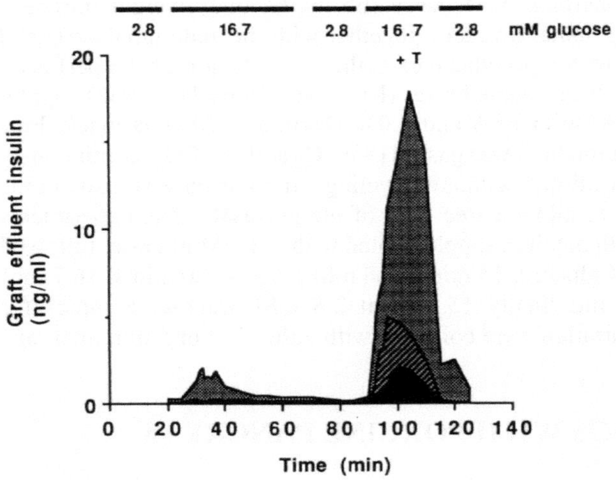

Figure 1. Mean values of the insulin concentration in the effluent medium, collected from perfused graft-bearings kidneys of nude mice, two months (black area; n = 4), four months (hatched area; n = 5) and six months (dotted area; n = 7) after transplantation of ≈ 600 porcine ICC. The grafts were perfused at different intervals with a low or high glucose concentration as indicated, and also with addition of 10 mM theophylline (T).

The insulin secretion of the ICC implanted into normoglycemic nude mice has been assessed at different time points by the kidney perfusion technique (Fig. 1). The grafts did not respond to an acute elevation in the glucose concentration two and four months posttransplantation. However, at six months a glucose response was observed. Addition of 10 mM theophylline to a high-glucose medium caused an enhanced insulin secretion already at 2 months, but the response was much more pronounced at 6 months. It should be noted that the grafted cells were able to down-regulate the insulin release, when the glucose concentration was lowered at the end of the perfusion experiment. Implantation of such ICC to alloxan-diabetic nude mice restored normoglycemia within 2-3 months (Korsgren et al., 1991; Liu et al., 1991). Moreover, in the latter animals there was a normal glucose-response at an earlier time point than in normoglycemic recipients (Korsgren et al., 1991). It thus seems as if hyperglycemia or the diabetic in vivo environment promotes the differentiation/maturation of fetal porcine β-cells. In this context it should be noted that a high glucose concentration (28 mM) stimulated the formation of ICC compared with the number formed at 11.1 mM glucose. However, the insulin content of the ICC was decreased in the former group (Korsgren at al., 1989).

An interesting feature of the porcine ICC implanted into normal nude mice was that the porcine ICC maintained the blood glucose concentration at a level prevailing in the pig (3-5 mM), rather than that of the nude mice (8-10 mM) (Korsgren et al., 1991). This might be of benefit if using the porcine ICC as xenografts in humans, when considering the normal blood glucose level in man.

Since the glucose metabolism is a prerequisite for an adequate glucose-induced insulin secretion in adult β-cells (Malaisse, 1983), we have studied the nutrient demands of fetal porcine β-cells (Sandler et al., 1992). For this purpose ICC were produced in medium RPMI 1640 + 10% human serum. Short-term incubation experiments were subsequently performed on day 5 of culture. It was found that the ICC D-[5-^{3}H]glucose utilization increased by 75% in islets incubated at 16.7 mM glucose compared with 4.2 mM glucose. A similar increase was observed for D-[6-^{14}C]glucose oxidation rates. The ICC exhibited a high rate of L-[U-^{14}C]glutamine oxidation. Glucose failed to further increase a high basal oxygen uptake and also to change the ATP content and ATP/ADP ratio in the ICC. Examination of ICC transplanted into nude mice, however, showed an increase in the graft ATP concentration with increasing time in vivo.

From experiments performed with fetal rat islets, it has been suggested that the attenuated glucose-induced insulin release in fetal β-cells depends on an immature glucose metabolism. This leads to a decreased synthesis of cellular ATP, and an insufficient closure of the ATP-regulated K^+-channels present in the cell membrane (Rorsman et al., 1989; Hole et al., 1988). The resulting deficient depolarization of the cell membrane will thus not open the voltage-dependent Ca^{2+}-channels, which is required for stimulation of insulin secretion. We observed that glucose did not increase the ATP content or the ATP/ADP ratio in ICC, which would explain the lacking insulin response to glucose. However, 8 weeks after grafting in vivo the ATP concentrations in the ICC grafts had increased (Sandler et al., 1992) in parallel with a maturation of the insulin secretory pattern (Korsgren et al., 1993).

Effects of Nicotinamide on the Function of Fetal Porcine ICC

At harvest 4-5 days after culture porcine ICC contain insulin-, glucagon-, somatostatin and PP-positive cells scattered among a majority of non-stained cells when evaluated by immunocytochemistry. The ICC show a notable capacity to synthesize insulin, but an insulin secretory response to an elevation of the ambient glucose concentration was not observed (Korsgren et al., 1988; Korsgren et al., 1993a; Korsgren et al., 1993b). It was therefore considered worthwhile to explore in vitro putative compounds that could stimulate fetal β-cell replication or differentiation.

One mode of affecting cellular differentation and replication in several cell types is by influencing poly(ADP-ribosylation) reactions (Ueda and Hayashi, 1985). This can be achieved by adding an inhibitor of the enzyme poly(ADP-ribose) polymerase (PARP), e.g. nicotinamide or 3-aminobenzamide. Previous studies have demonstrated that treatment of partially pancreatectomized rats with nicotinamide induced β-cell regeneration in the pancreatic remnant (Yonemura et al., 1984), and newly diagnosed IDDM patients treated with nicotinamide showed an extended remission period (Vague et al., 1987) We found that rates of DNA replication increased in adult mouse islets cultured in media supplemented with nicotinamide (Sandler and Andersson, 1986) and also that the cell replication in syngeneically grafted adult mouse islets was increased in animals given nicotinamide (Sandler and Andersson 1988). Addition of nicotinamide to cultures of human fetal pancreatic explants increased both the yield and insulin content of ICC (Sandler et al., 1989; Otonkoski et al., 1993).

Against this background we tested the effect of supplementation of nicotinamide (NIC; 10 mM) to primary cultures of porcine ICC (Korsgren et al., 1993b). Light microscopical examinations of ICC on day 4 of culture showed that NIC caused more than a doubling in the frequency of insulin-positive cells, whereas the rate of β-cell replication was unaffected. The insulin release in vitro after glucose stimulation was, however, essentially unchanged. Transplantation of ICC into diabetic nude mice revealed that ICC developing in medium supplemented with NIC were able to nomalize the hyperglycemia of the recipients at less than half the time required for control ICC. Examinations of the grafts 4-8 weeks after implantation showed that the insulin content was much higher in the NIC group than the control group, and at this stage a glucose response had been attained in vivo when the grafts were perfused. These findings strongly argue in favour of the view that NIC can stimulate differentiation of fetal porcine β-cells.

The mechanism of this action is not fully understood. A role for PARP is hypothesized, but it can not be excluded that NIC also acts as a protective agent for the β-cells against deleterious conditions in the in vitro milieu. Indeed, NIC can prevent β-cell toxic and inhibitory actions induced by streptozotocin and the cytokine interleukin-1β (Schein et al., 1967; Sandler et al., 1983, Cetkovic-Cvrlje et al., 1993; Andersen et al., 1994). We have therefore presently assessed the PARP activity (Fig. 2). Addition of NIC for 5 days led to a

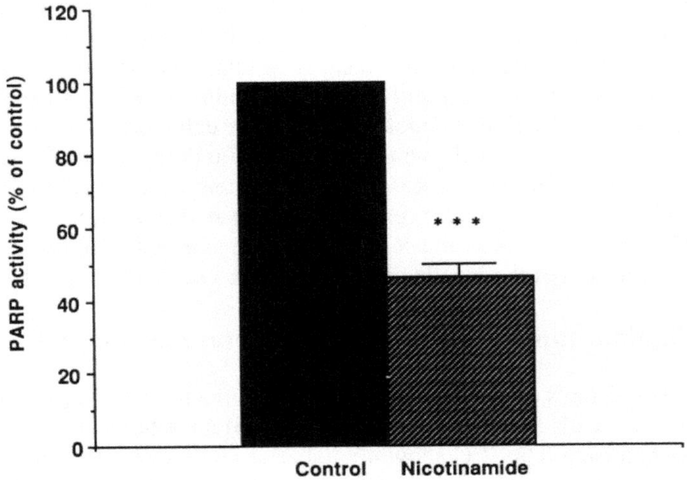

Figure 2. Poly(ADP-ribose) polymerase (PARP) activity in porcine ICC cultured in the presence of 10 mM NIC for 5 days. The activity of the control group was 1216 ± 325 dpm/100 ICC x 1 h. Values are means ± SEM for 4 experiments. *** denotes P<0.001 vs the control group, using Student's paired t-test.

more than 50% inhibition of the PARP activity. This magnitude of the inhibition of PARP is likely to influence cell differentiation of ICC, although the inhibition of PARP by 10 mM NIC is more pronounced in adult rat islet cells (Reddy, Salari-Lak and Sandler; unpublished data).

In a subsequent study we have screened several other putative inducers of β-cell differention and replication for their effects on porcine ICC in vitro (Korsgren et al., 1993a). It was found that also 200 ng/ml dexamethasone (DEX) and 2 mM sodium butyrate (BUT) increased the insulin content of the ICC. A comparison between the insulin contents of ICC cultured in the presence of 1% human serum plus DEX, NIC or BUT during the initial four days, and after a subsequent four day culture period in medium supplemented with 10% human serum only, demonstrated that DEX and BUT doubled the insulin content, compared with the control group cultured with addition of 1% human serum addition during the first four days (Korsgren et al., 1993a). The same groups of ICC plus NIC addition were also studied concerning their capacity to secrete insulin after stimulation (Fig. 3). NIC induced a minute insulin response after stimulation by 16.7 mM glucose. On the other hand, after stimulation with glucose in the presence of the phosphodiesterase inhibitor theophylline, a marked response was observed in the ICC cultured with NIC and BUT, whereas DEX did not mediate this effect. In the case of DEX this suggests that a heightened insulin content of the ICC does not necessarily correlate with a higher capacity to secrete insulin. Combinations of DEX, BUT and NIC have also been investigsgated, but they did not show a better insulin response than that observed with NIC alone (Korsgren et al., 1993a).

Effects of Immune Suppression on the Survival of Fetal Porcine ICC Transplanted to Mice

Two weeks after transplantation of ICC to normal C57BL/6 mice, receiving saline administration, a strong rejection of the graft had occurred. This was morphologically evidenced by a low ranking grade (1-2) , as defined above, and a very low insulin content of the graft. In C57BL/6 nude mice grafted with a similar amount of ICC, the graft insulin

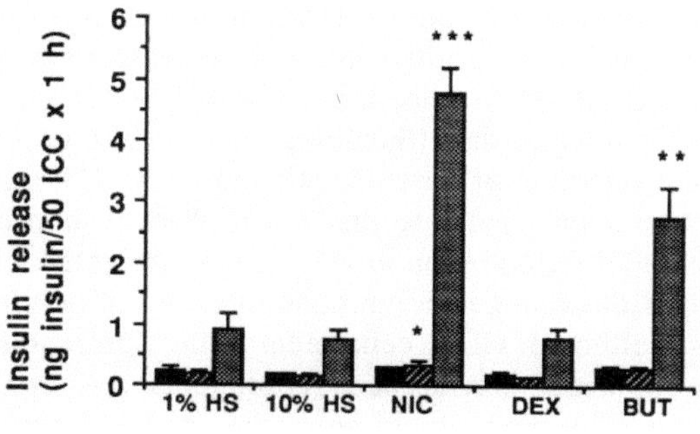

Figure 3. Insulin release of ICC exposed to 1.7 mM glucose (black bars), 16.7 mM glucose and 16.7 mM glucose + 5 mM theophylline. The ICC had been cultured for four days in medium as indicated under the bars, and for another four days in medium supplemented with 10% HS. Values are means ± SEM for 5 experiments. *, ** and *** denote $P<0.05$, $P<0.01$ and $p<0.001$ vs the corresponding incubation condition of the 1% HS group, using Student's paired t-test. Data are adapted from (Korsgren et al., 1993a), with the permission of the publisher.

content increased over a two-week period about 7-fold compared with the value on the day of implantation (≈ 400 ng insulin/graft). Treatment of normal C57BL/6 mice with CsA was not effective in prevention of graft rejection (Fig. 4; ranking grade: 1-2) and loss of the insulin content. On the other hand, both DSG (Fig. 5; ranking grade: 3-4) and CYP (ranking grade: 3-4) were found to markedly preserve the graft morphology and graft insulin content (DSG ≈ 2700 ng insulin/graft and CYP ≈ 1700 ng insulin/graft). Also treatment with

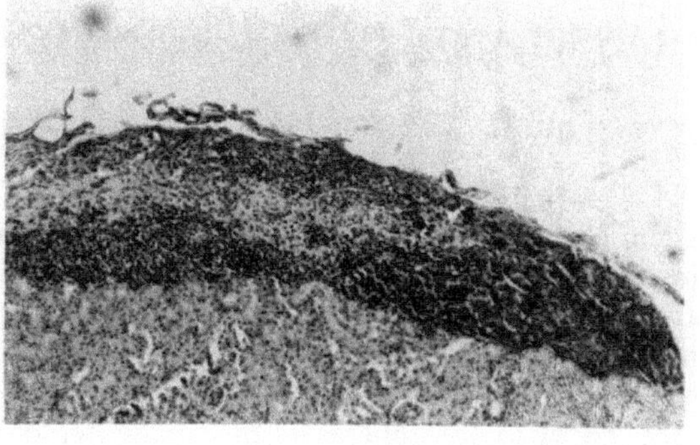

Figure 4. Light micrograph, on day 14, of ICC implanted beneath the kidney capsule of a normal C57BL/6 mouse treated with CsA. A marked mononuclear cell infiltration and only a few endocrine-like cells can bee seen; morphological rank 1. Hematoxylin-eosin; original magnification x110, reduced 82.5%.

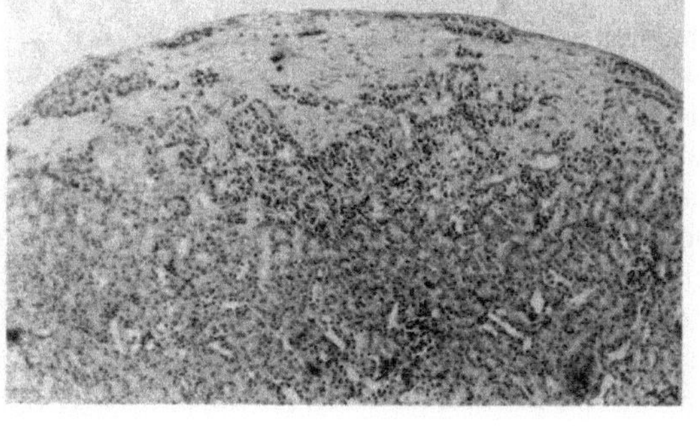

Figure 5. Light micrograph, on day 14, of ICC implanted beneath the kidney capsule of a normal C57BL/6 mouse treated with DSG. An intact graft with several endocrine-like cells and a very minor mononuclear infiltration is observed; morpholgical rank 4. Hematoxylin-eosin; original magnification x110, reduced 82.5%.

RS-61443 reduced the morphological signs of rejection of the ICC (ranking grade: 2-3) and in parallel insulin was retained in the grafts, but not to the extent observed with DSG.

The morphological findings in mice treated with DSG and CsA referred to above agree with our previously published data (Sandberg et al., 1993). Especially DSG seems to be effective in preventing rejection of porcine cells grafted to C57BL/6 mice. In addition the insulin content measurements indicate that these immunosuppressive drugs did not interfer with the growth and differentiation in vivo of the implanted fetal endocrine cells.

The exact nature of the xenogeneic immune rejection of porcine cells implanted in mice is largely unknown, although $CD4^+$ cells seem to be a prerequisite for this response (Auchincloss, 1990). In line with this it has been reported that rejection of fetal pig proislets in mice can be counteracted by monoclonal antibodies directed against the CD4 antigen (Wilson et al., 1989). The fact that DSG, which inhibits macrophage functions (Thomson and Starzl, 1993), was effective in the present experiments suggests that antigen presentation by macrophages might be a site for immune intervention in this xenograft model. Moreover, the xenograft rejection process appears to be very specific to the porcine cells, since experiments in which porcine ICC and isolated syngeneic islets were mixed and implanted beneath the kidney capsule of C57BL/6 mice indicated that the porcine ICC are rejected, whereas the mouse islets are retained (Korsgren and Jansson, 1994). However, there was some functional inhibition of the insulin secretion in these experiments, which could imply that soluble factors released during the xenogeneic rejection also impaired the syngeneic islets. One possibility is that cytokines inhibited the insulin secretion, since in vitro studies have demonstrated pronounced effects of cytokines on islet functions (Sandler et al. 1991; Sandler et al. 1994; Rabinovitch, 1993). In similar experiments with mixed islet grafts in mice and rats an allogeneic rejection of the syngeneic islets does not seem to cause a functional impairment (Sutton et al., 1989; Korsgren and Jansson, 1994).

TRANSPLANTATION OF PORCINE ICC TO IDDM PATIENTS

Assessement of Potential Risks of Grafting Porcine ICC to Humans

A number of experimental studies have been undertaken in order to assess the potential risks of grafting fetal porcine ICC to human recipients. In this context the risk that the xenogeneic material could elicit a coagulopathy in the recipient was examined. To address this issue anesthetized dogs (Swedish Foxhounds weighing 20-30 kg) were injected into the portal vein with ≈ 1 ml of ICC or ≈ 3 ml of minced porcine fetal pancreas (Tollemar et al., 1992). The dogs were studied acutely (0-2 h after injection) and up to 1 month after injection. A minor abberation of hepatic hemodynamics, and a small increase in plasma fibrinopeptide A, which could be prevented by heparin administration, was observed acutely. In contrast injection of minced adult porcine pancreas induced a marked coagulopathy.

Another potential hazard is the risk of transferring microorganisms from the pig to the human recipient. A comprehensive screening program of pregnant sows (serology, blood and endometrium cultures), primary ICC cultures and nude mice grafted with ICC, has therefore been worked out (Björersdorff et al., 1992; Bjöersdorff et al., 1994). Some pregnant sows had antibodies to Leptospira interrogans (3%) and Aspergillus fumigatus (56%), but no signs of active infection with these organisms were seen. It was also found that some sows had bacteria in the endometrium, whilst these bacteria were not found in the ICC cultures subsequently prepared. Bacteria (Corynebacterium spp and Lactobacillus spp), but no viruses, fungi or mycoplasma were found in 2/53 culture dishes of ICC. The brains of grafted mice were morphologically examined 9-23 months after ICC grafting under the kidney capsule, but no changes suggestive of prions could be seen. These results suggest that microorganisms can be identified by proper screening procedures, and the risk of transmission of such microoganisms from pig to man can be minimized.

Porcine ICC cells could acutely succumb due to lysis induced by antibody-dependent cellular cytotoxicity (ADCC) induced by natural human anti-porcine antibodies. However, in vitro experiments demonstrated that IgG-mediated ADCC against ICC cells was relatively weak, whilst porcine peripheral blood lymphocytes, obtained from adult pigs, elicited a stronger ADDC (Satake et al., 1993). The porcine ICC cells were also resistant to complement-dependent antibody-mediated cytotoxicity by human serum in vitro (Satake et al., 1993). These circumstances would argue against a hyperacute rejection of porcine ICC grafted into man. Moreover, previous observations have suggested that non-vascularized, cellular xenografts are not sensitive to hyperacute rejection and that the intensity of the T-cell-dependent response in vitro to xenogeneic antigen presenting cells is relatively weak (Sachs and Bach, 1990; Gill 1992). Also the cellular human anti-porcine xenoreactivity has been studied in vitro. The observations were interpreted to indicate as if the xenoreaction shared characteristics with allogeneic responses, although some differences existed (Kumagai-Braesch et al., 1993).

Xenotransplantation of Fetal Porcine ICC to Patients with IDDM

Against the background given above of the extensive safety tests, the curative effects of the ICC in experimentally diabetic animals, and the possiblitiy of an attenuated xenogeneic immune response in man, a clinical trial was performed in a limited number of patients with IDDM. After ethical approval, altogether ten patients received an intraportal injection of 200 000 to 1 million porcine ICC previously cultured in the presence of 10 mM NIC (Groth et al., 1992; Groth et al., 1994). In six of the patients the infusion of ICC was performed through a catheter placed in the portal vein by percutaneous transhepatic puncture and in two patients via a mesenteric vein exposed through a small laparatomy. In the two remaining patients, both of whom were about to receive a kidney graft, a corresponding number of ICC was placed in a pocket beneath the renal capsule just after the kidney had been revascularized in the recipient. All patients received conventional immune suppressive treatment with CsA, prednisolone and azathioprine due to previous or simultaneous kidney transplantation. At the time of xenotransplantation this treatment was supplemented with antithymocyte globulin or DSG. Graft function was monitored by radioimmunological measurements of urinary C-peptide excretion using an antibody with proven specificity to porcine C-peptide.

Of the patients who had received porcine ICC four showed excretion of small amounts of porcine C-peptide in the urine for up to 200 days after transplantation. The highest excretion recorded, 4 nmol/24 h, was about 20% of the human C-peptide level seen in normal individuals. One kidney biopsy, obtained three weeks after transplantation, showed small clusters of epithelioid cells, some of which stained positively for insulin, glucagon or chromogranin (Tibell et al., 1994b). There was, however, no amelioration of the insulin need in any of the patients.

Irrespective of the various tested immunosuppressive treatments, specific xenoantibodies of both IgM and IgG type were formed (Satake et al, 1994). The highest titers were found after 30-50 days, and they were maintained at a high level for at least 100 days. High titers of ADCC activity against porcine lymphoblasts were found in all patients. The authors consider this humoral response to be distinctly different from that observed in patients transplanted with allogeneic grafts. The humoral immune response as compared to the cellular response therefore appeared to be of greater importance for the rejection of the porcine ICC in man, than could be anticipated from the preceding in vitro experiments (Satake et al., 1993). The binding specificities of the IgM- and IgG-xenoantibodies to glycosphingolipid have been studied in more detail (Rydberg et al., 1994). Strong binding was observed to a "linear blood group B" structure, which thus might be an important target for the antibodies in this xenotransplantation model.

These studies show that porcine ICC survive for several months after transplantation to patients on insulin treatment and conventional immunosuppression. The cells eventually seemed to succumb to immune rejection and/or lack of adequate engraftment. There were no indications that the procedures applied involved any health hazards, but a more lasting and larger insulin production is needed. More knowledge of the mechanism and control of xenorejection is obviously warranted and this should be achieved by animal experiments.

ACKNOWLEDGEMENTS

Own work referred to in this chapter was supported by grants from the Swedish Medical Research Council (12P-9287; 12P-10739; 19P-8982; 12X-109; 12X-8273; 12X-9273), the Juvenile Diabetes Foundation International, the Swedish Diabetes Association, the Swedish Childhood Diabetes Fund, the Novo-Nordic Insulin Fund, and the Family Ernfors Fund.

REFERENCES

Alumets, J., Håkanson, R., and Sundler, F., 1985, Ontogeny of endocrine cells in porcine gut and pancreas. An immunocytochemical study, *Gastroenterology* 85: 1359-1372.

Andersen, H. U., Jørgensen, K. H., Egeberg, J., Mandrup-Poulsen, T., and Nerup, J., 1994, Nicotinamide prevents interleukin-1 effects on accumulated insulin release and nitric oxide production in rat islets of Langerhans, *Diabetes* 43:770-777.

Andersson, A., and Sandler, S., 1992, Fetal pancreatic transplantation, *Transplant. Rev.* 6:20-38.

Auchincloss, H., 1990, Xenografting: a review, *Transplant. Rev.* 4:14-27.

Benjamin, R. C., and Gill, D., 1980, ADP-ribosylation in mammalian cell ghosts, *J. Biol. Chem.* 255:10493-10501.

Bjöersdorff, A., Korsgren, O., Andersson, A., Tollemar, J., Malmborg, A.-S., Ehrnst, A., and Groth, C.-G., 1992, Microbiologic screening as a preparatory step for clinical xenografting of porcine fetal islet-like cell clusters, *Transplant. Proc.* 24:674-676.

Bjöersdorff, A., Korsgren, O., Feinstein, R., Andersson, A., Tollemar, J., Malmborg, A.-S., Ehrnst, A., and Groth, C.-G., 1994, Microbiologial characterization of porcine fetal islet-like cell clusters for clinical xenografting, *Xenotransplantion* In press.

Brown, J., Molnar, I. G., Clark, W., and Mullen, Y., 1974, Control of experimental diabetes mellitus in rats by transplantation of fetal pancreas, *Science* 184:1377-1379.

Cetkovic-Cvrlje, M., Sandler, S., and Eizirik, D. L., 1993, Nicotinamide and dexamethasone inhibit interleukin-1-induced nitric oxide production by RINm5F cells without decreasing messenger ribonucleic acid expression for nitric oxide synthase, *Endocrinology* 133:1739-1743.

DeKrijger, R. R., Aanstoot, H. J., Kranenburg, G., Reinhard, M., Visser, W. J., and Bruining, G. J., 1992, The midgestational human fetal pancreas contains cells coexpressing islet hormones, *Dev. Biol.* 153:368-375.

Eisenbarth, G. S., 1986, Type I diabetes mellitus. A chronic autoimmune disease, *N. Engl. J. Med.* 314:1360-1368.

Gepts, W., 1965, Pathological anatomy of the pancreas in juvenile diabetes mellitus, *Diabetes* 14:619-633.

Gill, R. G., 1992, The role of direct and indirect antigen presentation in the response to islet xenografts, *Transplant. Proc.* 24:642-643.

Gill, R. G., and Lafferty, K. J., 1989, The role of islet transplantation in the treatment of insulin-dependent diabetes mellitus, *Immunol. Allergy Clin. North Am.* 9:165-186.

Gray, D. W. R., McShane, P., Grant, A., and Morris, P. J., 1984, A method for isolation of islets of Langerhans from the human pancreas, *Diabetes* 33:1055-1061.

Groth, C.-G., Korsgren, O., Tibell, A., Tollemar, J., Möller, E., Bolinder, J., Östman, J., Reinholt, F. P., Hellerström, C., and Andersson, A., 1994, Transplantation of porcine fetal pancreas to diabetic patients: biochemical and histological evidence of xenograft survival, *Lancet* In press

Groth, C.-G., Korsgren, O., Andersson, A., Hellerström, C., Bjöersdorff, A., Tibell, A., Tollemar, J., Bolinder, J., Östman, J., Kumagai, M, and Möller, E., 1992, Evidence of xenograft function in a diabetic patient grafted with porcine fetal pancreas, *Transplant. Proc.* 24:972-973.

Heding, L. G., 1972, Determination of total serum insulin (IRI) in insulin-treated patients, *Diabetologia* 8:260-266.

Hellerström, C., Lewis, N. J., Borg, H., Johnson, R., and Freinkel, N, 1979, Method for large-scale isolation of pancreatic islets by tissue culture of fetal rat pancreas, *Diabetes* 28:769-776.

Hinegardner, R. T., 1971, An improved fluorometric assay for DNA, *Anal. Biochem.* 39:197-201.

Hole R.L., Pian-Smith M. C. M., and Sharp G.W.G., 1988, Development of the biphasic response to glucose in fetal and neonatal rat pancreas, *Am. J. Physiol.* 254: E167-E174.

Kissane, J. M., and Robins, E., 1958, The fluorometric measurement of deoxyribonucleic acid in animal tissues with special reference to the central nervous system, *J. Biol. Chem.* 233:184-188.

Krebs, H. A., and Henseleit, K., 1932, Untersuchungen über die Harnstoffbildung im Tierkörper, *Hoppe-Seylers Z. Physiol. Chem.* 210:33-66.

Korsgren, O., Andersson, A., and Sandler, S., 1993a, In vitro screening of putative compounds inducing fetal porcine pancreatic β-cell differentiation: implications for cell transplantation in insulin-dependent diabetes mellitus, *Upsala J. Med. Sci.* 98:39-52.

Korsgren, O., Andersson, A., and Sandler, S., 1993b, Pretreatment of fetal porcine pancreas in culture with nicotinamide accelerates reversal of diabetes after transplantation to nude mice, *Surgery* 113:205-214.

Korsgren, O., and Jansson, L, 1994, Characterization of mixed syngeneic-allogeneic and syngeneic-xenogeneic islet-graft rejections in mice. Evidence of functional impairment of the remaining syngeneic islets in xenograft rejections, *J. Clin. Invest.* 93:1113-1119.

Korsgren, O., Jansson, L., and Andersson, A., 1989, Effects of hyperglycemia on function of isolated mouse pancreatic islets transplanted under the kidney capsule, *Diabetes* 38:510-515.

Korsgren, O., Jansson, L., Eizirik, D., Andersson, A., 1991, Functional and morphological differentiation of fetal porcine islet-like cell clusters after transplantation into nude mice, *Diabetologia* 34:379-386.

Korsgren, O., Sandler, S., Jansson, L., Groth, C.-G., Hellerström, C., and Andersson, A., 1989, Effects of culture conditions on formation and hormone content of fetal porcine isletlike cell clusters, *Diabetes* 38(Suppl. 1): 209-212.

Korsgren, O., Sandler, S., Schnell Landström, A., Jansson, L., and Andersson, A., 1988, Large-scale production of fetal porcine pancreatic isletlike cell clusters. An experimental tool for studies of islet cell differentiation and xenotransplantation, *Transplantation* 45: 509-514.

Kumagai-Braesch, M., Satake, M., Korsgren, O., Andersson, A., and Möller, E., 1993, Characterization of cellular human anti-porcine xenoreactivity, *Clin. Transplant.* 7:273-280.

Liu, X., Federlin, K. F., Bretzel, R. G., Hering, H. J., and Brendel, M. D., 1991, Persistent reversal of diabetes by transplantation of fetal pig proislets into nude mice, *Diabetes* 40:858-866.

Lukinius, A., Ericsson, J. L. E., Grimelius, L., and Korsgren O., 1992, Ultrastructural studies of the ontogeny of fetal human and porcine pancreas, with special reference to colocalization of the four major islet hormones, *Dev. Biol.* 153:376-385.

Malaisse, W. J., 1983, Insulin release: the fuel concept, *Diabete Metab.* 119:313-320.

Otonkoski, T., Beattie, G. M., Mally, M. I., Ricordi, C., and Hayek, A., 1993, Nicotinamide is a potent inducer of endocrine differentiation in cultured human fetal pancreatic cells, *J. Clin. Invest.* 92:1459-1466.

Rabinovitch, A., 1993, Role of cytokines in IDDM pathogenesis and islet β-cell destruction, *Diabetes Rev.* 1:215-240

Ricordi, C., Lacy, P.E., Finke, E.H., Olack, B.J., and Scharp, D. W, 1988, Automated method for isolation of human pancreatic islets, *Diabetes* 37:413-420.

Robertson, P.R., 1992, Pancreatic and islet transplantation for diabetes - cures or curiosities?, *N. Engl. J. Med.* 327:1861-1868.

Rorsman P., Arkhammar P., Bokvist K., Hellerström C., Nilsson T., Welsh M., Welsh N., and Berggren P.-O., 1989, Failure of glucose to elicit a normal insulin secretory repsonse in fetal pancreatic beta cells results from glucose insensitivity of the ATP-regulated K^+ channels, *Proc. Natl. Acad. Sci. USA* 86: 4505-4509.

Rydberg, L., Cairns, T. D. H., Groth, C.-G., Gustavsson, M. L., Karlsson, E. C., Möller, E., Satake, M., Tibell, A., Samuelsson, B. E., 1994, Specificities of human IgM and IgG anticarbohydrate xenoantbodies found in the sera of diabetic patients grafted with fetal pig islets, *Xenotransplantation* 1:69-79.

Sachs, D. H., and Bach, F. H., 1990, Immunology of xenograft rejection, *Hum. Immunol.* 28:245-251.

Sandberg, J.-O., Korsgren, O., Groth, C.-G., and Andersson, A., 1993, 15-deoxyspergualin prolongs pancreatic islet allo- and xenograft survival in mice, *Pharmacol. Toxicol.* 73: 24-28.

Sandler, S., and Andersson, A., 1986, Long-term effects of exposure of pancreatic islets to nicotinamide in vitro on DNA synthesis, metabolism and B-cell function, *Diabetologia* 29:199-202.

Sandler, S. and Andersson, A., 1988, Nicotinamide treatment stimulates cell replication in transplanted pancreatic islets, *Transplantation* 46:30-31.

Sandler, S., Andersson, A., Korsgren, O., Tollemar, J., Peterson, B., Groth, C.-G., and Hellerström, C., 1989, Tissue culture of human fetal pancreas. Effects of nicotinamide on insulin production and formation of isletlike cell clusters, *Diabetes* 38(Suppl. 1):168-171.

Sandler, S., Andersson, A., Schnell, A., Mellgren, A., Tollemar, J., Borg, H., Peterson, B., Groth, C.-G., and Hellerström, C., 1985, Tissue culture of human fetal pancreas. Development of and function of B-cells in vitro and transplantation of explants to nude mice, *Diabetes* 34:1113-1119

Sandler, S., Eizirik, D. L., Sternesjö, J., and Welsh, N., Role of cytokines in regulation of pancreatic B-cell function., 1994, *Biochem. Soc. Trans.* 22:26-30.

Sandler, S., Eizirik, D. L., Svensson, C., Strandell, E., Welsh, M., and Welsh, N., 1991, Biochemical and molecular actions of interleukin 1 on pancreatic β–cells, *Autoimmunity* 10: 241-253.

Sandler, S., Welsh, M., and Andersson, A., Streptozotocin-induced impairment of islet B-cell metabolism and its prevention by a hydroxyl radical scavenger and inhibitors of poly(ADP-ribose) synthtase, *Acta Pharmacol. Toxicol.* 53:392-400.

Satake, M., Kumagai-Braesch, M., Kawagishi, N., Tibell, A., Groth, C.-G., and Möller, E., 1994, Kinetics and character of xenoantibody formation in diabetic patients transplanted with fetal porcine islet cell clusters, *Xenotransplantation* 1:24-35.

Satake, M., Kumagai-Braesch, M., Korsgren, O., Andersson, A., and Möller, E., 1993, Characterization of humoral human anti-porcine xenoreactivity, *Clin. Transplant.* 7:281-288.

Scharp, D. W., Lacy, P.E., Santiago, J. V., McCullough, C. S., Weide, L. G., Falqui, L., Marchetti, P., Gingerich, R. L., Jaffe, A. S., Cryer, P. E., Anderson, C. B., and Flye, M W., 1990, Insulin independence after islet transplantation into type 1 diabetic patient, *Diabetes* 39:515-518.

Schein, P. S., Cooney, D. A., Vernon, M. L., 1967, The use of nicotinamide to modify the toxicity of streptozotocin diabets without loss of antitumor activity, *Cancer Res.* 37:2324-2332.

Sutton, R., Gray, D. W., McShane, P., Dallman, M. J., and Morris, P. J., 1989, The susceptibility and the absence of susceptibility of pancreatic islet β cells to nonspecific immune destruction in mixed strain islets grafted beneath the renal capsule in the rat, *J. Exp. Med.* 170:751-762.

Teitelman, G., 1993, On the origin of pancreatic endocrine cells, proliferation and neoplastic transformation, *Tumor Biol.* 14:167-173.

Teitelman, G., and Lee, J. K., Cell lineage analysis of pancreatic islet cell development: glucagon and insulin cells arise from catecholaminergic precursors present in the pancreatic duct, *Dev. Biol.* 121:454-466.

Thomson, A. W., and Starzl, T. E., 1993, New immunosuppressive drugs: mechanistic insights and potential therapeutic advances, *Immunol. Rev.* 136: 71-138

Tibell, A., Groth, C.-G., Möller, E., Korsgren, O., Andersson, A., and Hellerström, C., 1994a, Pig-to-man islet transplantation in eight patients, *Transplant. Proc.* 26:762-763.

Tibell, A., Reinholt, F. P., Korsgren, O., Andersson, A., Hellerström, C., Möller, E., and Groth, C.-G., 1994b, Morphological identification of porcine islet cells three weeks after transplantation into a diabetic patient, *Transplant. Proc.* 26:1121.

Tollemar, J., Groth, C.-G., Korsgren, O., Andersson, A., Blombäck, M, and Olsson, P., 1992, Injection of xenogeneic endocrine pancreatic tissue into the portal vein - Effects on coagulation, liver function, and hepatic hemodynamics. A study in the pig-to-dog model, *Transplantation* 53:139-142.

Ueda, K., and Hayashi, O., 1985, ADP-ribosylation, *Annu. Rev. Biochem.* 54:73-100.

Vague, Ph., Vialettes, B., Lassman-Vague, V., and Vallo, J., 1987; Nicotinamide may extend remission phase in insulin-dependent diabetes, *Lancet* i:619-620.

Warnock, G. L., Kneteman, N. H., Ryan, E., Seelis, R. E. A., Rabinovitch, A., and Rajotte, R. V., 1991, Normoglycemia after transplantation of freshly isolated and cryopreserved pancreatic islets in type 1 insulin-dependent diabetes mellitus, *Diabetologia* 34:55-58.

Wilson, J. D., Simeonovic, C. J., Ting, J. H., and Ceredig, R., 1989, Role of $CD4^+$ T-lymphocytes in rejection by mice of fetal pig proislet xenografts, *Diabetes* 38(Suppl. 1):217-219.

Yonemura, Y., Takashima, T., Miwa, K., Miyasaki, I., Yamamoto, H., and Okamoto, H., 1984, Amelioration of diabetes mellitus in partially pancreatectomized rats by poly(ADP-ribose) synthetase inhibitors. Evidence of islet B-cell regeneration, *Diabetes* 33:401-404.

5

BASIC BIOLOGY OF PIG FETAL PANCREAS AND ITS USE AS AN ALLOGRAFT

Bernard E. Tuch,[†*] Ann M. Simpson,[*] Murray S.R. Smith,[|] Patrick Waugh,[|] Anthony J. Weinhaus,[*] Jian Tu,[*] and Margaret Rose[#]

[†] Department of Endocrinology
Prince of Wales Hospital
Sydney, New South Wales, Australia
[|] School of Anatomy
The University of New South Wales
Sydney, New South Wales, Australia
[#] Department of Surgery
Prince Henry Hospital
Sydney, New South Wales, Australia

Diabetes is a chronic disorder of metabolism, which has the potential to result in the development of microvascular complications, such as retinopathy and nephropathy, many years after the onset of the disease process. This is particularly relevant to insulin-dependent diabetes, which affects the young, with blindness and renal failure occurring early in life, rather than at an advanced age, which can occur in non-insulin dependent diabetes. Until insulin dependent diabetes can be prevented, or cured by means of gene transfer, pancreatic transplantation is probably the most likely means at our disposal to normalize blood glucose levels, and thus prevent the occurrence of complications.

TRANSPLANTATION OF HUMAN FETAL PANCREAS

Over the past decade experiments to reverse diabetes have been undertaken in humans by transplanting human fetal pancreatic tissue which is capable of secreting insulin (1). Human fetal pancreatic tissue will grow and its insulin content increase (2), with blood glucose levels being normalized when the tissue was grafted into diabetic athymic mice (3,4). The time required for reversal of diabetes varied from 1-5 months, this time being essential not only for the number of insulin-producing ß cells to reach a critical number, but also for these cells to reach maturity particularly in regard to their ability to release insulin in response to physiological stimuli, such as glucose (5). In the diabetic athymic rat, which is 8 times

[*]Correspondence to: Bernard Tuch, Department of Endocrinology, Prince of Wales Hospital, Randwick, New South Wales 2031, Australia. FAX: 61 - 2 - 314 5003.

the size of the athymic mouse, xenografted human fetal pancreas took a similar period of time to normalize blood glucose levels (6). Further, transplantation of similar sized units of human fetal pancreas resulted in reversal of diabetes in the rat and mouse after the same period of engraftment (7), suggesting that maturation of endocrine tissue was more critical than the mass of tissue in the determination of reversal of diabetes.

Grafting of the human fetal pancreas, which has been so successful in the immunoincompetent mouse and rat (3,4,6) has been attempted in diabetic patients. While numerous claims have been made by a variety of investigators (8,9), convincing evidence is available to demonstrate that the tissue will survive for at least 12 months when transplanted to immunosuppressed recipients (10), and that some insulin was secreted from the graft (11,12). Claims that recipients are able to cease their need for exogenous insulin have yet to be substantiated. One of the reasons for the lack of success was probably that the number of cells grafted was too few to make an impact on the patients' diabetic control (10). Further human trials will involve the utilization of many human fetal pancreases, perhaps 12 or more, for each recipient. This amount of tissue, even with the use of cryopreservation to stockpile organs (13), is far in excess of that presently available from most Western sources to satisfy the needs of more than a handful of insulin-dependent diabetic individuals.

TRANSPLANTATION OF PIG FETAL PANCREATIC TISSUE

It was for this reason that our group along with a number of others (14-17) turned attention to utilizing tissue from the pig fetal pancreas (Figure 1). Like the human fetal pancreas, the pig fetal pancreas contains a much greater percentage of ß cells than that found in the adult. It has vast growth potential, and, at least early in gestation, has few of the exocrine enzymes, which digest tissues (18), that are such a problem with the adult pancreas. As with the human fetal pancreas, transplantation of the pig fetal pancreas into immunoincompetent diabetic mice results in growth of the graft and reversal of diabetes after 1-4 months, regardless of the form in which the fetal cells are transplanted; as either pancreatic explants (15) or islet-like cell clusters [ICCs] (14,16). ICCs are clusters of what are probably mostly epithelial cells that form as discrete units when the pancreatic explants are digested

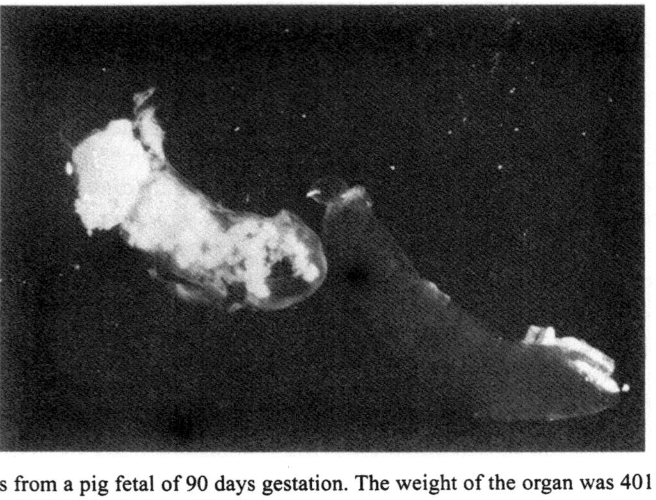

Figure 1. Pancreas from a pig fetal of 90 days gestation. The weight of the organ was 401 mg. It is attached to the fetal spleen which is the darker of the two organs.

with collagenase (19). Recently these experiments have been extended into immunocompetent mice, transiently immunosuppressed with anti-CD4 antibody, with successful reversal of diabetes (17,20).

Pig fetal pancreas, both as explants and partly characterized collagenase digests, has been allografted into the omentum of inbred mini pigs, with survival of ß cells for 10 months (21) and possibly some graft function (22) when cyclosporin and azathioprine were used to immunosuppress the recipients. Both the donor and recipient in these experiments had the same MHC antigens, but minor differences in non-MHC antigens. Transplants between outbred animals, which were MHC incompatible, have not been successful despite the use of the above immunosuppressive agents in doses similar to those used to prevent rejection of solid organs in humans (18).

Recent experiments xenografting pig fetal ICCs beneath the renal capsule of uraemic diabetic humans have been carried out in 2 patients, with survival of α and ß cells for three weeks in one patient (23). Despite immunosuppression using cyclosporin, azathioprine, prednisone, and 15-deoxyspergualin, the endocrine cells were observed to undergo rejection, as judged by the presence of a mixed inflammatory infiltrate around the cells and in the renal graft. Histological survival could not be demonstrated when up to 520,000 ICCs, obtained from the litters of three pregnant sows (24), were injected into the portal vein of 8 immunosuppressed diabetic patients, who had previously received a renal transplant (25). These grafts produced a small amount of C-peptide (co-secreted with insulin) in the urine of three recipients, but this hormone was never detectable in blood and the insulin requirements of the recipients remained unchanged.

The present pattern of poor results is similar to the results of allografting adult islets into diabetic humans in the 1980's, a technique that only in this decade achieved success in reversing diabetes, for at least 12 months in one out of every ten recipients, with another 30% retaining some graft function at this time (26). Before further human trials with pig fetal pancreas are attempted, it is important to demonstrate that this tissue can reverse diabetes in an allograft model. Such a model offers an advantage over the isograft, since it will demonstrate not only the innate capacity of the tissue to grow and mature in a large animal, but that rejection can be prevented in this species. Prevention of allograft rejection in pigs is likely to be different from the process involved in preventing the destruction of pancreatic tissue xenografted in humans; regardless, we would argue that failure of an allograft to function must make it less likely that a xenograft will be successful. The history of tissue transplantation has basically followed this order of events demonstrating success with an allograft before the xenograft was attempted.

Preparations of Pig Fetal Pancreas

Pregnant sows used in the following experiments were of 76-110 days gestational age (term is usually at 114 days) and were killed either at a piggery or an abattoir; fetuses were transported on ice and reached the Endocrinology Laboratory at the Prince of Wales Hospital within 4 hours of removal from the uterus. Three forms of pig fetal pancreas have been created from the original tissue for possible transplantation to reverse diabetes, these being (a) 1 mm^3 explants, (b) ICCs, and (c) endocrine-rich monolayers.

A. One mm^3 Explants. These are obtained by dicing the pig fetal pancreas with fine scissors. Such tissue secretes insulin in response to agents that increase levels of cyclic AMP and the oral hypoglycaemic agent, tolbutamide, but not to glucose, arginine or leucine (15). Explants, usually maintained in organ culture for several days before transplantation, have been shown to normalize blood glucose levels in diabetic athymic (15) and immunosup-

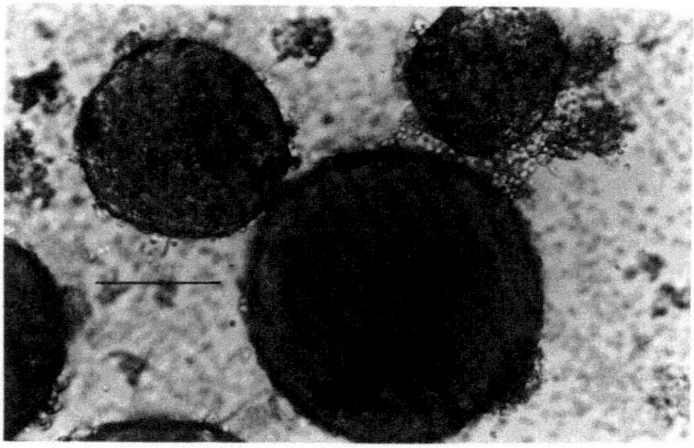

Figure 2. Islet-like cell clusters obtained by digestion of pig fetal pancreas at 90 days gestation. The diameter of the larger ICC is 111 μm, and of the smaller two, 80 and 56 μm. Scale bar: 50 μm.

pressed NOD mice (20) when grafted beneath the renal capsule. Explants consist of clusters of epithelial cells, a number of which are endocrine cells, and mesenchymal tissue.

B. Islet-Like Cell Clusters. ICCs are formed by partial collagenase digestion of explants of the pig fetal pancreas. Collagenase P (Boehringer-Mannheim) was used at a concentration of 3 mg/mL, with the tissue being vigorously stirred for 10-15 minutes. Initially after digestion clusters of cells are found with no particular symmetry. These clusters round up to form ICCs after a culture period of 48-72 hours. When transplanted beneath the renal capsule, ICCs have been shown to reverse diabetes in athymic mice (14,16) and rats (27), and immunosuppressed CBA mice (17). It is in this form that pig fetal pancreas has been xenografted in humans (23,25).

Morphology. Histological examination of pig fetal ICCs (Figure 2) shows that they consist mostly of epithelial cells, with about 10% of cells in the ICC being endocrine, ß cells predominating over α, δ and pancreatic polypeptide cells; the remaining cells are probably exocrine. The endocrine cells are found in small groups throughout the ICC, but predominate at the periphery. This is best observed with laser scanning confocal microscopy after the ICCs have been stained with a primary antibody to insulin and a fluorescent second antibody (Figure 3). The percentage of ß cells in any single ICC has been shown to vary from zero to 13% (median: 2.4%), demonstrating the heterogenous nature of the developing tissue. There are also a number of endothelial cells in the ICCs and a few mesenchymal cells. The lack of mesenchymal cells makes the use of ICCs very attractive because 40% of the original fetal pancreas consists of fibrous tissue.

Electronmicroscopic analysis of the ICC (Figure 4a & b) confirms the presence of numerous acinar cells containing zymogen granules and a smaller number of endocrine cells. Comparison of this picture with that of the intact pig fetal pancreas (Figure 5) show that ICCs are present as *progenitor epithelial balls [PEBs]* in the intact fetal pancreas. In fact, these PEBs form the majority of non-mesenchymal cells in the intact pancreas, there being no islets (our own observation and 15), unlike the situation with the human fetal pancreas (28). The observation that the source of ICCs is from existing structures within the pancreas is new despite a decade of experiments transplanting ICCs internationally. The PEB consists of a mixture of endocrine and exocrine cells, the former being

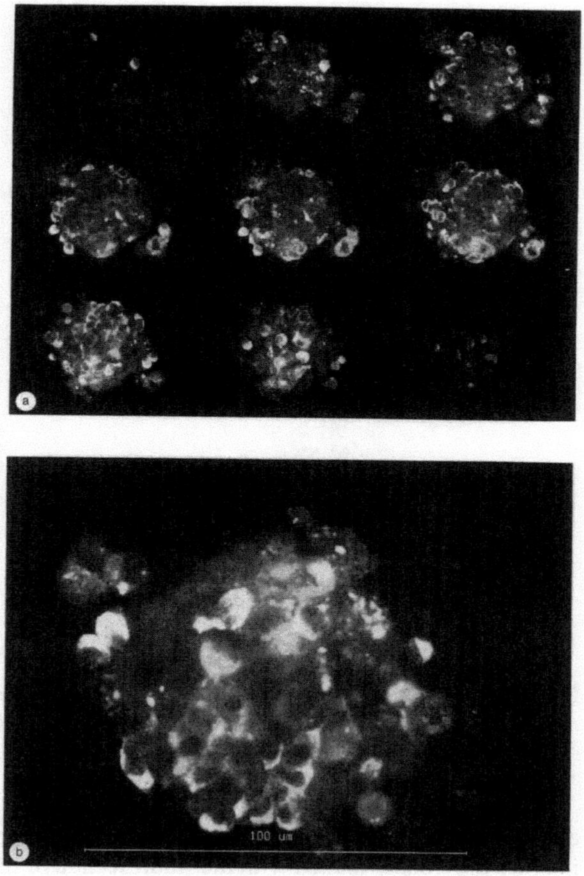

Figure 3. Laser scanning confocal microscopic analysis of pig fetal ICCs. (a) is a scantile view of an ICC examined in different planes from the top to its bottom. (b) is an enlargement of an ICC in one plane. The yellow represents insulin reacting with a guinea pig anti-insulin antibody and an anti-guinea pig immunoglobulin attached to fluorescein isothiocyanate. Scale bar: 100 μm.

characterized by small granules containing the pancreatic hormones, and the latter by much larger granules, the zymogen granules which contain proenzymes. Endocrine cells are frequently adjacent to capillaries; exocrine cells border a lumen. A PEB is either adjacent to another PEB or surrounded by mesenchymal tissue, the amount varying, depending upon the developmental age of the pancreas. Examination of the fetal pancreas towards the end of gestation indicates that the endocrine cells from different PEBs are attracted to one another, thereby creating a mature islet (1% of an adult pancreas), while the exocrine cells in each PEB becomes an acinus, which is the basic structure of the exocrine pancreas (99% of an adult pancreas).

Synthesis and secretion of hormones. ICCs are capable of synthesizing insulin in response to glucose, and can release it when challenged with agents that activate cyclic AMP (19). Glucose is not a stimulus for secretion, probably because of immaturity of enzymes involved in its metabolism. The enzymes involved are probably those in the glycolytic and allied pathways, which allow production of ATP, the key factor in the process of membrane depolarization and eventual secretion of insulin. Activity of glucokinase, a key enzyme in the glycolytic pathway, is diminished in pig fetal ICCs, the Vmax being 20% of that of adult pig islets (Table 1). The affinity of the enzyme for glucose is likewise reduced. Also the activity and affinity of hexokinase are also reduced (Table 1). It is not surprising, therefore, that glyceraldehyde, a more distal metabolite in the glycolytic pathway, is unable to allow

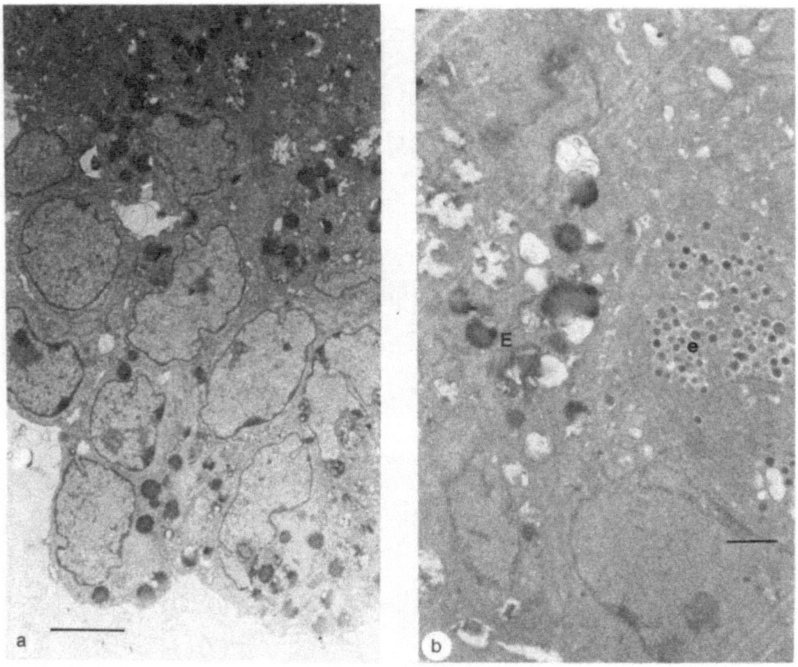

Figure 4. Electronmicroscopic views of an ICC. (a) demonstrates exocrine cells containing large dark staining zymogen granules. Scale bar: 5μm. (b) is a higher magnification demonstrating an endocrine cell (e) alongside an exocrine cell (E). The endocrine cell is characterized by the presence of small electrondense granules with a light staining halo. Scale bar: 1μm.

entry of extracellular Ca^{2+} which results in insulin secretion. Figure 6 demonstrates this effect in ICCs previously loaded with the fluorescent dye fura 2. In contrast, the citric acid cycle, a pathway which is much more efficient than the glycolytic pathway in generating ATP, appears to be intact. Leucine, which enters this pathway at its beginning with the formation of acetyl CoA, does allow entry of extracellular Ca^{2+} (Figure 6).

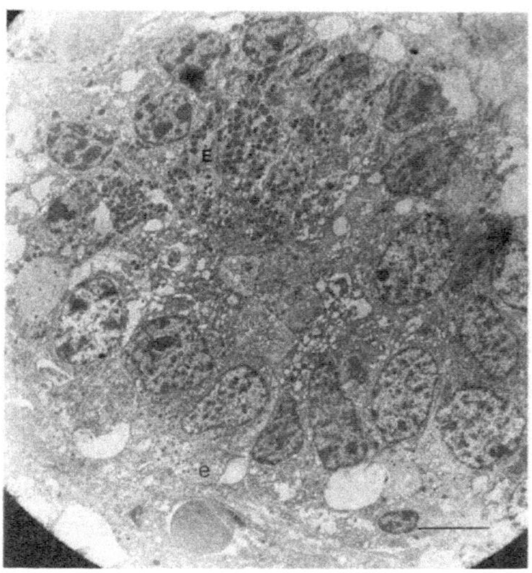

Figure 5. Electronmicroscopic view of a pig fetal pancreas age 90 days. Note the presence of endocrine (e) and exocrine (E) cells as were observed in the ICC (Figure 4). The packing density of the zymogen granules is much greater in the fetal pancreas than in the ICCs. Scale bar: 5 μm.

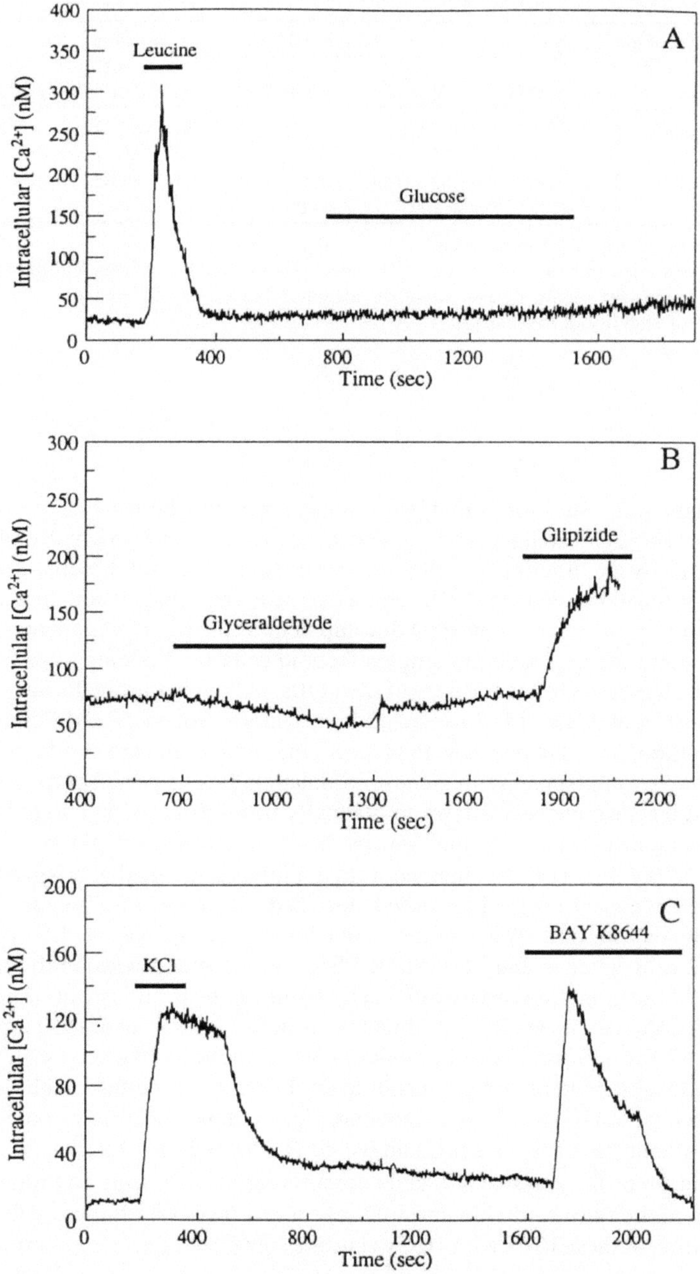

Figure 6. Effect of nutrients glucose, (Panel A), glyceraldehyde (Panel B) and leucine (panel A); as well as effectors of the ATP-dependent K^+ and voltage-activated Ca^{2+} surface channels glipizide (panel B), KCl (panel C) and BAY K8644 (panel C) on $[Ca^{2+}]_i$ in pig fetal ICCs previously loaded with the fluorescent dye fura-2. The black bar indicates the period during which the reagents were added. The concentration of each reagent was: glucose 20 mM, glyceraldehyde 20 mM, leucine 20 mM, glipizide 50 μM, KCl 20 mM, and BAY K8644 2 μM. The basal perifusion solution contained 2 mM glucose.

Table 1. Glucokinase and Hexokinase Activity in Pig Fetal ICCs and Adult Pig Islets

Islets	Glucokinase (GK) Vmax*	Glucokinase (GK) Km (mM)	Hexokinase (HK) Vmax*	Hexokinase (HK) Km (mM)	Glucokinase (% of phosphorylation)†	Lactate dehydrogenase‡
Adult	76.54 ± 7.45	5.29 ± 0.82	156.34 ± 27.88	.015 ± .002	34.28±5.25	72.67 ± 8.80
Fetal	15.21 ± 3.52	19.25 ± 1.1	65.83 ± 18.04	.036 ± .005	23.21±5.65	123.10 ± 23.17
P	<< 0.01	<< 0.01	<< 0.05	<< 0.01		

Values are the mean ± SEM of 4-5 experiments.
Lactate dehydrogenase is a measure of viability of the islets. Though fetal islets were cultured for 4 days and adult islets only overnight before measurement of phosphorylation, the difference in results cannot be explained by loss of viability of the fetal islets.
*nmol/mg protein/h.
† $\left(\frac{GK}{GK + HK}\right) \times 100$
‡unit/mg protein.

Transplantation. One month after being transplanted into the athymic mouse 50% of the cells present in an ICC remain undifferentiated, but by 2 months virtually all cells have differentiated, mostly into ß cells (14). Other endocrine cells - α, γ, and PP cells - are still present but in the main in small numbers (14). The endocrine cells are arranged both in islets and small clusters, in a similar pattern to the normal development of the pig fetal pancreas. Ducts are a prominent feature of the grafts, comprising epithelioid cells and budding from these cells are the ß cells. Exocrine tissue is not a feature of the grafts, although a few cells have been shown to stain positively for amylase (14). In association with this morphological differentiation is the biochemical maturation of the response to glucose. Pig fetal ß cells are similar to human fetal ß cells in that they are unresponsive to glucose stimulation. Over a period of months after ICCs are transplanted ß cells have been shown to gradually become responsive to glucose (14,16), and this results in normalization of blood glucose levels of diabetic recipients.

Up to 100,000 ICCs can be obtained from the litter of an 100 day pregnant sow. Fewer ICCs are obtained if the culture medium used is enriched with amino acids (29 and unpublished observations by our group). The medium used by our group was RPMI 1640 medium containing 11.2 mM glucose and 20 mM HEPES, supplemented with antibiotics and 10% heat-inactivated human pooled serum. Fetal calf serum can be used instead of human serum, but the yield of ICCs is reduced (29). The diameter of ICCs varies from 33-600 μm, the median being between 67 and 113 μm (Table 2), which is less than the average size of a normal adult islet (150 μm). Insulin content varies depending on the period of culture, with there being an inverse relationship between these two parameters. For example, the insulin content of 20 ICCs on the 3rd day of culture is 5.4 ± 1.2 mU and on the 7th day 0.94 ± 0.1 mU.

It is important to note that the cells comprising the ICCs are immunogenic. They stimulate pig lymphocytes to divide and multiply when mixed with these cells (Figure 7). Gamma irradiation of these ICCs with 10 Gy causes a significant decrease in immunogenicity (Figure 7).

C. Endocrine-Rich Monolayers. If the digestion of explants is continued for 20-25 minutes instead of the 10-15 minutes for formation of ICCs, a single cell suspension will form which can be plated into culture flasks. Fibroblasts can be removed by reculturing the cells that have not attached to the flask after 24 hours, most of the fibroblasts having already plated down by this time. The concentration of fetal calf serum in the culture medium is changed from 5% initially to 7% after 4 days to assist in the preferential growth of epithelial

Table 2. Diameter of ICCs Obtained from Pig Fetal Pancreas at Different Stages of Gestation

	Diameter of ICCs (μm)					
Gestational age (days)	mean	SEM	minimum	maximum	median	no. counted
88	142	13	50	600	100	80
100	77	6	33	333	67	60
100 *	87	5	33	200	83	60
110	145	8	38	472	113	120
110	80	4	40	200	80	90

*culture medium contained 6 times normal concentration of amino acids

cells. Cultures of these cells are maintained for two weeks, in order for them to reach confluence. The number of endocrine cells that can be obtained from any one litter is between 10^8 and 10^9 after culture, 19% being ß cells (30).

The ß cells in these monolayers are capable of synthesizing, storing and secreting insulin (31) in the same manner as ß cells in the ICC (19). The main stimuli for secretion are those that increase levels of cyclic AMP and Ca^{2+}, and activate the enzyme protein kinase C; glucose is not effective (30). In contrast, glucose stimulated insulin synthesis (30), probably at the level of translation, as has been described for ICCs (19). Cells in the monolayers are much less immunogenic than freshly prepared single cell suspensions from a pig fetal pancreas (30) [Figure 8]. This reduction in responsiveness of pig splenocytes in a mixed endocrine cell lymphocyte culture is probably because of the loss of antigen presenting cells.

It has yet to be demonstrated that endocrine-rich monolayers of pig fetal pancreas can normalize blood glucose levels in diabetic athymic mice. There is no reason to believe that this is not possible, since both of the other forms of pig fetal pancreas have demonstrated the capability to achieve normalization.

Allografting Pig Fetal Pancreas into Outbred Pigs

Although it has been demonstrated that pig fetal pancreas will survive when transplanted in minipigs across minor histocompatibility barriers (21), this has not been shown for outbred pigs where there are major histocompatibility barriers. We suggest that failure to demonstrate prolonged survival and function of such grafts makes it much less likely that xenografts of this tissue into humans will ever be successful. It is important to remember

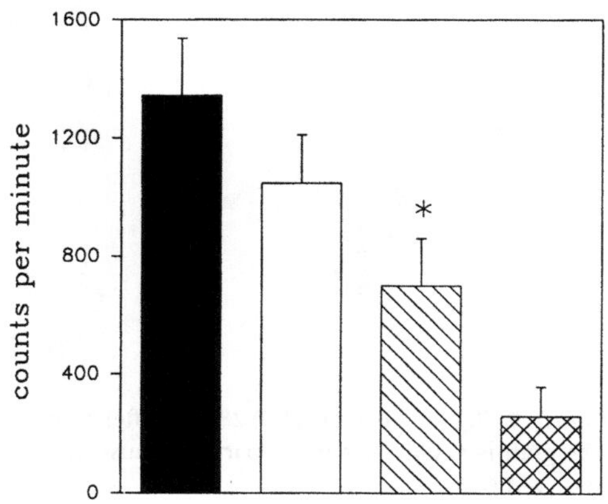

Figure 7. Effect of gamma irradiation of ICCs on their ability to stimulate pig lymphocytes. * P = 0.03 compared with ICCs not irradiated. Lymphocytes were obtained either from peripheral blood of juvenile pigs or from the spleen of pig fetals. Controls were the responder cells alone. Data are expressed as mean ± SEM.

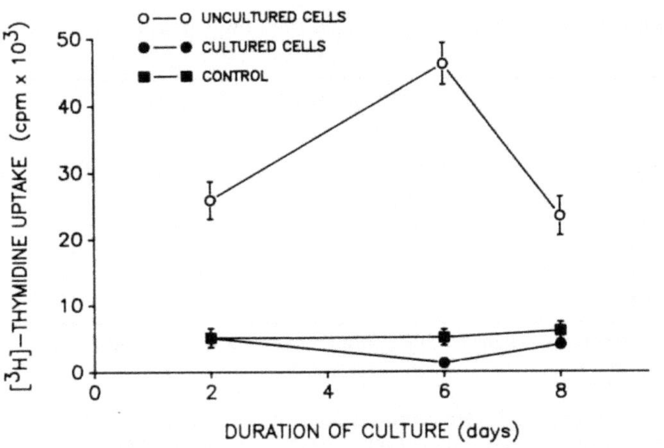

Figure 8. Proliferation of pig fetal splenocytes in response to stimulation by pig fetal pancreatic cells over a period of 8 days. The stimulator cells had either been cultured as monolayers for 14 days or were derived from a freshly collagenased uncultured cell suspension. Controls were responder lymphocytes alone. Values are expressed as mean ± SEM. Reproduced with kind permission of Williams and Wilkins from Simpson AM, Tuch BE, Vincent PC. Transplantation 1990; 49: 1133-7.

that immunological barriers that exist in the outbred allograft, although different from the xenograft, are extensive.

Site of transplantation. In recent experiments we have examined a number of different sites for transplanting pig fetal pancreas. We have confirmed that the omentum is a suitable site for transplanting fetal pancreatic cells, regardless of which form of cell preparation was used. Both ICCs and endocrine-rich monolayers have been used in these experiments. Pancreatic ducts and all four pancreatic endocrine cells - ß (insulin), α (glucagon), δ (somatostatin), and PP (pancreatic polypeptide) - engrafted and survived for up to 8 days when placed in a mesenteric pouch, the neck being tied off with a purse string

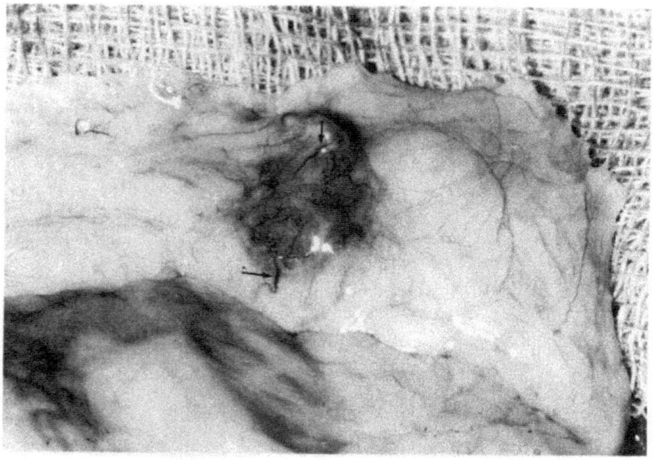

Figure 9. Pig fetal ICCs (5000) 28 days after being grafted as a plasma clot in the omentum of an outbred pig. The graft is visible as a mass, partly because of lymphocytic infiltration. Vascularization of the graft can be observed (→).

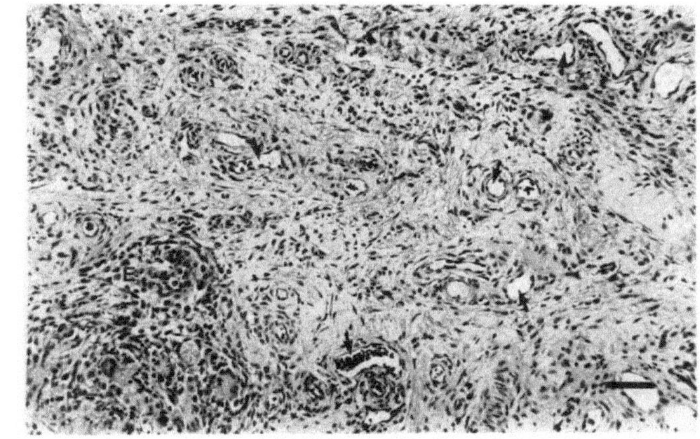

Figure 10. Microscopic view of pig fetal ICCs 4 days after being grafted in the omentum of an outbred immunosuppressed pig. Note the presence of numerous capillaries (→) around ducts. Some lymphocytic infiltration can be observed around surviving epithelial cells (E). Scale bar: 30 μm.

suture. Good vascularization has been observed both macroscopically (Figure 9) and microscopically (Figure 10). Lymphocytic infiltration was a marked feature of these initial grafts because no immunosuppression was used to prevent rejection. The omentum was chosen as the site of transplantation because it is a central site, with such sites being more optimal than peripheral ones (2), and has been used previously by other research groups (18,21,22). The liver was impracticable as a site for transplantation because of the difficulty in finding grafted tissue at the end of the experiment, and the spleen because of its normal component of lymphocytic tissue. In addition to the omentum, we have trialled the capsule of the kidney and the anterior peritoneal wall. Neither of these sites is immunologically privileged, and also it was technically very difficult to separate the kidney from its capsule to insert a graft.

Survival of ICCs in immunosuppressed recipients. We have demonstrated that up to 5000 ICCs will survive for at least 28 days when grafted as a plasma clot (31) into immunosuppressed outbred pigs, but lymphocytic infiltration has been observed to be a problem in many of the recipients (Figure 12). Cyclosporin, azathioprine and prednisolone were used to immunosuppress the recipients, and no immunomodulation of the ICCs was carried out in culture before transplantation. The regimen used by our group was:

- cyclosporin 3 mg/kg intravenously on day 0, followed by 45-60 mg/kg orally in two divided doses.
- azathioprine 2 mg/kg intravenously on day 0, followed by 2 mg/kg orally
- prednisolone 500 mg intravenously on day 0, followed by 0.5 mg/kg orally

Trough levels of cyclosporin in blood, that is, levels measured immediately before administration of the immunosuppressant, have been maintained mostly above 300 ng/mL (Figure 11). All pancreatic endocrine cell types (ß, α, δ, and PP) could be identified mostly as groups of cells budding from ducts (Figure 12). Lower doses of cyclosporin resulted in complete rejection of the graft by 28 days, with germinal centres being a typical feature of the heavy lymphocytic infiltrate observed at this time (Figure 13).

Side effects of immunosuppression. A general side effect of the heavy immunosuppressive therapy used was increased incidence of infection, antibiotics not being used

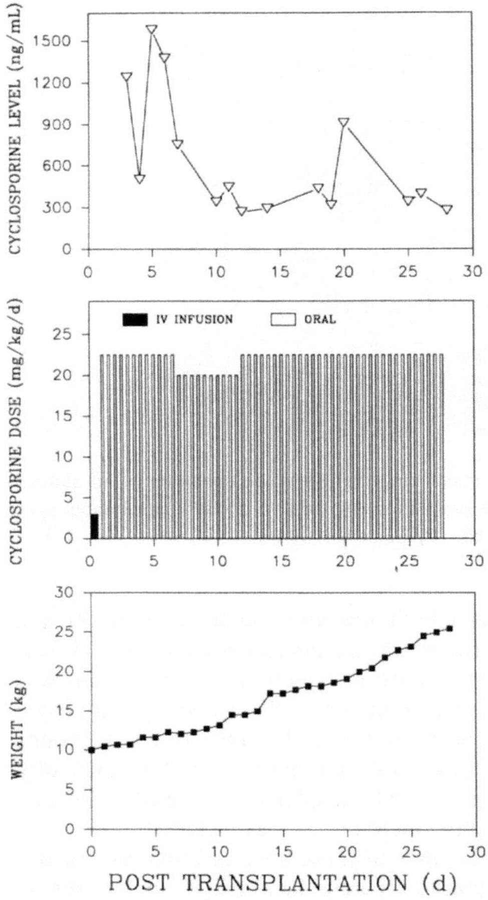

Figure 11. Flow chart of one recipient pig immunosuppressed with high concentrations of cyclosporin together with azathioprine and prednisolone. Note whole blood concentrations of cyclosporin are > 300 ng/mL. The monoclonal assay used measures mostly parent compound. No interference with weigh gain in this juvenile pig was observed.

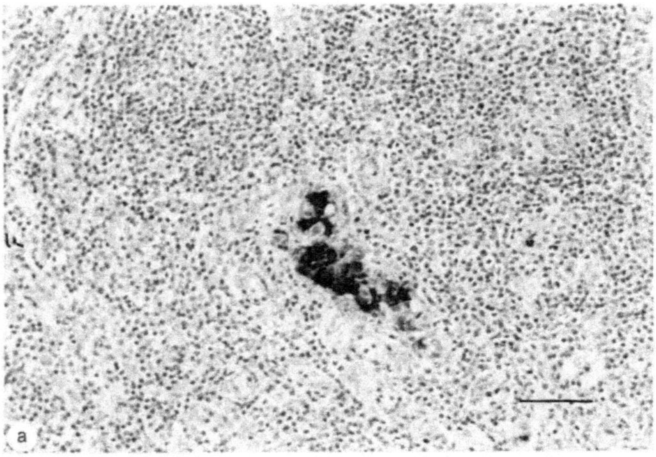

Figure 12. Survival of endocrine cells (a) ß cells; (b) α cells; (c) δ cells [→]; and (d) pancreatic polypeptide cells [→] 28 days after 5000 ICCs were grafted in the omentum of an immunosuppressed pig. The endocrine cells, which are darkly stained by the immunoperoxidase technique, are present in small clusters. Ducts can also be observed. Large numbers of lymphocytes are present around the endocrine cells and ducts. Scale bar: 40 μm for (a) and 20 μm for (b), (c), and (d).

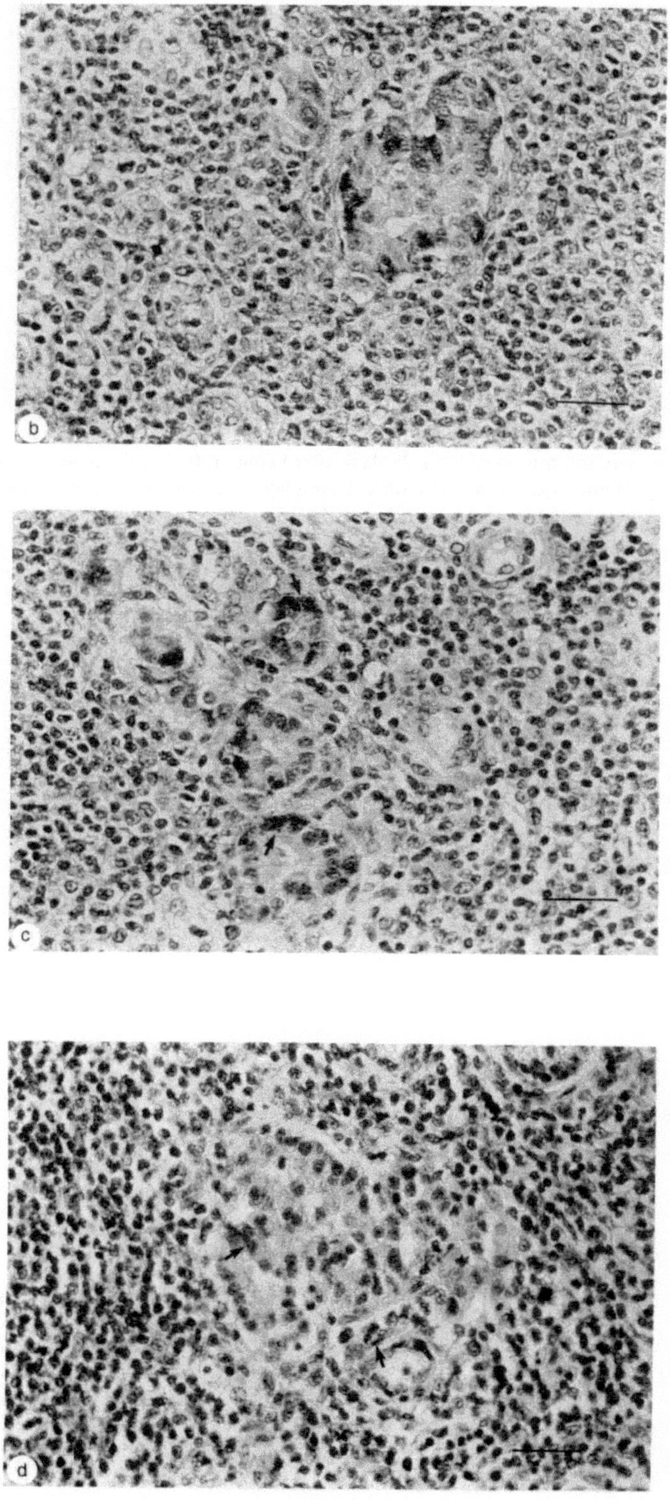
b
c
d

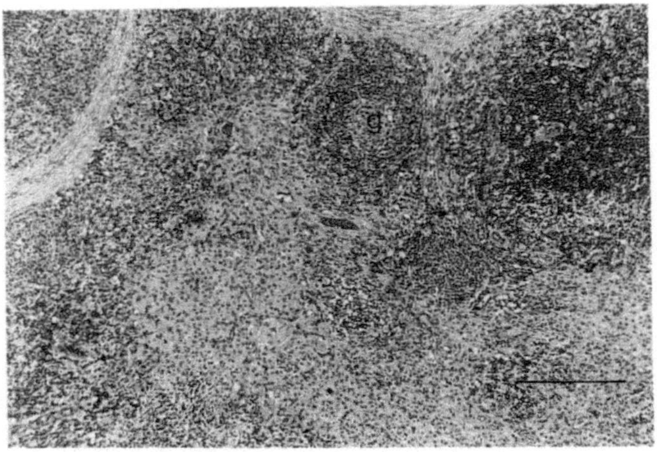

Figure 13. Lymphocytic infiltration of ICCs 28 days after being grafted in the omentum of an immunosuppressed outbred pig. While most of the cells were T lymphocytes, there were a number of B lymphocytes, which are clustered in germinal centers (g). Scale bar: 50 μm.

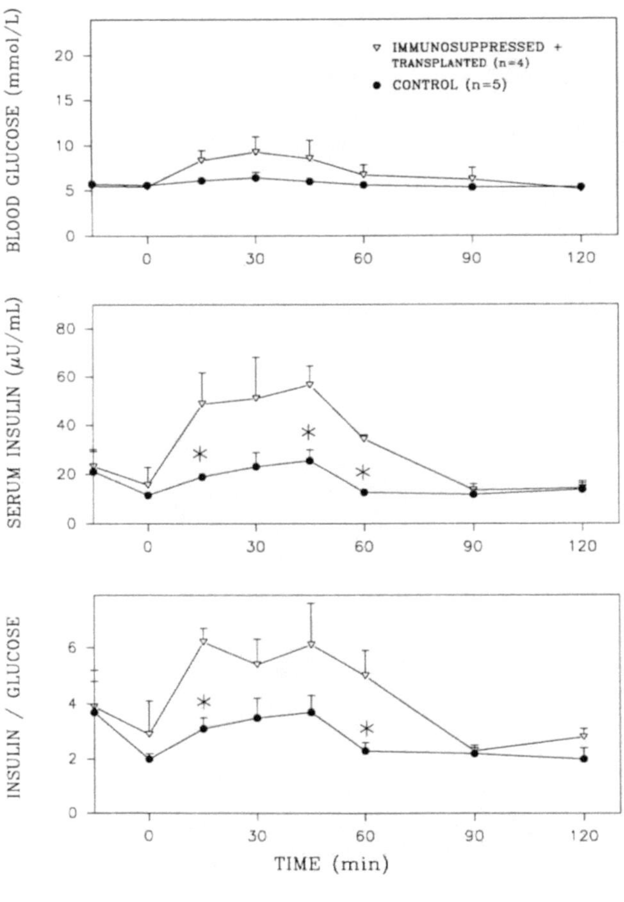

Figure 14. Oral glucose tolerance tests performed after an overnight fast on both immunosuppressed and non-immunosuppressed pigs. Glucose (2 g/kg) was delivered orally through a nipple, and blood removed periodically from a catheter in the jugular vein. * $P < 0.05$.

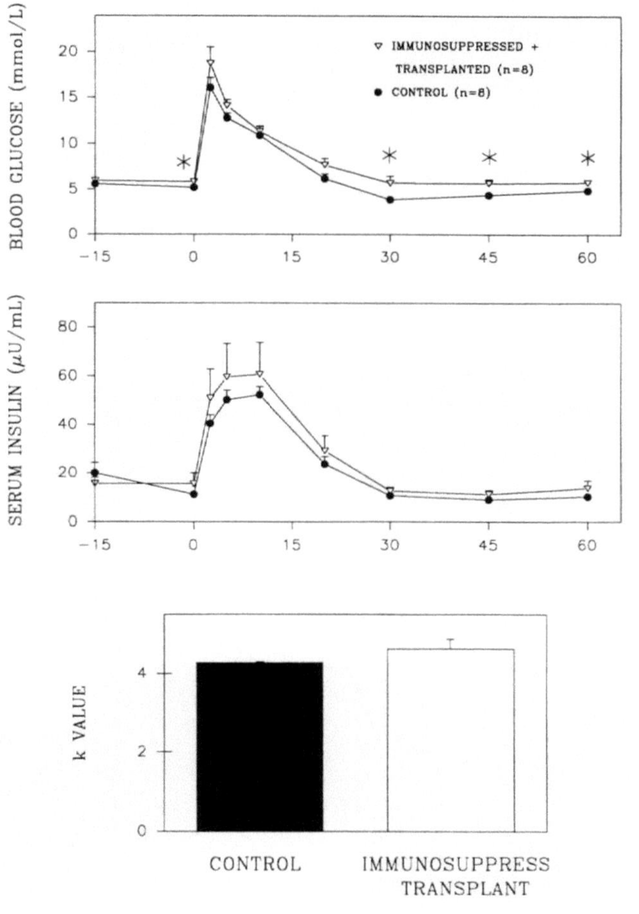

Figure 15. Intravenous glucose tolerance tests performed after an overnight fast on both immunosuppressed and non-immunosuppressed pigs. Glucose (0.5 g/kg) was injected rapidly into the jugular vein, with blood samples collected from the same vein commencing 4 minutes later. * $P < 0.05$. The k value is the rate of disappearance of glucose (%/min).

prophylactically. Unlike the expected result in humans high concentrations of cyclosporin in the pig did not adversely affect the liver or kidney, either in terms of the blood levels of liver enzymes, bilirubin, albumin, and creatinine or histologically at post mortem. Further, azathioprine did not cause bone marrow toxicity. There was, however, synergism between the effects of cyclosporin and the 500 mg bolus of prednisolone given at the time of transplantation, probably as a result of competition for cytochrome P450 in the liver. As a result the trough level of cyclosporin on the morning after grafting was often very high (5000 ng/mL). No adverse effect on weight gain was observed from the immunosuppressive agents used.

Oral and intravenous glucose tolerance tests carried out on immunosuppressed transplanted pigs showed that insulin resistance was a feature. This was most noticeable in the oral glucose tolerance tests (Figure 14) where the insulin levels were higher in the treated animals. Insulin secretion from the ß cell was not inhibited by cyclosporin (Figure 15) and the rate of disappearance of glucose (k) in the intravenous glucose tolerance tests being unaffected 4.63 ± 0.25, c.f., 4.28 ± 0.02.

Induction and management of diabetes. We have confirmed that diabetes can be induced by an intravenous infusion of 150 mg/kg of streptozotocin [STZ] (32). Vomiting, a side effect of STZ, was prevented by fasting the animals overnight before infusion of the

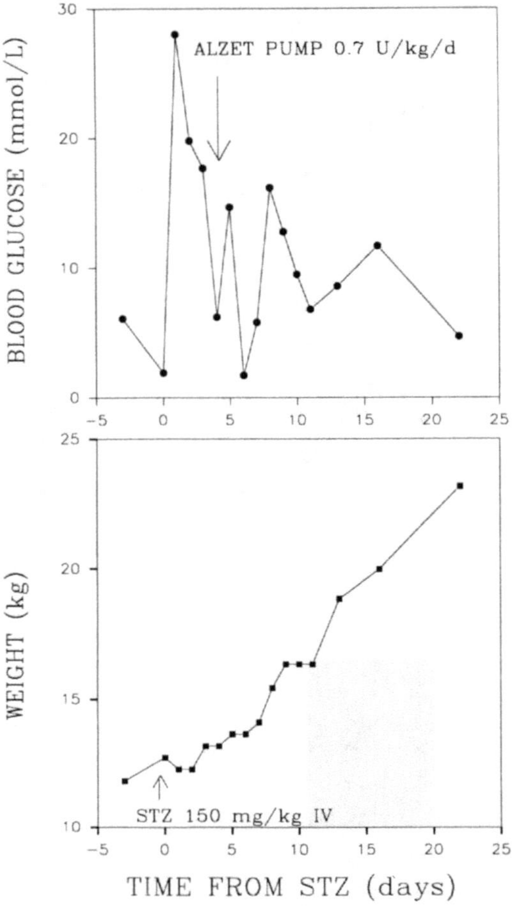

Figure 16. Blood glucose levels in a non-immunosuppressed pig made diabetic with streptozotocin. A mini-osmotic Alzet pump containing 200 units soluble insulin was placed subcutaneously 4 days later. Blood glucose levels obtained thereafter are imperfect, but not in a toxic range. The pig remained well, and continued to gain weight.

drug and giving mylanta with food. Hypoglycaemia due to insulin being released from the destroyed ß cells was avoided by giving the animals an infusion of 4% dextrose and N/5 saline.

In our studies we have shown that control of diabetic pigs can be quite difficult. This relates not only to the injection of insulin through pain sensitive skin, but also to the handling of the animals because of the effects of poor blood glucose control on their temperament. Adequate glycaemic control was achieved by inserting a large Alzet mini-osmotic pump subcutaneously containing sufficient quick acting insulin to last 4 weeks (Figure 16). It has been demonstrated that it is essential to add glutamine (7 mg/mL) to this to prevent aggregation (33). Since it is expected that fetal grafts will not function for several months, pumps will need to be replaced monthly.

THE FUTURE

Consistent prevention of the pig fetal pancreas allograft in outbred pigs has yet to be achieved. There is reason to believe that *in vitro* immunomodulation, for example, with γ irradiation (Figure 7) or ultraviolet-B irradiation (34) before the ICCs are grafted may be beneficial since responsiveness of lymphocytes in islet lymphocyte cultures is reduced. Alternatives include supplementation with yet another immunosuppressive agent, such as 15-deoxyspergualin, which suppresses activation of infiltrating cells not adequately covered by the other agents used; or the use of monoclonal antibodies which attach to and kill lymphocytes. Currently there is only one such antibody, against CD8 positive lymphocytes (35); its application should result in the destruction of most lymphocytes since in the pig the majority of them are both CD8 and CD4 positive (36). Regardless of what steps are taken, the history of transplantation suggests that it is likely to be necessary to demonstrate that pig fetal pancreas can be successfully allografted into outbred pigs if xenografts of this tissue into humans is ever to result in reversal of diabetes.

ACKNOWLEDGMENTS

The technical assistance of Chitra de Silva, Sandy Beynon, Julia Beretov and Roma Gakas in looking after the pigs, carrying out the immunoassays, and histological staining of the tissue is gratefully acknowledged. We are also indebted to Jeffrey Hamdorf and Gregory Keogh for their surgical expertise with the pigs.

REFERENCES

1. Federlin, K., Bretzel, R.G., and Hering, B.J., 1991. Recent achievements in experimental and clinical islet transplantation. Diab. Med. 8: 5-12.
2. Tuch, B.E., Grigoriou, S., and Turtle, J.R., 1986. Growth and hormonal content of human fetal pancreas passaged in athymic mice. Diabetes 35: 464-469.
3. Tuch, B.E., Osgerby, K.J., and Turtle, J.R., 1988. Human fetal pancreas grafted into non-diabetic nude mice normalizes blood glucose levels once diabetes is induced. Transplantation 46: 608-611.
4. Hullett, D.A., Falany, J.L., Love, R.B., Burlingham, W.J., Pan, M., and Sollinger, H.W., 1987. Human fetal pancreas - a potential source for transplantation. Transplantation 43: 18-22.
5. Tuch, B.E., 1991. Reversal of diabetes by human fetal pancreas: Optimization of requirements in the hyperglycaemic nude mouse. Transplantation 51: 557-562.
6. Tuch, B.E., Monk, R.S., and Beretov, J., 1991. Reversal of diabetes in athymic rats by transplantation of human fetal pancreas. Transplantation 52: 172-175.
7. Tuch, B.E., 1992. Reversal of diabetes by the human fetal ß cell: message from the athymic rat. Diab. Nutr. Metab. 5 (Suppl. 3): 75-78.
8. Hu, Y-f., Gu, Z-f., Zhang, H-d., and Ye, R-s., 1992. Fetal islet transplantation in China. Transplant. Proc. 24: 1998-1999.
9. Shumakov, V.I., Bljumkin, V.N., Ignatenko, S.N., Skaletsky, N.N., Slovesnova, T.A., and Babikova, R.A., 1987. The principal results of pancreatic islet cell culture transplantation in diabetes mellitus patients. Transplant. Proc. 19: 2372.
10. Tuch, B.E., Sheil, A.R.G., Ng, A.B.P., Trent, R.J., and Turtle, J.R., 1988. Recovery of human fetal pancreas after one year of implantation in the diabetic patient. Transplantation 46: 865-870.
11. Groth, C.G., Andersson, A., Björken, C., Gunnarsson, R., Hellerström, C., Lundgren, G., Petersson, B., Swenne, I., and Östman, J., 1980. Attempts at transplantation of fetal pancreas to diabetic patients. Transplant. Proc. 12 (Suppl. 2); 208-212.
12. Farkas, G., Szabo, M., and Voros, P., 1992. Ten years' clinical experience of fetal islet transplantation. Transplant. Proc. 24: 2954-2955.
13. Hullett, D.A., Bethke, K.P., Landry, A.S., Leonard, D.K., and Sollinger, H.W., 1989. Successful long-term cryopreservation of human fetal pancreas. Diabetes 38 (Suppl. 1): 284.
14. Korsgren, O., Jansson, L., Eizirik, D., and Andersson, A., 1991. Functional and morphological differentiation of fetal porcine islet-like cell clusters after transplantation into nude mice. Diabetologia 34: 379-386.

15. Thompson, S.C., and Mandel, T.E., 1990. Fetal pig pancreas: Preparation and assessment of tissue for transplantation, and its *in vivo* development and function in athymic (nude) mice. Transplantation 49: 571-581.
16. Liu, X., Federlin, K.F., Bretzel, R.G., Hering, B.J., and Brendel, M.D., 1991. Persistent reversal of diabetes by transplantation of fetal pig proislets into nude mice. Diabetes 40: 858-866.
17. Simeonovic, C.J., Ceredig, R., and Wilson, J.D., 1990. Effect of GK1.5 monoclonal antibody dosage on survival of pig proislet xenografts in $CD4^+$ T cell-depleted mice. Transplantation 49: 849-856.
18. Korsgren, O., Sandler, S., Landström, A.S., Jansson, L., and Andersson, A., 1988. Large-scale production of fetal porcine pancreatic isletlike cell clusters. Transplantation 45: 509-514.
19. Mandel, T.E., and Koulmanda, M., 1994. Xenotransplantation of fetal pig pancreas and reversal of diabetes in spontaneously diabetic NOD mice. Transplant. Proc. in press.
20. Mullen, Y., Nagata, M., Matsuo, S., Taura, Y., and Miyazawa, K., 1990. Effective treatment regimes against fetal islet rejection in miniature swine with or without a combined kidney allograft. Horm. Metab. Res. Suppl. 25: 190-192.
21. Mullen, Y., Taura, Y., Ozawa, A., Miyazawa, K., Shiogama, T., Matsuo, S., Nagata, M., Takasugi, M., Klandorf, H., Tsunoda, T., Terada, M., Motojima, K., and Clare-Salzler, M., 1989. Reversal of experimental diabetes in miniature swine by fetal pancreas allografts. Transplant. Proc. 21: 2671-2672.
22. Mullen, Y., 1988. Fetal pancreas transplantation for treatment of type I diabetes: miniature swine model. In *Fetal Islet Transplantation*, eds. Peterson CM, Jovanovic-Peterson L, Formby B. Springer Verlag, New York pp. 111-125.
23. Tibell, A., Reinholt, F.P., Korsgren, O., Andersson, A., Hellerström, C., Möller, E., and Groth, C-G., 1994. Morphological identification of porcine islet cells 3 weeks after transplantation into a diabetic patient. Transplant. Proc. 26: 1121.
24. Andersson, A., Groth, C.G., Korsgren, O., Tibell, A., Tollemar, J., Kumagai, M., Möller, E., Bolinder, J., Östman, J., Bjöersdorff, A., and Hellerström, C., 1992. Transplantation of porcine fetal islet-like cell clusters to three diabetic patients. Transplant. Proc. 24: 677-678.
25. Tibell, A., Groth, C.G., Möller, E., Korsgren, O., Andersson, A., and Hellerström, C., 1994. Pig-to-human islet transplantation in 8 patients. Transplant Proc 26: 762-763.
26. International Islet Transplant Registry, eds. Hering, B.J., Geier, C., Schultz, A.O., Bretzel, R.G., and Federlin, K., Dept Medicine, Justus-Liebig-University of Giessen 1994; 4: 16-18.
27. Korsgren, O., and Jansson, L., 1994. Porcine islet-like cell clusters cure diabetic nude rats when transplanted under the kidney capsule, but not when implanted into the liver or spleen. Cell Transplant. 3: 49-54.
28. Tuch, B.E., 1992. Clinical results of transplanting fetal pancreas. In *Fetal tissue transplants in medicine*, ed. Edwards, R.G.. Cambridge University Press, Cambridge pp. 215-237.
29. Korsgren, O., Sandler, S., Jansson, L., Groth, C-G., Hellerström, C., and Andersson, A., 1989. Effects of culture conditions on formation and hormone content of fetal porcine isletlike cell clusters. Diabetes 38 (Suppl. 1): 209-212.
30. Simpson, A.M., Tuch, B.E., and Vincent, P.C., 1990. Tissue culture of pig fetal pancreas. Transplantation 49: 1133-1137.
31. Simeonovic, C.J., Brown, D.J., Teittinen, K.U.S., and Wilson, J.D., 1992. Preparation and transplantation of fetal proislets. In *Pancreatic islet cell transplantation*, ed. Ricordi, C.. RG Landes Co, Austin pp. 238-248.
32. Wilson, J.D., Dhall, D.P., Simeonovic, C.J., and Lafferty, K.J., 1986. Induction and management of diabetes mellitus in the pig. Aust. J. Exp. Biol. Med. Sci. 64: 489-500.
33. Bringer, J., Heldt, A., and Grodsky, G.M., 1981. Prevention of insulin aggregation by dicarboxylic amino acids during prolonged infusion. Diabetes 30: 83-85.
34. Benhamou, P.Y., Stein, E., and Mullen, Y., 1994. Effect of ultraviolet-B irradiation on the function and immunogenicity of fetal porcine islets. Transplant. Proc. 26: 705.
35. Suzuki, T., Sundt III, T.M., Mixon, A., and Sachs, D.H., 1990. *In vivo* treatment with antiporcine T cell antibodies. Transplantation 50: 76-81.
36. Saalmüller, A., Reddehase, M.J., Bühring, H-J., Jonjic, S., and Koszinowski, U.H., 1987. Simultaneous expression of CD4 and CD8 antigens by a substantial proportion of resting porcine T lymphocytes. Eur. J. Immunol. 17: 1297-1301.

6

COMBINED TRANSPLANTATION OF ADULT AND FETAL ISLETS FOR IMPROVEMENT OF GRAFT FUNCTION: PROSPECTIVE APPROACH FOR DIABETES TREATMENT

Yoko Mullen

Department of Surgery, UCLA School of Medicine and
VA Medical Center, West Los Angeles
Diabetes Research Center
675 Circle Drive South
Los Angeles, California 90024-7036

The major threat of diabetes mellitus is the progressive development of debilitating complications. Current treatment modalities remain suboptimal as evidenced by persistent, significant morbidity and mortality (1, 2). More than twenty years ago, our group pioneered fetal pancreatic islet transplantation for treatment of type 1 diabetes (3). Our working hypothesis has been that diabetic complications can be prevented if blood glucose levels are tightly controlled by physiological mechanisms. The lessons we have learned from the Diabetes Control and Complications Trial (4) support this hypothesis. The islets of Langerhans isolated from the pancreas can be transplanted into diabetic patients with a minimally invasive technique. The transplanted islets release insulin in response to high glucose stimuli by homeostatic mechanisms and thus can provide the best control of blood glucose (5). Furthermore, successful islet transplantation will free the patients from the repeated blood glucose monitoring, insulin injections, and improve the quality of life. In order to achieve this goal, pancreatic islet transplantation must ultimately fulfill the following three requirements: Transplanted islets 1) will have their effect on hyperglycemia soon after transplantation, 2) will provide long-lasting insulin independence, preferably life-time, and 3) will survive without continuous use of immunosuppressive agents.

CURRENT STATUS OF CLINICAL ISLET TRANSPLANTATION

Most clinical islet transplantations have used donor islets prepared from the adult human pancreas. The major advantages of adult islets are that 1) a large number of islets can be isolated from the organ and even a single pancreas can provide a sufficient number of islets for transplantation and 2) the transplanted islets can function within a short period after transplantation and demonstrate their ability in controlling hyperglycemia. The International

Fetal Islet Transplantation
Edited by C. M. Peterson, L. Jovanovic-Peterson, and B. Formby, Plenum Press, New York, 1995

Islet Transplantation Registry reported positive serum C-peptide (indicative of viable grafts) for more than 1 month in 80% of the recipients who received combined islet and kidney transplants during 1990-1992 (6,7). Twenty five percent of these became free of insulin injections. However, in 60% of the recipients this insulin independence lasted less than one month. To date, over 200 adult islet transplantations have been performed world-wide. Among those, only 16 recipients achieved insulin independence for longer than 1 month. Insulin independence has, at best, lasted for a maximum of three years. Thus, unlike pancreatic organ transplants or islet autografts, the function of adult islet allografts in patients with type 1 diabetes gradually declines. These results are attributed primarily to an insufficient number of donor islets and to the quality of transplanted islets (6,7).

The currently recommended number of islets for type 1 diabetic recipients is >6,000 IEQ (islet number equivalent to 150 um in diameter) per kg of recipient's body weight (8). This number of islets can normalize hyperglycemia or significantly reduce daily insulin requirements shortly after transplantation, leading to insulin independence in some cases or providing better control of blood glucose. However, this islet number, 6000 IEQ/kg of body weight or 500,000 IEQ per patient, is considerably lower than that present in the pancreas. In our data, the number of islets counted in the collagenase-digested pancreatic tissue (before islet isolation) is well over a million (9). Therefore, the islet number used for transplantation is approximately half of that in the pancreas. Based on this, the transplanted islets may have to overwork in controlling blood glucose, although the number of β cells required to control blood glucose is not known. Furthermore, islets transplanted into type 1 diabetic recipients are exposed to additional insults associated with both alloimmune and autoimmune responses and immunosuppressive agents, cyclosporine and steroids.

The success rate of islet autografts in the patients, whose pancreas was removed due to severe pancreatitis, is considerably higher and their function continues for many years (10). The higher success rate of these islet autografts may be accounted for by: 1) islet autografts do not suffer immunological insults, including the adverse effect of immunosuppressants and 2) most of autotransplantation uses a crude preparation of islets, instead of a highly purified islet preparations used for allografts in type I diabetics. Fully differentiated, purified adult islets may have a disadvantage of a limited proliferative capacity and life-span. It is not known how long β cells live and whether β cells are replaced by newly generated islets in the pancreas of normal individuals. A study in partially pancreatectomized rats suggests that new β cells are generated in the adult pancreas (11). We also observed, in streptozotocin-injected pigs, the presence of unusually large islets that consist of many β cells (12). "Honeymoon" periods observed in patients with newly diagnosed diabetes may also indicate β cell regeneration (or hypertrophy) in the pancreas. Furthermore, the insulin independence achieved many months after islet transplantation also suggests that there is β cell regeneration in transplanted adult islets (6,8). Therefore, it may be possible that in the pancreas β/islet cells are replaced, from time to time, by newly formed cells and that β cells may not live throughout the life time. In rodents, cells that stain for insulin or glucagon are often found in the ductal epithelium of newborn pancreata transplanted into diabetic animals (13). The newly formed islets in the 90% pancreatectomized rats are generated from the duct epithelium (11). During the islet isolation process from the adult human pancreas, we have observed single cells, that are positively stained with dithizone (a staining for β cells), among the ductal epithelial cells (14). These lines of evidence suggest that the ductal epithelium contains islet stem cells. If islets are generated, depending on needs, from pancreatic ducts, transplanted islets carefully isolated from other pancreatic components would have a considerable disadvantage, whereas the crude islet preparations used for autografts would have a greater advantage. At the University of Minnesota, the crude islet preparations were transplanted into two type 1 diabetic recipients. One of the two became insulin independent 326 days after transplantation that has continued for nearly two years (8). If this insulin independence lasts for many years, this would indicate the distinct advantage of the crude islet preparation for transplantation. Care must be taken, however, to solve other problems associated with this approach, including portal hypertension and stronger alloimmune reactions.

ADVANTAGES AND DISADVANTAGES OF FETAL PANCREAS IN TRANSPLANTATION

We have conducted systematic investigations, initially in inbred strains of rats and subsequently in the NIH miniature swine, to assess the feasibility of fetal pancreas transplantation for treatment of insulin-dependent diabetes. Our studies, as well as others, have demonstrated several advantages of fetal pancreas as donor tissue. The most distinct advantage is the tremendous capacity for continuous growth, differentiation, and maturation of the endocrine pancreas (islets) from stem cells (3,15). Fetal islets are neither fully formed nor fully functional. Fetal β cells do not respond to high glucose stimuli with an insulin release until they have reached the gestational age close to birth: 21 days in rodents (16), >100 days in pigs (the gestation period is 114 days) (17), and >25 weeks in humans (18). After reaching this age, the β cell responsiveness rapidly increases and there is the release of a sufficient amount of insulin for reversal of hyperglycemia. Fetal pancreatic tissue continuously grows and proliferates following transplantation. Because of this ability, one or even part of a pancreas can reverse diabetes in an adult rat or mouse and provide long-lasting graft function (19-21). In rats, a single pancreas from a 17 day fetus can reverse severe diabetes, induced by streptozotocin, in an adult rat. The optimal growth and function can be obtained when hyperglycemia is carefully controlled for 3 weeks (19). A single fetal pancreas transplant can also support metabolic needs during pregnancy in rats that were made severely diabetic with an intravenous injection of 90 mg/kg streptozotocin (20). After diabetes was reversed by a single fetal pancreas transplant, these rats were mated, carried out normal pregnancy, gave a birth, raised pups and remained normoglycemia after parturition. These results demonstrated the reserved capacity of a single fetal pancreas. Fetal pancreata of a large animal species, swine, also continuously grow and proliferate after transplantation, and normalize blood glucose in streptozotocin-induced diabetic pigs. A well grown graft was observed after 400 days in a diabetic pig that had been continuously treated with cyclosporine (12). This graft contained a large mass of β cells. Likewise, islets of the human fetal pancreas continuously proliferate and mature both in culture and in vivo in athymic mice (18, 21-23). Because of this ability, human fetal pancreas allografts would provide long-term β cell function to control hyperglycemia under appropriate conditions.

During fetal development, the endocrine pancreas precedes the exocrine pancreas. Insulin is detected in the fetal pancreas at an early stage of gestation (24). The exocrine elements, chymotrypsinogen and trypsinogen, become detectable after 18 day gestation in rats (25), after 55 days in pigs (26), and after 18-20 weeks in humans (27). Following transplantation, a whole pancreas taken from the appropriate developmental age becomes a pure endocrine organ without exocrine elements. In rats, this gestational age is found to be before the appearance of the exocrine components, especially trypsinogen (<18 day of gestation). The pancreas from older fetuses often develops a cystic formation at the graft site and the transplant's function is variable (16). Although the best growth and proliferation of islets is achieved with an intact fetal pancreatic tissue, these abilities are preserved even after the organ is collagenase digested (28,29). After collagenase digestion, the purification of islets is unnecessary, and total digested tissues can be transplanted or cultured. Fetal islets continuously proliferate and grow from the collagenase digested tissue.

The considerable disadvantage of the fetal pancreas in clinical transplantation is that the transplant does not function immediately to control or affect hyperglycemia. There will be no clear indication of graft function, except possible positive serum C-peptide, for many months. Although fetal pancreas transplants can reverse diabetes in rats within 10 days under appropriate conditions (16), in pigs it takes at least two months before detecting some effect on daily insulin requirements, despite their ability in subsequently achieving insulin independence (28, 29). Following transplantation, fetal islets need time to proliferate, grow and mature to attain a normal insulin response. At least 3-4 months would be required for human fetal β cells to show some clinical indications (23). In the clinical situation, this waiting period would be very frustrating, especially without knowing its outcome, as we have experienced with fetal islet transplantation in pigs. Another potential problem is the need for a large number of donor pancreata to provide a sufficient β cell function. In rats, a single fetal pancreas can sufficiently grow to control hyperglycemia within a relatively short (3-4 weeks) period after transplantation (16, 19). In severely diabetic pigs four pancreata from 50 day fetuses or the same number of collagenase digested tissue from 60 day fetuses had very little effect on blood glucose: daily insulin requirements reduced only transiently from 15-20 U to 10 U and then increased to the pretransplant level (28). Despite of this, a viable graft containing β cells was detected by histological examination. The pancreas of pigs reaches the adult size in less than one year. Therefore, the islet number in the pancreas reaches an adult level within one year. In humans, it takes for more than 12-13 years for the pancreas to reach the adult size and adult islet number. Therefore, it would take many years, even under the best condition, for human fetal islets to grow to supply a sufficient amount of insulin. Even if multiple fetal pancreata are transplanted, it may take many years to achieve the optimal function.

BENEFITS OF COMBINED TRANSPLANTATION OF ADULT AND FETAL ISLETS

In vivo, well controlled blood glucose, especially during the earlier stages of transplantation, helps the optimal growth and proliferation of immature β cells in the fetal pancreas (16, 19). When hyperglycemia is controlled by daily insulin injections, normoglycemia returns in diabetic rodents within 2-3 weeks. If daily insulin injections are not given, it takes 5-6 weeks to normalize blood glucose or the grafts often fail to reverse diabetes with the same number of donor pancreata. In organ culture growth factors, including insulin, promote active proliferation of fetal islet cells (30). When both adult and fetal islets are combined and used as donor tissue for transplantation into type 1 diabetics, adult islets produce insulin shortly after transplantation. Adult islets, at best, eliminate the need for daily insulin injections and reverse hyperglycemia, thus providing a better environment and a sufficient time for the optimal growth and maturation of fetal islets. Even at its worst, transplanted adult islets together with daily insulin injections provide better control of hyperglycemia, thus giving fetal β cells a better opportunity for their development. Human fetal β cells start to respond to high glucose stimulation after 25 weeks of gestation. The amount of released insulin increases rapidly as the gestation period advances (18). Therefore, after growing for several months, fetal β cells would start to share the workload with adult islet transplants. At the same time, new β cells and islets would be continuously generated in the fetal pancreatic graft.

The presence of both fetal and adult islets may also be beneficial in providing each other with growth factors. Insulin may have a direct impact on β cell regeneration (30). Therefore, insulin produced by co-transplanted adult islets can be beneficial for fetal β cell growth. There are a number of other growth factors that promote insulin production and DNA synthesis of adult and fetal islets (30). A growing number of reports suggests that endogenous production of growth factors in the pancreas, including insulin-like growth factor I and II (IGF I and II), may contribute to β cell proliferation (31). Both IFGs are present in human fetal pancreas. In the tissue obtained early in the second trimester, the duct and islet cells stain positively for IGF-II, and a similar pattern is obtained for IGF-binding proteins as well (32). IGFs are also present in β cells of cultured fetal pancreas (33) and appear to be actively synthesized (34). During the development of rats, IGF-I, IGF-II and their specific binding proteins are expressed in the pancreas: IGF-II is the predominant peptide of fetal and neonatal pancreas and is highest in 18 day fetal pancreas, but it is no longer detectable in the 14 day or older postnatal pancreas. IGF-I mRNA is also present throughout the pancreas, but in a low amount during fetal life. It becomes predominant around the time of weaning, but is only found in the exocrine tissue of the adult pancreas. It has been also reported that when IGF-I and IGF-II were added to fetal islet culture media, DNA synthesis increases in 24 hours, all of the proliferating cells are stained for insulin (31). Exogenous IGF-I stimulates DNA synthesis in cultured human fetal islets (35), and IGF-II promotes both β cell proliferation and function (36). These observations suggest that IGFs exert a paracrine/autocrine action on fetal beta cell growth. Based on these data, it would be reasonable to speculate that 1) IGFs, especially IGF-II, are produced by fetal human pancreatic cells in culture and after transplantation, 2) endogenous and exogenous IGFs play an important role as growth and differentiation promoters for fetal β cells in culture and after transplantation, and 3) the paracrine effects of IGFs are important for the regeneration of adult islet cells. It is possible that highly purified, isolated adult islets may have little ability to produce these growth factors, since pancreatic acinar cells appear to involve the growth factor production. The adult pancreas of rats contains IGF-I only in acinar cells, but no detectable IGF-II. In combined islet transplantation, the paracrine effects of IGFs or other potentially effective growth factors produced by the fetal pancreatic tissue may also influence adult islet regeneration.

We recently used donor tissue of combined adult and fetal islets for transplantation into the thymus of NIH minipigs made diabetic by total pancreatectomy (37). Donor tissue consisted of islets isolated from 1-2 adult pancreata and collagenase-digested fetal pancreatic tissues from multiple farm pigs. Combined adult and fetal islets were transplanted into the cervical lobes of the thymus and the recipient was treated only with anti-lymphocyte serum for 5 days starting the day of transplantation. No insulin injections were given for more than 4 months after transplantation. Following transplantation, blood glucose of all eight pigs was maintained lower than 200 mg/dl for at least one month. Thereafter, fasting blood glucose levels of two long-lived pigs gradually increased, but maintained at levels below 300 mg/dl for four to six months. Results of serum C-peptide levels were interesting, and provided the basis in speculating on the functions of adult and fetal β cells. Serum C-peptide levels were at the lower level of the normal range for 30-40 days after transplantation. This C-peptide level corresponded to fasting blood glucose levels (<200 mg/dl). Thereafter, serum C-peptides were detectable but the levels had significantly dropped and blood glucose gradually rose. Interestingly, serum C-peptide levels again increased after 2-3 months, reaching close to the previous level. C-peptide levels had again declined gradually, but maintained at a low, but detectable level for nearly 200 days in one pig and 300 days in another. We attributed the initial control of hyperglycemia and the first C-peptide peak primarily to the activity of adult islets, and the second peak to the activity of fetal islets. However, fetal β cells were not able to control blood glucose sufficiently. The above assumptions are reasonable, since our results in pigs that received total pancreatectomy and were transplanted with adult islets alone, have repeatedly shown that the function of adult islets is irreversible once it starts to decline (38). Although our interpretation of the results is speculative and well defined experiments are necessary, the results in two long-lived pigs have demonstrated that fetal β cells can continuously proliferate and produce insulin in severely diabetic pigs when hyperglycemia is controlled by co-transplanted adult islets. Although not directly related to the subject discussed in this section, the goal of our intrathymic islet transplantation performed in pigs is directed to the third requirement for clinical islet transplantation; to develop a procedure that allows islet allografts without a need for continuous use of immunosuppressant.

SUMMARY

A sufficient number of high quality islets from the adult pancreas can normalize blood glucose within a short period after transplantation. However, the function of adult islet allografts in type 1 diabetic recipients gradually declines. Although many factors may be involved, this limitation may be attributable to exhaustion of β cells and the limited ability of adult islets to regenerate new islets. Unlike adult islets, immature fetal β cells cannot reverse hyperglycemia soon after transplantation and need time to mature and to respond to high glucose levels with insulin release. However, the distinct advantage of fetal islets is their capacity for continuous growth, proliferation, and maturation after transplantation. Because of these unique characteristics, donor tissue consisting of both adult and fetal islets would compensate the shortcomings of each and would fulfill the fundamental requirements for clinical transplantation.

REFERENCES

1. Report from the Center for Disease Control, 1990, M.M.W.R. 39;809
2. Sutherland, D.E., 1991, Clinical Review 25; Current status of pancreas transplantation, J. Clin. Endocrinol. Metab. 73;461-3
3. Brown, J., Molnar, I.G., Clark, W.R., Mullen, Y., 1974, Control of experimental diabetes in rats by transplantation of fetal pancreas, Science 184;1377-9
4. Santiago, J.V., 1993, Lessons from the Diabetes Control and Complications Trial. Diabetes 42;1549-54
5. Scharp, D.W., Lacy, P.E., McLear, M., Longwith, J., Olack, B., 1992, The bioburden of 590 consecutive human pancreases for islets- transplant results. Transplant. Proc. 24;974-5
6. Hering, B.J., Geier, C., Schultz, A.O., Bretzel, R.G., Federlin, K., 1993, Islet Transplant Registry Report
7. Brunicardi, F.C., Mullen, Y., 1993, Conference Report- Critical issues in clinical islet transplantation. Pancreas 9;281-90
8. Hering, B.J., Geier, C., Schultz, A.O., Bretzel, R.G., Federlin, K., 1994, Islet Transplant Registry Report
9. Mullen Y, Une S., unpublished observations
10. Sutherland, D.E., Gores, P.F., Farney, A.C., Wahoff, D.C.,Matas, A.J., Dunn, D.L., Gruessner, R.W., Najarian, J.S., 1993, Evaluation of kidney, pancreas, and islet transplantation for patients with diabetes at the University of Minnesota, Am. J. Surg. 166;456-91
11. Brockenbrough, J.S., Weir, G.C., Bonner-Weir, S., 1988, Descordance of exocrine and endocrine growth after 90% pancreatectomy in rats. Diabetes 37;232-6
12. Taura, Y., Matsuo, S., Mullen, Y., unpublished results
13. Terada, M., Salzler, M., Lennartz, K., Mullen, Y., 1988, The effect of H-2 compatibility on pancreatic beta cell survival in the nonobese diabetic mouse. Transplantation 45;622-627
14. Mullen, Y., Watt, P.C., unpublished data
15. Peterson, C.(ed.), 1988 Fetal Pancreas Transplantation, Springer Verlag, NY
16. Brown, J., Clark, W.R., Molnar, I.G., Mullen, Y., 1976, Fetal pancreas transplantation for reversal of streptozotocin-induced diabetes in rats, Diabetes 25;56-64
17. Tsunoda, T., Furui, H., Klandorf, H., Soon-Shiong, P., Mullen, Y., 1989, Functional maturation of porcine fetal pancreatic explants, Transplant. Proc. 21;1190-2

18. Shiogama, T., Mullen, Y., Hansen, K., Tsunoda, T., Stein, E., 1989, Cryopreservation of human fetal pancreatic tissues- Growth and functional maturation of tissues grafted into athymic mice, Horm. Metab. Res. 25;239-41
19. Mullen, Y., Clark, W.R., Molnar, I.G., Brown, J., 1977, Complete reversal of experimental diabetes mellitus in rats by a single fetal pancreas, Science 195;68-70
20. Brown, J., Heininger, D., Kuret, J., Mullen, Y., 1982, Normal response to pregnancy in rats cured of streptozotocin diabetes by transplantation of one fetal pancreas, Diabetologia 22;273-5
21. Mandel, T.E., 1984, Transplantation of organ-cultured fetal pancreas: Experimental studies and potential clinical application in diabetes mellitus. World J. Surg. 8:158-168
22. Tuch, B.E., Monk, R.S., Beretov, J., 1991, Reversal of diabetes in athymic rats by transplantation of human fetal pancreas, Transplantation 52;172-5
23. Tuch, B.E., 1991, Reversal of diabetes by human fetal pancreas. Optimization of requirements in the hyperglycemic nude mouse, Transplantation 51;557-62
24. Clark, W.R., Rutter, W.J., 1972, Synthesis and accumulation of insulin in the fetal rat pancreas. Dev. Biol. 29;468-81
25. Brown, J., Clark, W.R., Makoff, R.K., Weisman, H., Kemp, J.A., Mullen, Y., 1978, Pancreas transplantation for diabetes mellitus, Ann. Inter. Med. 89;951-965
26. Sasaki, N., Yoneda, K., Bigger, C., Brown, J., Mullen, Y., 1984, Fetal pancreas transplantation in miniature swine. 1. Developmental characteristics of fetal pig pancreases. Transplantation 38;335-346
27. Mullen, Y., Brown, J., unpublished results.
28. Mullen, Y., Taura, Y., Ozawa, A., Miyazawa, T., Shiogama, T., Matsuo, S., Nagata, M., Takasugi, M., Klandorf, H., Tsunoda, T., Terada, M., Motojima, K., Clare-Salzler, M., 1989, Reversal of experimental diabetes in miniature swine by fetal pancreas allografts, Transplant. Proc. 21;1196-8
29. Korsgren, O., Jansson, L., Eizirik, D., Andersson, A., 1991, Functional and morphological differentiation of fetal porcine islet-like cell clusters after transplantation into nude mice, Diabetologia 34;379-86
30. Nielsen, J.H., Moldrup, A., Billestrup, N., Petersen, E.D., Allevato, G., Stahl, M., 1992, The role of growth hormone and prolactin in β cell growth and regeneration. pp9-17, in Pancreatic Islet Cell Regeneration and Growth, Vinik, A.I. (ed), Plenum Press, N.Y.
31. Hill, D.J., Hogg, J., 1992, Expression of insulin-like growth factors and their binding proteins during pancreatic development in rat, and modulation of IGF actions on rat islet DNA. pp113-122, in Pancreatic Islet Cell Regeneration and Growth, Vinik, A.I. (ed), Plenum Press, N.Y.
32. Hill, D.J., Clemnons, D.R., Wilson, S., Han, V.K.M., Strain, A.J., Milner, R.D.G., 1989, Immunological distribution of one form of IGF binding protein and IGF peptides in human fetal tissue, J. Mol. Endocrinol. 2;31-38
33. Hill, D.J., Frazer, A., Swenne, I., Wirdnam, K., Milner, R.D.G., 1987, Somatostomedin-C in the human fetal pancreas: Cellular localization and release during organ culture. Diabetes 36;465-71
34. Han, V.K.M., Lund, P.K., Lee, D.C., D'Ercole, A.J., 1988, Expression of somatomedin/IGF in the human fetus: Identification, characterization and tissue distribution. J. Clin. Endocrinol. Metab. 66;422
35. Otonkoski, T., Tnip, M., Wong, I., Simell, O., 1988, Effect of growth hormone and IGF on endocrine function of human fetal islet-like cell clusters during long-term culture. Diabetes 37;1678-83
36. Hullett, D.A., Smith, L., Sollinger, H.W., 1994, Enhancement of proislet functional viability with growth factor. Transplant. Proc.26;709-10
37. Kenmochi, T., Miyamoto, M., Nakagawa, Y., Une, S., Benhamou, P.Y., Mullen, Y., 1994, Successful intrathymic allografts of porcine pancreatic islets without continuous immunosuppression. Transplant. Proc. 27; (in press)
38. Nomura Y, Yamaguchi T, Watanabe Y, Mullen Y., unpublished results.

7

STUDIES ON PRETREATMENT OF HUMAN FETAL ISLET IN VITRO AND CLINICAL ISLET TRANSPLANTATION IN CHINA

Yuan-Feng Hu, Jing-Juan Xu, Wei-Ping Dong, Yu-Fei Wang, Hong-De Zhang, Sheng-Rong Zhong and Yu Li

Diabetes Research Laboratory
Shanghai First People's Hospital, Shanghai Medical University
190 North Suzhou Road, Shanghai 200085
The People's Republic of China

We have been undertaking the studies on experimental islet transplantation since 1978 and clinical islet transplantation with short-term cultured human fetal islet tissue in patients with insulin-dependent (type I) diabetes mellitus since 1981 (1-4). On entrustment of the Ministry of Health, we have sponsored several special courses from 1984 to 1986 to popularize islet transplantation in China. The National Cooperating Group for study of Islet Transplantation was established in 1985. There has been great progress in clinical islet transplantation in China in recent years (5-7). According to the data of the Islet Transplant Registry of the National cooperating Group, as of the end of 1991, there were 939 patients with type I diabetes altogether having received islet grafts in 59 hospitals all over China, 835 of them with integral data. This article will present the influences of pretreatment in vitro on the immunogenecity of human fetal islet and an analysis of the clinical data of 835 diabetics with islet grafts.

MATERIALS AND METHODS

Human Fetal Pancreases

The pancreases of human fetuses with gestational age of 18-24 wk were obtained just after delivery using water-bag induction. The tissue culture procedures were completed within 2 hours after the delivery.

Isolation and Purification of Fetal Islets

The enzymatic isolation of fetal islets, described previously (8), was briefly reviewed as follows: the minced pancreatic fragments in Hanks solution containing 0.5 mg/ml collagenase (type V, Sigma) PH 7.8, were incubated in 38°C water bath for 8 min, the enzymatic digestion was stopped with ice-cold Hanks solution containing 10% neonatal calf serum (NCS), after centrifugating, the digests were purified by discontinuous density gradient of Ficoll, the islets were washed 3 times in Hanks solution, then incubated with medium RPMI 1640 containing 20% NCS as planned for mixed lymphocyte islet cultures.

Pretreatment Methods

1. 37°C Culture: The fetal pancreas was minced into fragments of about 1 mm^3 in size, and then placed in medium RPMI 1640 supplemented with 20% NCS, 100 u/ml penicillin and 100 ug/ml streptomycin, PH 7.2, incubated in cell incubator (Napco, U.S.A.), at 37°C, 95% air / 5% CO_2, for 1 wk.
2. 24°C Culture: The pancreatic fragments were suspended in 1640 medium and incubated in Cell Incubator, at 24°C, 95% air / 5% CO_2, for 1 wk.
3. Cryopreservation: The pancreatic fragments were placed in 1640 medium and incubated at 37°C for 2 days, and then collected in 2 ml ampules, medium 1640 containing 10% DMSO (Baker Chemical Co.) was added, equilibrating at 4°C for 30 min, then cooled at a rate of 0.3°C/min to -80°C with programmed freezer, and put into liquid nitrogen for 2 days. After rewarming, the islet tissues were diluted with cold Hanks solution step by step, and collected after centrifugating and incubated in 1640 medium at 37°C for 2 days.

Assessment of Islet Immunogenecity

1. Mixed Lymphocyte Islet Cultures (MLICs): The human fetal islet as stimulator (100 islets/well) and normal adult lymphocyte as responder ($1x10^5$ cells/well) were cultured in triplicate in 96 well culture plate with medium 1640 for 5 days, ^{3}H-thymidine (Shanghai Atomic Nucleus Institute) was added to the cells and incubated for further 18h, the cells were collected on glass filter paper and cpm counts were performed by Beckman LS-3800 Liquid Scintillator. Stimulation index was calculated according to the following formula:

SI = cpm(responders+stimulators) / cpm(responders)

2. HLA-DR Positive Cell Assay: Fetal islet tissues were embedded in O.C.T., cryostat sections were prepared, then fixed with acetone, Anti-Human HLA-DR monoclonal antibody (DAKO-HLA-DR, Dakopatts) was added and stained with immunohistochemical technique using ABC Kit (Vector Laboratories). HLA-DR Positive nucleated cells in 10 high power fields of each sample were counted and expressed as mean value. The HLA-DR Positive cells of adult cadaver pancreas was assayed similarly.

3. Lymphoid Cell Assay: Cryostat sections of fetal islet tissue were prepared as above, anti-human Leucocyte common Antigen monoclonal antibody (DAKO LCA, Dakopatts) was added, and stained with ABC kit. LCA positive cells in 10 HP fields of each sample were counted and expressed as mean value.

Subjects

As of the end of 1991, 939 patients with type I diabetes received islet transplants in 59 hospitals all over China. The source and preparation of all islet grafts were identical with those of ours (3,5), 835 of them with integral data were analyzed in this study.

Amongst 835 patients with type I diabetes, 458 were male and 377 were female, with mean age at onset of 23.23±11.14yr (1-63yr) and mean duration of diabetes of 6.90±4.49yr (1-35yr).

Islet Grafts

The preparation of the islet grafts was described elsewhere (3,5) and reviewed briefly as follows: Fetal pancreases were obtained just after delivery by water bag induction. After removing the capsular and vascular tissues in cold Hanks solution, the pancreas was minced into fragments of about 1 mm3 in size and then placed in 1640 medium supplemented with 10% HEPES, 20% fetal calf serum and 50 ug/ml gentamycin, and incubated in cell incubator at 37°C, 95% air / 5% CO_2 for 1-2 wk. The medium was changed every other day.

Transplanting Approaches

Of these 835 recipients, 471 (56.41%) were transplanted intraperitoneally, 310 (37.13%) intramuscularly, 25 (2.99%) intrahepatically, 12 (1.44%) intracerebrally, 10 (1.20%) under pancreatic capsule, 4 (0.48%) in bone marrow, and 3 (0.36%) in the periphery of kidney.

Immunosuppressive Agents

After transplantation, 30 recipients (3.59%) took 1-3 doses of anti-human thymocyte globulin (AHTG), 75 (8.98%) took short course of glucocorticoid, 14 (1.68%) azathioprine, 3 (0.36%) cyclophosphamide, 3 (0.36%) cyclosporin A, 268 (32.10%) Chinese traditional medicines, and 442 (52.93%) had not taken any immunosuppressive agents.

Follow-Up

After transplantation, 835 recipients were followed up for 15.98±14.92 mo (1.5-92 mo), 351 (42.04%) for more than 1 yr, 94 (11.26%) >2 yr, and 91 (10.90%) >3 yr.

Criteria of Transplanting Effect

Effective: Insulin requirement reduced by more than 25% compared to that pretransplant, diabetes controlled well, and fasting serum C-peptide level enhanced significantly.

Ineffective: Insulin requirement reduced by less than 25% compared to that pretransplant, diabetes control improved or not, and fasting serum C-peptide level did not have any significant increment.

Statistical Analysis

All data were expressed as mean±SD, and statistical significance was analyzed by student's t test for paired data.

RESULTS

Influences of Pretreatments on Islet Immunogenecity

1. Mixed Lymphocyte Islet Culture (MLICs): The results of MLICs demonstrated that the stimulation index of fetal islet tissue following different pretreatments were reduced significantly compared to those of the unpretreated, $p<0.05-0.01$,

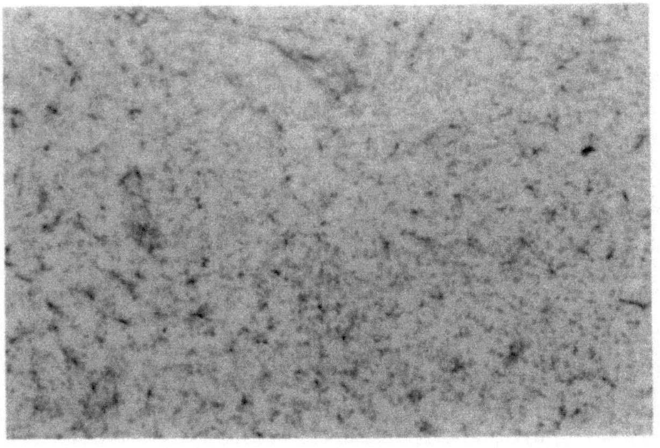

Figure 1. DR positive cells in adult pancreatic tissue; original magnification 100X, reduced 66%.

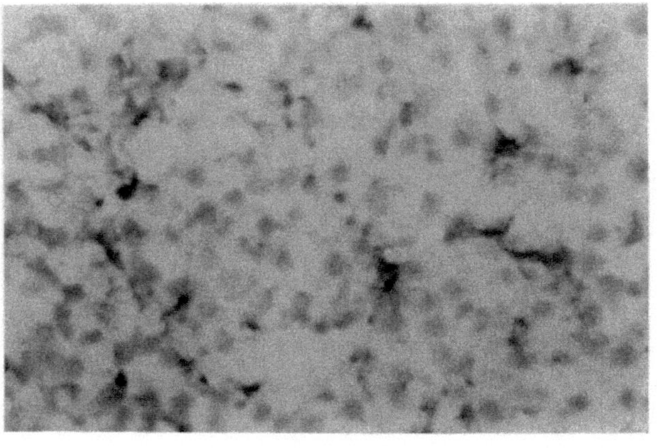

Figure 2. DR positive cells in adult pancreatic tissue; original magnification 400X, reduced 66%.

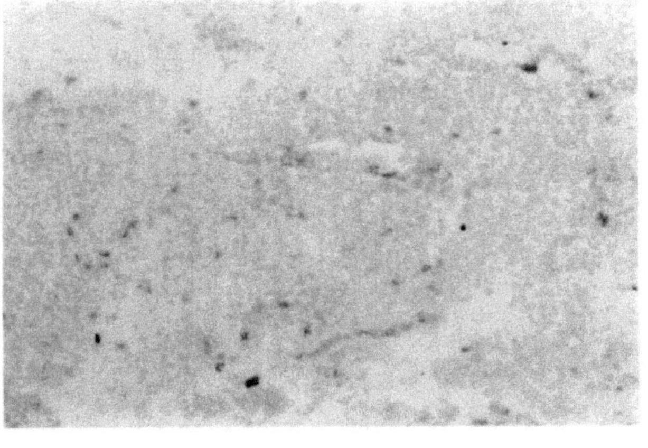

Figure 3. DR positive cells in fetal pancreatic tissue; original magnification 100X, reduced 66%.

Table 1. The SI of islet tissue cultured at 37°C was significantly increased compared to that of cultured at 24°C, $p<0.01$.

2. HLA-DR Positive Cell Assay: The HLA-DR positive cell count of fetal islet tissue following different pretreatments was significantly less than those of the unpretreated, $p<0.001$, Table 1, Figs. 5-7.

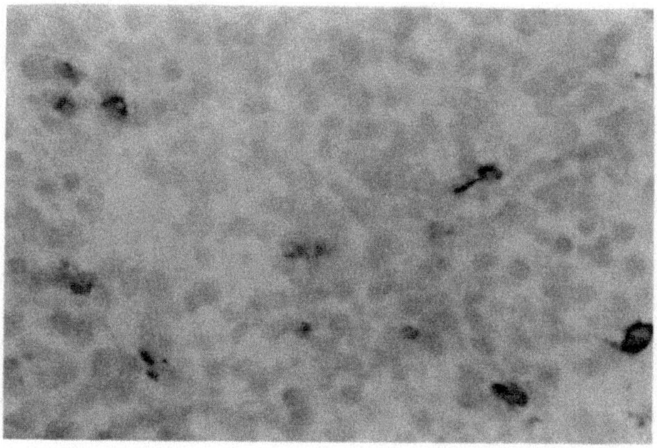

Figure 4. DR positive cells in fetal pancreatic tissue; original magnification 400X, reduced 66%.

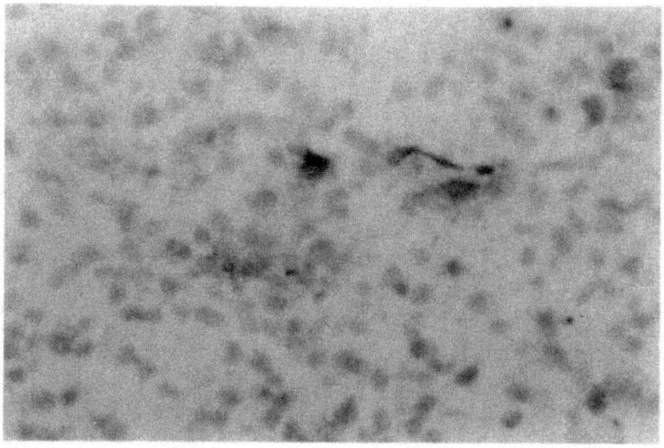

Figure 5. DR positive cells in fetal islet tissue pretreated with 37°C culture; original magnification 400X, reduced 66%.

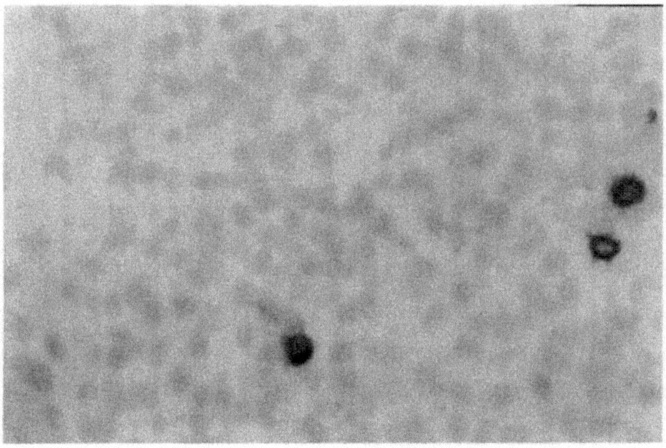

Figure 6. DR positive cells in fetal islet tissue pretreated with 24°C culture; original magnification 400X, reduced 66%.

The HLA-DR positive cell count of the adult cadaver pancreatic tissue (n=6) was markedly increased compared to that of fetal pancreas (n=5), 35.50±4.36 vs 16.36±2.95, p<0.001, Figs. 1-4.

3. Lymphoid Cell Assay: The LCA Positive cell (mainly lymphoid cell) count of the fetal islet tissue following different pretreatments was significantly less than those of the unpretreated, p<0.001, Table 1.

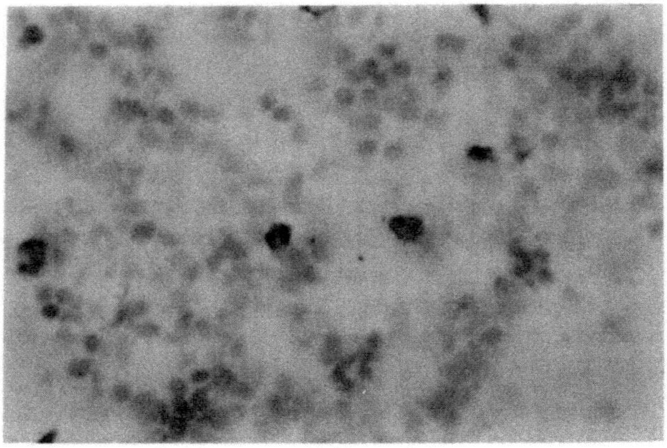

Figure 7. DR positive cells in fetal islet tissue pretreated with cryopreservation; original magnification 400X, reduced 66%.

Table 1. Influences of Pretreatments on Islet Immunogenecity

Pretreatment	Stimulation Index	DR+ Cell Count	Lymphoid Cell Count
Control (unpretreated)	22.24±11.05 (n=6)	16.36±2.95 (n=5)	13.44±1.50 (n=5)
37°C Culture	3.25±1.15* (n=6)	4.04±0.48*** (n=5)	4.48±1.37*** (n=5)
24°C Culture	1.57±0.46** (n=6)	2.24±0.20*** (n=5)	3.30±1.12*** (n=5)
Cryopreservation	2.03±0.68** (n=6)	2.58±0.40*** (n=5)	3.54±1.0*** (n=5)

* $P< 0.05$ ** $P< 0.01$ *** $P< 0.001$

Transplanting Effect

After islet transplantation in 835 patients with type I diabetes, 723 (86.59%) were proved to be effective and 112 (13.41%) ineffective. The islet grafts of the effective cases began to take effect at 1-113 days (15.78±12.84 days) following the transplantation. Thereafter, hypoglycemia of a variable degree would occur repeatedly, and insulin dosage should be reduced accordingly. The mean insulin requirements, fasting and postprandial plasma glucose concentrations of the effective cases decreased significantly compared to those pretransplant, $p<0.001$, and fasting serum C-peptide levels enhanced markedly in comparison with those pretransplant, $p<0.001$, Table 2. 59 (7.07%) diabetic patients became

Table 2. Transplanting Effect of 723 Effective Recipients

	Insulin Requir. (u/d)	Plasma Glucose (mmol/L) fasting	Plasma Glucose (mmol/L) postprand.	Fasting C-peptide (pmol/L)
Pretransplant	51.38±17.76 (719)	13.87±5.61 (719)	18.26±7.72 (586)	62.8±95.4 (408)
Posttransplant	24.20±13.13 (689)	9.16±3.38 (682)	11.82±4.31 (472)	176.5±162.5 (371)
P	< 0.001	< 0.001	< 0.001	< 0.001

Table 3. Transplanting Effect of 59 Diabetics Having Become Insulin Independent

	Pretransplant	Posttransplant	P
Insulin Requir. (u/d)	47.03±17.78 (59)	0	
Plasma Glucose			
Fasting (mmol/L)	13.74±4.87 (59)	8.32±2.71 (59)	< 0.001
Postprand.(mmol/L)	19.68±6.35 (39)	10.58±2.67 (34)	< 0.001
Serum C-peptide			
Fasting (pmol/L)	112±148 (27)	309±212 (31)	< 0.001
Postprand.(pmol/L)	261±163 (8)	532±188 (12)	< 0.01

insulin independent and remained for 1.5-86 mo (13.56±17.55 mo), their fasting and postprandial serum C-peptide levels increased significantly compared to those pretransplant, p<0.01-0.001, and the fasting and postprandial plasma glucose concentrations reduced significantly in comparison with those pretransplant, p<0.001, Table 3.

Immunosuppressive Agents and Transplanting Effect

There were no significant differences in the transplanting effect between the recipients taking different immunosuppressive agents and those without any immunosuppressive agents, Table 4.

Implanting Site and Transplanting Effect

Besides the much lower effect of islet transplants in bone marrow, there were no significant differences in the transplanting effect between the different sites of implantation, Table 5.

COMPLICATIONS AND ADVERSE REACTIONS

Besides incision infection in 5 cases after islet transplantation, there were no other complications or any serious adverse reactions.

Table 4. Immunosuppressive Agents and Transplanting Effect

		Effective	
Agents	Cases	Cases	%
AHTG	30	30	100
Glucocorticoid	75	67	89.33
Azathioprine	14	13	92.86
CSA	3	1	33.33
Cyclophosphamide	3	3	100
Traditional Chinese Medicine	268	228	85.07
None	442	381	86.2

Table 5. Implanting Site and Transplanting Effect

		Effective	
Sites	Cases	Cases	%
Lesser Omental Cavity	471	409	86.84
Muscle	310	264	85.16
Liver	25	25	100
Brain	12	11	91.67
Under Pancreatic Capsule	10	9	90
Bone Marrow	4	2	50
Renal Periphery	3	3	100

DISCUSSION

MHC-II antigen is considered to play an important role in islet allograft rejection, and class II antigen is considered to be present on the dendritic cells including lymphocytes, macrophages and capillary endothelial cells, whereas islet cells are likely devoid of class II antigen (9,10). There are studies showing that pretreatment of islet grafts in vitro with conventional tissue culture, 24°C culture, or cryopreservation might reduce those antigen bearing cells and the islet immunogenecity, and prolong the survival of islet allo- or xenografts (9-15). Our recent study on the influences of pretreatment in vitro on the immunogenecity of human fetal islet demonstrated that the stimulation index of islet tissue pretreated in MLICs was significantly reduced compared to that of unpretreated, $p<0.05$-0.01, the HLA-DR positive cells and lymphoid cells of islet tissue pretreated were decreased markedly in comparison with those of unpretreated, $p<0.001$, indicating that the pretreatment, in particular, with 24°C culture or cryopreservation may lessen significantly the immunogenecity of human fetal islet, and may thereby improved the acceptance and survival of those islet grafts.

835 patients with type I diabetes were transplanted with short-term cultured human fetal islet tissue, 723 (86.59%) were proved to be effective, 59 of them became insulin independent and remained for 1.5-86 mo. This series of type I diabetic subjects with islet transplants seems to be currently the largest series of clinical islet transplantation with better results in the world.

The source and preparation of islet grafts are the key factors for a successful islet transplantation. Human fetal pancreas could be used without islet separation for transplantation owing to the abundance of islet tissues and poor differentiation of acinar tissues. The fetal islet tissue maintains its normal capacity of growth and proliferation after transplantation and furthermore, the immunogenecity of fetal islets seems to be much less than that of adult islets. Therefore, human fetal pancreas seems to be the ideal donor tissue for islet transplantation. The water-bag induction used in present study to terminate the mid-term pregnancy through its physical and mechanical stimulation to initiate and promote contraction of the pregnant uterus and induce the delivery would not exert any harmful influences on the fetal tissue and so, the water-bag induction is much more beneficial to keeping good quality of fetal pancreas than any kind of drug induction. The results of our previous study[3] indicated that short-term culture of human fetal pancreas seems to be the ideal preparation method of donor islet tissue. The tissue culture not only promotes the proliferation and development of fetal pancreatic islet and the rapid degeneration of the acinar tissue, but also decreases the immunogenecity of fetal islets and benefits the accumulation and preservation of donor tissues, the assay of viability and sterility.

The implanting site may have certain effects on the islet transplantation. However, there were no significant differences in the transplanting effect between the implantation of islet grafts in different sites in the present study. We suggest that the lesser omental cavity seems to be the ideal site for islet transplantation, because the abundant blood supply of the omentum is beneficial to the growth of the islet grafts, while insulin release into the portal system is in accord with the physiological pathway of insulin secretion, and the omental cavity is wide enough for implantation of the grafts. In addition, the surgical procedure is very simple and safe.

Immune rejection of islet transplant is a crucial factor resulting in failure of islet transplantation. The immunogenecity of fetal islets was reported to be much less than that of the adult and might be further reduced through tissue culture (11,12,14,16). The data of our recent study showed that the HLA-DR positive cells of human fetal islet tissue were significantly less than those of the adult pancreas, 16.36 ± 2.95 vs 35.5 ± 4.36, $p<0.001$, and the immunogenecity and MHC-II antigen presenting cells of fetal islet following 1 wk culture at 37°C were decreased significantly compared to those of the unpretreated, $p<0.05$-0.001. The islet grafts in 442 diabetic recipients without any immunosuppressive agents of this series could survive for a long period of time, indicating that the immunogenecity of pretreated fetal islet grafts was so markedly decreased that the immunosuppressive agents was likely not needed for its survival. However, the fetal islets still had residual class II antigen bearing cells following the pretreatment with either 24°C culture or cryopreservation and furthermore, the islet graft might still be destroyed by the autoimmune mechanism of the recipient. We suggest that a short course of AHTG therapy may be needed for the long term survival of human fetal islet grafts, but the chronic immunosuppression seems to be unnecessary.

REFERENCES

1. Hu Y.F., Zhang H., Zhang H.D., et al: Experimental studies on islet allotransplantation in 114 alloxan-induced diabetic rats. Chinese J Organ Transplant 1981; 2:77-81
2. Hu Y.F., Zhang H., Zhang H.D., et al: Clinical studies on islet transplantation in 20 patients with insulin-dependent diabetes mellitus. Chinese J Intern Med 1983; 22:288-292
3. Hu Y.F., Zhang H., Zhang H.D., et al: Culture of human pancreas and islet transplantation in 24 patients with type I diabetes mellitus. Chinese Med J (Engl. Ed.) 1985; 98:236-243
4. Hu Y.F., Zhang H., Zhang H.D., et al: Islet transplantation in 39 patients with insulin-dependent diabetes mellitus. in Advanced Model for the Therapy of Insulin-dependent Diabetes. Ed. Brunetti P. and Waldhausl W.K. Raven Press, New York 1987, pp.309-313
5. Hu Y.F., Cheng R.L., Shao A.H., et al: The Influence of islet transplantation on metabolic abnormalities and diabetic complications. Horm Metabol Res 1989; 21:198-202
6. Hu Y.F., Gu Z.F., Zhang H.D. and Ye R.S.: Fetal islet cell transplantation in China. Transplant Proc 1989; 21:2605-2607
7. Hu Y.F., Gu Z.F., Zhang H.D. and Ye R.S.: Fetal islet transplantation in 755 patients with insulin-dependent diabetes mellitus in China. Diab Nutr.& Metabol 1992; 5(Suppl 1):199-202
8. Hu Y.F., Wang Y.F., Ding Y.M., et al: Monolayer culture of human fetal pancreatic islet cells. Chinese J Organ Transplant 1990, 11:158-160
9. Faustman D, Lacy P.E. and Davie J.M.: Transplantation without immunosuppression. Diabetes 1982; 31(Suppl 4):11-14
10. Alejandro R., Shienold F.L., Hajek S.V., et al: Immunocytochemical localization of HLA-DR in human islet of langerhans. Diabetes 1982; 31(Suppl 4):17-22
11. Mandel T.E., Hoffman L., Collier S., Carter W.M. and Koulmanda M.: Organ culture of fetal mouse and fetal human pancreatic islet for allografting. Diabetes 1982; 31(Suppl 4):39-47

12. Rabinovitch A., Alejandro R., Noel J.,Brunschwig J.P. and Ryan U.S.: Tissue culture reduces Ia-antigen-bearing cells in rat islets and prolongs islet allografts survival. Diabetes 1982; 31(Suppl 4):48-54
13. Markmann J.K., Tomasxewski J., Posselt A.M., et al: The effect of islet culture in vitro at 24 degree C on graft survival and MHC antigen expression. Transplantation 1990; 49:272-277
14. Lacy P.E., Davie J.M., Finke E.H.: Prolongation of islet allografts survival following in vitro culture (24°C) single injection of ALS. science 1979; 204:312-313
15. Mark S.C., Garth L.W., Norman M.K.: The effect of cryopreservation on the survival and MHC antigen expression on murine islet grafts. Transplantation 1993; 55:159-163
16. Eloy R., Doillon C., Inbois P.: Fetal pancreatic transplantation: Review of experimental data. Transplant Proc 1980; 12(Suppl 2):179-185

8

THE USE OF HUMAN FETAL ISLET TISSUE FOR ADJUNCTIVE TREATMENT IN INSULIN-DEPENDENT DIABETIC PATIENTS: THE CASE FOR "PARTIAL SUCCESS"

Lois Jovanovic-Peterson,* Bent Formby, Alison Okada Wollitzer, and Charles M. Peterson

Sansum Medical Research Foundation
2219 Bath Street
Santa Barbara, California 93105

In 1922, Mrs. Thompson pleaded with doctors in Toronto to save her dying child. Banting and Best (1) had recently shown that a pancreatic extract could lower blood glucose in diabetic dogs, but never before had the hypoglycemic hormone, insulin, been given to a human being. Leonard Thompson thus became the first person to receive insulin. He not only recovered but grew into his third decade, eventually dying from pneumonia.

The commercial availability of insulin instantly converted diabetes from an acute disease to a chronic disease with manifestations including retinopathy, neuropathy, cardiovascular disease, cerebrovascular disease, peripheral vascular disease, nephropathy, myopathy, and impotence. Since that time, there has been a great debate over the etiology of diabetic complications. Although animal studies clearly showed glucose as the villain in the development of complications of diabetes, many clinicians believed that human diabetic complications were a result of the diabetic state *per se*, while others argued it was directly related to the level of hyperglycemia.

The recently published results of the Diabetes Control and Complications Trial (DCCT, 2) clearly showed that long-term normoglycemia reduces diabetic complications. The DCCT report documented a significant amelioration of eye, kidney, and neurological sequelae of diabetes in both the primary and secondary intervention wings of the study (2). Retinopathy risk decreased by 76% in those patients with no evidence of retinopathy at the start of the trial. For those patients who had minimal evidence of retinopathy there was a 54% improvement in progression of eye disease. Nephropathy improved such that patients in the intensive care group had a 54% decrease in the onset of proteinuria over the ten years of the study. Neuropathy onset was 60% less in the intensive care group. These improvements occurred with a modest improvement in mean blood glucose concentrations as evidenced by

*(805) 682-7638; FAX (805) 682-3332.

Fetal Islet Transplantation
Edited by C. M. Peterson, L. Jovanovic-Peterson, and B. Formby, Plenum Press, New York, 1995

hemoglobin A_{1c} values of approximately 9% in the standard therapy group and 7% in the intensive therapy group.

The improvements in the intensive care group, however, came with a three-fold increase in risk of severe hypoglycemia, a 1.6-fold increase in a significant weight gain and an increased risk (180 events in the insulin pump group) of severe infections. Thus the results of the DCCT emphasize the difficulty of maintaining normoglycemia with subcutaneously injected insulin. The precise integration of injection times and dosages with meal plans, exercise needs, metabolic needs and stress related changes is nearly impossible.

Patients with residual endogenously secreted insulin as manifested by C-peptide levels have better blood glucose control with less hyper- and hypoglycemia (3). These clinical observations provide an impetus for benign strategies designed to improve blood glucose control through transplantation of insulin secreting tissue even though these efforts may fall short of a "cure" in terms of insulin independence. The amelioration of "brittle diabetes" in which the blood glucose levels swing rapidly from severe hypo- to hyperglycemia, frequently and without apparent reason, into "easy diabetes" in which the blood glucose levels can be stabilized with a minimum of attention and effort on the part of the patient and the health care team, is a valid objective until a "cure" is found. Thus studies of human fetal pancreatic tissue as a potential source of insulin secretory tissue which may convert "brittle diabetes" to "easy diabetes" have become increasingly important.

History

The idea of using fetal pancreata as a source of insulin secreting tissue is not new. A number of investigators including Banting have favored the use of fetal tissue at one time or another because of the relative lack of development of exocrine tissue in the fetal environment and hence a relative enrichment of endocrine cells with lessened possibility of enzymatic digestion of insulin or insulin containing cells (1). In 1928, the human fetal pancreas was first used for transplantation purposes (4). In that year Fichera placed pancreatic tissue from three fetuses into various sites in an 18 year old male with diabetes mellitus. The experiment failed in that the recipient died in diabetic coma three days later.

Despite these inauspicious beginnings, a resurgence in interest in the procedure of fetal islet or whole pancreas transplantation began in about 1977 (5). The impetus for this renewed consideration of an abandoned procedure lay in the high morbidity and mortality associated with vascularized transplants performed in man, and the experiments of Brown and coworkers that documented that implantation of fetal rat pancreas could reverse experimental diabetes in adult animals (6-8). To date, perhaps as many as 4000 transplants of fetal pancreatic tissue into man have taken place, mostly in the People's Republic of China and the former Soviet Union (9,10).

Studies of Isolation, Storage, Shipment, and Function In Vitro

Dr. Brown's group was also the first to demonstrate that the histologically complex rodent fetal pancreas could be cryopreserved, stored indefinitely and used to successfully reverse diabetes after transplantation and that such an approach might be feasible in humans (11,12). Since that time, a great deal of effort in a number of laboratories has been devoted to the study of the optimum source and handling of potentially transplantable human fetal tissue (4, 5, 13-18). Such studies are particularly important since the ß-cell content of a single human fetal pancreas is not sufficient to immediately normalize the hyperglycemia of an adult diabetic recipient. Therefore, successful transplantation must either await significant expansion and differentiation of the implanted fetal ß-cell mass or material collected from more than one fetus needs to be implanted at a single procedure into a milieu that fosters growth and secretory maturation of the tissue.

Tissue Retrieval

Theoretically, if there were a way to procure fetal tissue in which the tissue underwent the least deterioration, the tissue would be obtained from elective abortions performed without the introduction of solutions which first destroy the products of conception. When normal saline or prostaglandins are used, there may be a 24-48 hour period of decay before the uterus is emptied. The procedure of dilation and extraction does not affect the viability of the aborted pancreatic tissue since no instillation is used, and thus the yield of insulin secreting cells maximized. The optimal retrieval procedure would be to obtain the tissue within minutes of extraction and place it in culture medium. The loss of viable tissue would thus be minimized. Our methodology was substantially adopted by the National Disease Research Interchange when it became involved in fetal tissue procurement from 1984 to 1987 (14).

Culture Condition Experiments

Our first experiments were designed to optimize our yield of tissue with the maximal insulin secretion potential. Two variables of interest were culture conditions and gestational age of the tissue (13,14,20,21).

Fetal human pancreases were obtained from 49 aborted fetuses ranging in gestational age from 14 to 24 weeks. Each abortion was induced by laminaria dilatation of the cervical canal 12 to 16 hours before mechanical expulsion of the fetus. Within 10 minutes, the pancreas was removed aseptically and immediately processed for tissue culture. About one-tenth of each pancreas was used for morphologic studies to confirm that the fetal pancreas was retrieved in each case. Eight fetal pancreases were divided into two equal parts and cultured under two different conditions.

Each pancreas was divided into about one mm^3 pieces and one half of each was cultured in 50 ml Falcon flasks in F-10 (HAM) solution (Gibco Laboratories, Grand Island, NY, USA) supplemented with 10% fetal calf serum. The flasks were maintained at 37°C in a gas phase of 5% CO_2 in humidified air for a period of 23 days. The medium was changed every second day. The other half of each of the eight fetal pancreata was cultured in Dulbecco's modified Eagle's medium supplemented with 10% fetal calf serum and 1 g/L (100 mg/dl) glucose. The flasks were maintained at room temperature. In these eight pancreata we performed a glucose challenge test (200 mg/dl glucose) with an incubation time of thirty minutes.

Aliquots from each medium change were frozen and stored at -20°C for subsequent insulin radioimmunoassay using human insulin standards. All media from each organ were assayed at the same time. The insulin content measured were IU per ml culture medium. Statistical analyses were carried out using Students' t test for paired or unpaired data where applicable.

The culture medium, O_2 and temperature had a significant influence on the insulin secretion. In Dulbecco's solution with high oxygen as well as in F-10, the insulin secretions on day 2 of culture was similar. On day 4, the insulin secretion of the specimens in Dulbecco's solution was already significantly higher ($P \leq 0.0001$) and remained higher until day 21 ($P \leq 0.0001$). An additional eight fetal pancreata were incubated for 30 minutes in 200 mg/dl glucose on day 6 and 7 of culture; thereafter, on days 8-10, the glucose concentration was again 100 mg/dl. The insulin concentration in the incubation media increased significantly from day 6 to 7 (P≤0.0001). Despite the cessation of the high glucose stimulus, the insulin content in the culture medium rose significantly during the following days (P≤0.01).

Gestational Age Experiments

We investigated four age groups of fetal pancreata during a 23 day culture period to answer the question of gestational age and insulin secretion potential. The four age groups were divided as follows: Group I 14 to 16 weeks gestation (n=8), Group II 17 to 9 weeks gestation (n=9), Group III 20 to 22 weeks gestation (n=7), and Group IV 23 to 24 weeks gestation (n=9).

Insulin secretion was dependent on gestational age only during the first four days in culture. Group IV had a significantly higher insulin content on day 2 and 4 when compared to Groups I and II (P≤0.01). Fetal pancreata of the age groups I and II showed a significant increase in insulin secretion from day 4 to 8 (P≤0.0001), which was lacking in the older age groups (III and IV). During the culture period from day 9 through 23, insulin release was similar in all age groups. There were wide variations of insulin secretion in all investigated groups.

These data show that fetal human islets can secrete insulin in vitro over prolonged periods. The amounts of insulin produced depend on the gestational age only during the first days in culture. From day 6 on there were no differences in the insulin concentrations between the investigated age groups. Tissue of younger gestational age seems to be more suitable for in vitro culture as a significant increase was observed from day 4 to day 8 only in the gestational age groups of 14-16 weeks and 17-19 weeks. Whether this effect is even more pronounced in tissue with a gestational age of less than 14 weeks has yet to be established. The transplantation data from Usadel, et al. (16) supposes that fetal pancreata of less than 12 weeks gestational age are more viable in an in vivo culture compared to older tissue.

The type of culture medium had a significant influence on the insulin secretion of the tissue in vitro. In Dulbecco's solution with a high oxygen gas phase, the hormone levels were significantly higher within the first 21 days in culture. Farkas and Ferenc (17) recently showed in an 18 week culture period of 5 human fetal pancreata, an almost continuous insulin release during the first 12 weeks and less variations between the investigated pancreata. Mandel and Georgiou (18) on the other hand, reported a continuous increase of insulin secretion in 4 out of 5 fetal pancreata during a 25 day culture period. We found wide variations, but there was a consistent decrease in insulin secretion as a typical behavior of human fetal pancreata during prolonged culture under the above conditions. Increase or steady insulin release after 8 days in culture was only seen in exceptional cases. In addition, we were able to show a further rise in insulin content in the medium with higher glucose concentrations.

Other parameters that may affect the outcome of human fetal islet transplantation are the duration of cold storage (since the site of isolation of human fetal tissue and the transplantation team may be widely separated) and the gestational age of the fetal donor. In vitro studies were therefore again undertaken with human fetal pancreatic tissue to determine (a) viability of human fetal pancreatic islets after cold storage at 0° to +2°C from 18 to 144 hours and (b) the effect of gestational age on *in vitro* insulin secretory capacity (14).

Viability expressed by the insulin secretory capacity was assessed by insulin responses to 2 successive 1 hr static batch incubations. The first incubation (F1) was in low glucose (2 mM) medium (KRB pH 7.40 containing 24 mM HEPES, 2 mM glucose, and 0.3% bovine serum albumin at 37°C in an atmosphere of 95% O_2/5% CO_2) to stabilize the basal secretion while the second incubation (F2) included 25 mM glucose and 1 mM 3-isobutyl-1-methylxanthine (IBMX) as potentiator. The fractional stimulatory ratio (FSR defined as F2/F1) and trypan blue exclusion rates (15) of isolated fetal islets were used as indexes of viability. Our most important observation was that cold storage of whole pancreata up to 144 hr did not alter insulin secretory capacity (FSR-values), but the percentage of dead islets indicated by trypan blue uptake increased. Microscopic examination of dithizone stained islets showed intact and well demarcated variable sized islets. Electron microscopic examination revealed islets with well preserved endocrine cells after cold storage for 18 hr followed by culture for 48 hr. Fetal islets isolated from pancreata of 16-18 weeks gestational age were found to have a 2-fold increase in FSR-values when compared to islets isolated from pancreata of 19-24 weeks of gestational age. Taken together, these data document that human fetal pancreatic tissue is viable under conditions of storage on ice as whole tissue for periods up to 144 hr. This finding is of importance because the site of isolation and the transplantation team may be widely separated. Also of importance is our observation that if short periods of ischemia at room temperature occur, e.g., during transportation without cooling, it can cause significant damage to the functional capacity of the fetal tissue. The implication of and the reasons for the increased fractional secretion of insulin noted in the fetal islets isolated from fetuses of 16-18 weeks of gestational age, are not clear. While the conditions utilized to potentiate insulin secretion, i.e., the addition of IBMX, were not physiologic, the transient sensitivity to stimulus-secretion coupling may be of significance during ontogeny. It still remains to be determined whether islets isolated from fetuses between 16-18 weeks gestational age will have allograft advantage.

Animal Studies

We chose to perform our first transplantation studies in a model which would swiftly reject tissue, because if our processing procedures delayed rejection in this model, such an approach might be applicable to human transplantation. We concluded from the *in vitro* experiments detailed above, that the pancreata from fetuses before 19 weeks of gestation produced the highest concentration of insulin secretion.

The initial xenograft studies involved 20 Wistar rats made diabetic with an injection of streptozotocin (20). Pancreatic fetal tissue was transplanted immediately (N=10), or after a 2 day culture period (N=10), beneath the kidney capsule. A 2 day culture period before transplantation had a statistically significant prolongational effect on the lifetime of the grafted tissue. In rats receiving fresh tissue, there was a drop in mean blood glucose from 336 mg/dl prior to transplantation to 199 mg/dl on day 1. Transplantation of cultured tissue led to a significant lowering of blood glucose from a pre-transplant value of 315 mg/dl to a day 1 post-transplant value of 213 mg/dl. Mean blood glucose (350 mg/dl) in the rats receiving cultured tissue returned to a plateau value more slowly (17 days cultured as opposed to 8 days fresh). The blood glucose levels in the rats which received the cultured tissue remained significantly lower than their pre-transplant glucose values or than the mean blood glucose in the rats which received the freshly transplanted tissue. This difference was significant for up to 50 days ($P \leq 0.001$).

Based on experiments such as these, we initiated a study of islet cell transplantation into Type I insulin dependent diabetic patients (21). Our studies were based on the literature and our belief that optimally, fetal islet transplantation could be offered to diabetic patients who were not immunosuppressed and who were early in their disease process.

Human Studies: Studies in the early 1980s

Several ethical issues surrounding the retrieval process had to be addressed prior to the initiation of our studies. Our initial work was in New York City. In order to obtain tissue for our first studies in animals using human fetal tissue, the simple questions of consent from the mother and the confidentiality of the consent process needed to be answered (22). After two years of deliberation in three institutional ethics committees (Beth Israel Hospital, Cornell University Medical Center, and Rockefeller University), a consensus was agreed upon. We, as investigators, could not request permission from the mothers, for such an approach might be construed as coercion regarding the decision to have an abortion. Instead, the floor nurse presented the consent form for the abortion to the mother. The form gave three choices as to the disposal of the tissue:

1. Allow the hospital to dispose of all tissue in the usual fashion after pathological examination,
2. Return the abortus for a burial, or
3. Allow researchers to use the tissue in experiments which may lead to discoveries of better treatments for persons with chronic diseases.

The mothers were told that under Option 3 the investigators would be allowed to study the tissue but no names would be attached. The nurse who obtained the consents noted a 92% rate of approval from the first 100 women. The patients underwent the abortion under general anesthesia and thus never met the investigator who did not enter the operating suite, but stayed in a sterile receiving alcove off of the operating room.

Patient Selection and Tissue Preparation

Type I diabetic men were chosen for the initial studies to eliminate a number of ethical questions related to women with reproductive potential. In view of the toxicity of hyperglycemia for fetal islets, targets for glycemic control were a glycohemoglobin level less than 7% and mean blood glucose levels less than 140 mg/dl. No endogenous insulin secretion was documented by a C-peptide level less than 0.03 ng/ml following a Sustacal challenge test. The men were maintained normoglycemic prior to transplantation with the use of constant insulin infusion pump therapy (21). The four men chosen for this study had 7-23 years duration of diabetes and were between the ages of 24-55.

To assure the retrieval of non-infected tissue, only pancreases from women with negative tests for cytomegalovirus, syphilis, hepatitis, toxoplasmosis and rubella were used. Six to twelve fetal pancreata were prepared for each recipient. The fetal pancreata were dissected free in a sterile fashion within 15 min of the D and E procedure. The pancreata were minced into 1-2 mm^3 sections and placed into culture media consisting of 90% Dulbecco's and 10% recipient serum with added antibiotics. The tissue was cultured at 37°C with room air and 5% CO_2 for 48 hours. The media was tested serially for insulin concentration and for bacteriological contamination.

Surgical Procedure

Our criteria for choosing a site for implantation were as follows: A. The site needed to be superficial so as to minimize the trauma of the procedure. B. The site needed to have a easy access for venous sampling of pancreatic production of insulin. C. The site should have been reported previously to be adequate for the implantation of a glandular tissue.

The literature on the implantation of parathyroid tissue at the time of surgery for hyperparathyroidism advocated the use of the brachioradialis muscle of the non-dominant arm (23-25). Because parathyroid tissue and pancreatic tissue are histologically similar, we chose to implant our first two patients at that site. Although this site did allow for easy venous sampling via the brachial vein, the surface area available to place 6-12 pancreata was not sufficient. Therefore, the left lower abdominal quadrant was chosen for our next two patients.

Studies of Endocrine Function

To study both the basal and the meal related secretion of insulin, each patient underwent an endocrine assessment at weekly intervals for the first month post transplant, monthly for the next three months, and then quarterly for one year.

At 8 AM, after an overnight fast, the insulin pump was turned off. This technique allowed for a rate of rise of the blood glucose to be calculated. A truly insulin-dependent diabetic person, devoid of pancreatic secretion of insulin, will show a rise in blood glucose of 75-100 mg/dl per hour following the discontinuation of continuous subcutaneous insulin infusion (26). At 9 AM, 12 oz. of a liquid meal (Sustacal) composed of 6.1g/100 ml protein, 2.3 g/100 ml fat and 14g/100 ml carbohydrate, was given at each of the above-mentioned time points. Bloods for C-peptide and glucose were drawn at 8 AM, 9 AM, 9:30 AM, 10:00 AM, 10:30 AM, as per the protocol used for The Diabetes Control and Complications Trial (2).

All four patients had an increase in C-peptide secretion, along with a decrease in exogenous insulin requirement. No patient became insulin independent although some secretory capacity has persisted up to 5 years in one subject followed for that time period. At the peak of C-peptide secretion (1-3 weeks post implant), the total insulin requirement in these patients showed a drop between 71 and 100%. In addition, all four patients had an improvement of their glycemic levels from an initial group mean glycohemoglobin of 7.2% to a group mean of 6.0% by one month post transplant. By three months post transplant, the C-peptide response was markedly decreased, but still present and remained stable for one year and in one patient for 5 years. Over the five years of observation, this patient did have "easy diabetes" with maintenance of a HbA1c within the normal rage without significant hyper or hypoglycemia.

Studies of Immunological Function

Anticytoplasmic islet cell antibody titers were measured before the transplant and monthly thereafter. None of these patients increased their titer. Patient 4 had a weakly positive titer before transplantation which became negative during the year of follow-up (21).

Although we did not perform a complete panel of tests to assess immunological function, the clinical course of these patients implied that much of the initial function of the transplanted islets was lost over three months, yet some remained. The deterioration may have had an immunological basis, but it also may be due to necrosis of the tissue before sufficient vascularization has developed to insure adequate blood supply has developed or to lack of appropriate growth factors. Some of the functioning tissue did appear to survive. Thus either a subpopulation of cells is immunologically less antigenic, or was able to survive long enough for an adequate blood supply to develop. Further studies are needed to elucidate the mechanisms involved in the survival and loss of insulin secreting tissue.

The experiments up to 1988 documented that human fetal pancreatic fragment allografts can be performed in man and result in persistent secretion of C-peptide for up to five years without initiating an anamnestic response to anticytoplasmic islet cell antibodies. These studies also show that a simple surgical procedure of implanting the tissue under local anesthesia may suffice. Further work was needed to optimize survival of insulin secreting tissue. Nevertheless, these experiments provided hope that fetal tissue may serve as a replacement source of insulin secreting islet tissue in the person with Type I Diabetes Mellitus. From 1988 until January 23, 1993, we observed the moratorium on the use of fetal tissue for transplantation.

Studies after January 1993

Once the moratorium was lifted, re-initiating studies of fetal islet transplantation was still difficult due to limited procurement sources and funding. The results of The Diabetes Control and Complications Trial essentially mandated intensive care programs for all type I insulin dependent diabetic patients to decease the risk of complications of diabetes (2). Because of our studies prior to 1988 (13-15,20-21), we felt that human fetal islets may provide the endogenous insulin secretion needed to convert "brittle diabetes" into "easy diabetes" and thus make the task of providing intensive care programs to type I insulin dependent diabetic patients easier without the complications seen in the Diabetes Control and Complications Trial (2). We therefore took advantage of an opportunity to collaborate with Russian investigators at the Russian Institutes of Transplantology and Perinatology in Moscow, who had ongoing sources of human fetal islets and had published on the utility of this tissue as an adjunctive therapy for diabetes management (10,27). Once initial agreements were signed, the Russians released a press statement which was published in *The Los Angeles Times* and *The New York Times*. This news article elicited over 1000 written requests to be a volunteer to receive the tissue. Each potential volunteer was asked to complete a medical questionnaire and write an essay on the reasons he/she wished to receive an islet transplantation. After the eligible candidates were chosen based on their medical qualifications, twenty-four individuals were selected based on the humanistic qualities of the essay.

To begin these studies, approval had to be obtained from an Institutional Review Board for studies in human subjects constituted according to guidelines published in the Federal Register. To collaborate with Russian scientists, approval from the Centers for Disease Control and the Food and Drug Administration had to be received to bring tissue to this country from Russia as well as approval from the Russian Government. By July 31, 1994, all necessary approvals were obtained and the Russian scientists successfully transported to The Sansum Medical Research Foundation twenty-four "transplant units" to be injected into twenty-four patients.

The eligibility criteria for the twenty-four patients were: insulin dependent diabetes with less than 0.25 ng/ml C-peptide on a Sustacal Challenge test (the lower limits of the assay in most commercial laboratories); evidence of mild to moderate diabetic retinopathy (background to preproliferative retinopathy, not treated with laser); significant proteinuria (greater than 150 mg/day total protein and or greater than 50 mg/day microalbuminuria); and serum creatinine levels less than 4 mg/dl. The transplantation procedures occurred within six hours of the Russian's arrival with the tissue to minimize the time between cessation of optimal culture conditions and implantation. After the transplant procedure, which took less than 10 minutes per patient to inject the tissue, patients were monitored for two hours and then asked to remain in bed for two days.

In addition to studying the C-peptide response every week after the transplantation procedure, we had an opportunity to determine if the course of eye or kidney changes was altered by the procedure. Thus, we followed all the patients with kidney function testing and retinal fundus photography monthly over the next year.

Subsequent to the transplantation of the 24 patients with Russian tissue, we were able to transplant patients with tissue procured in The United States of America and processed in our laboratory. These patents were matched to the Russian tissue recipients for C-peptide level and eye and kidney status. The Russian approach has been to inject the tissue into the muscles of the abdomen with a syringe and needle, along with growth factors into the buttocks. Our approach was modified based on the collaboration with the Russian scientists such that we no longer needed to perform an incision but rather implanted the United States procured tissue by injecting the tissue above the abdominus rectus. In either case, the procedure was done under local anesthesia, and the recipient went home within 2 hours. From either approach, there has been only one skin rash due to an iodine allergy from the scrub solution and two suggestions of infection at the injection site, both easily treated with oral antibiotics without complications. Recipients were scheduled for follow-up visits weekly for 4 weeks, monthly for 3 visits, and every three months thereafter up to a year to monitor the results.

Evaluating "Partial Success"

Although optimally an islet transplantation procedure would eliminate the need for exogenous insulin injections to maintain normoglycemia, few would deny the need for adjunctive therapy to stabilize the chaotic swings of blood glucose levels typical of long-standing insulin-dependent diabetes mellitus. For safety reasons, many clinicians do not attempt to normalize the blood glucose in patients who have marked hypo- and hyperglycemia for fear that this attempt will potentiate the hypoglycemic episode and increase the danger to the patient. Thus, a treatment which stabilized the blood glucose levels and essentially acted as a buffer to the effects of insulin, would be a great contribution to diabetes care. Fetal islet cell transplantation, although it may not create insulin independence may provide the stabilizing factor necessary to maintain as near normal glycemia as is necessary to prevent complications without the danger of severe hypoglycemia.

A definition of "partial success" is necessary in order to evaluate the efficacy of the transplantation. As summarized in a chapter in this book, the participants of the Second International Fetal Islet Cell Transplantation Symposium established the criteria for partial success as follows:

1. A drop in insulin requirement of greater than 50% of a baseline dose expressed as units per kilogram (to account for a drop in insulin requirement merely due to weight loss) which maintains the blood glucose levels with an equivalent HbA_{1c} of equal or under 7.0%; and
2. An increase of 3 standard deviations above the baseline value based on the inter-assay coefficient of variation (CV) for the C-peptide assay in the range for the values under study is defined as an significant increase in C-peptide response. Based on an interassay CV of 16% in the low range, an increase over the course of the study of 48% would be significant. Based on an intra-assay CV of 8%, and increase of 24% above baseline in a given challenge test would constitute a significant and positive response to the test on that day.

Of the 24 patients who received tissue from Russia, 17 showed a significant rise of C-peptide above baseline (greater than 48% increase response) at some time during the 12 month observation period. Baseline C-peptide of the group was 0.106±0.089 pg/ml. The group as a whole had a rise of C-peptide at the 1 month time point to 0.179±0.160 pg/ml (P=0.058). At the 12 month time point the group mean was 0.151±0.086 (P=0.016).

At the time of writing, six patients who received tissue from from the United States have only completed the six month visit. Each has shown a significant rise above baseline by the criteria described above.

All patients had at least a 15% drop in insulin requirement. Four patients in the Russian group and 5 patients in the USA group had a 50% reduction in insulin requirement to 0.31 to 0.38 units per kilogram per day, down from an insulin requirement of 0.7-0.8 units per kilogram per day. The response of those patients who became pregnant was especially noteworthy and is described elsewhere in this volume.

Diabetic complications take five to seven years to significantly progress once there is evidence that the process has already started. Most of our transplant recipients had mild to moderate retinopathy and/or significant proteinuria (250 mg/24 hour protein). The natural history of diabetic complications suggests that a significant number would become visually impaired, require treatment or have end stage kidney disease in the next five years.

Our follow-up thus far has been too short to observe an impact of the islet cell transplant on the natural history of diabetic complications. Patients in both groups had a significant weight loss (1 to 3 kilograms) despite a significant decline in glycosylated hemoglobin (9.0% to 7.1%, $P \leq 0.01$). These findings contrast dramatically with the findings of the Diabetes Control and Complications Trial in which patients tended to gain weight concomitant with improvement in glucose control (2).

Although it is too soon to note a change in retinal or kidney status, there has been a significant decrease in blood pressure over time ($P \leq 0.01$). Our plan is to follow those patients who received the Russian procured and prepared tissue and the IDDM patients who received the United States procured tissue prepared in our laboratory over the coming years, in order to observe the effect of the islet cell transplantation on the natural history of retinopathy and nephropathy. Such follow-up will allow for the definition of potential adverse responses to the procedure, but may not suffice to delineate efficacy in view of the time required to study the cumulative incidence of these diabetic sequelae. Our hypothesis is that we shall observe the same if not a better outcome as the Diabetes Control and Complications Trial without the complications of hypoglycemia and weight gain. Only clinical trials of this nature will define the utility of fetal islet transplantation as well as provide a benchmark for studies of improved methods that are now being developed.

REFERENCES

1. Bliss, M., 1982, The Discovery of Insulin. Chicago, *The University of Chicago Press* 28-29.
2. Diabetes Control and Complications Trial Research Group, 1993, The effect of intensive treatment of diabetes on the development and progression of long term complications in insulin dependent diabetes mellitus, *New Eng. J. Med.* 329:977-986.
3. The DCCT Research Group 1987, Effects of Age, Duration and Treatment of Insulin-Dependent Diabetes Mellitus on Residual Beta Cell Function. Observations During Eligibility Testing for Diabetes Control and Complications Trial (DCCT),*J. Clin. Endocrinol Metab.* 65: 30-36.
4. Downing, R., 1984, Historical review of pancreatic islet transplantation, *World J. Surg.* 8: 137-142.
5. Sutherland DER. 1981, Pancreas and islet transplantaion II Clinical trials, *Diabetologia* 20: 435-450.
6. Brown, J., Clark, W.R., Molnar, I.G., and Mullen, Y.S., 1976, Fetal pancreas transplantation for reversal of streptozotocin-induced diabetes in rats, *Diabetes* 25:56-64.
7. Brown, J., Molnar, I.G., Clark, W., and Mullen, Y., 1974, Control of experimental diabetes mellitus in rats by transplantation of fetal pancreases, *Science* 184: 1377-1379.
8. Sutherland, DER., Goetz, F.C., and Najarian, J.S., 1981,Review of world's experience with pancreas and islet transplantation and results of intraperitoneal segmental pancreas transplantation from related and cadaver donors at Minnesota,*Transplant Proc.* 13: 291-297.
9. Hu,Y.F., 1985, Clinical studies on islet transplantation in 39 patients with insulin-dependent (type I) diabetes mellitus, Wuhan Int. Symp. Organ Transplant. 39-40.
10. Shumakov,V.I., Bljumkin, V.N., Ignatenko, S.N., 1986, The principal results of pancreatic islet cell culture transplantation in diabetes mellitus patients, Int. Congress Transplant Soc. 11: 40.
11. Kemp, J.A., Mullen, Y., Weisman,H., Nagata, and M., Matsuo, S., 1978, Reversal of diabetes in rats using fetal pancreases stored at -196C, *Transplantation* 26: 260-264.
12. Brown,J., Kemp, J.A., Hurt, S., Nagata, M., Matsuo, S., Taura, Y., and Miyazawa, K., 1980, Cryopreservation of Human Fetal Pancreas, *Diabetes* 29 Suppl. 1: 170-73.
13. Peterson, C.M., Jovanovic-Peterson, L., Formby, B., Gondos, B., Monda, L.M., Walker, L., Rashbaum, W.m., and Williams, K., 1989, Human fetal pancreas transplants, *J. Diabetes Complications* 3: 27-34.
14. Formby, B., Walker, L., and Peterson, C.M., 1987, Effects of duration of cold storage and gestational age on the insulin secretory capacity of human fetal pancreatic islets, Diabetes Rsrch. 4 13-116.

15. Formby, B., Walker, L., and Peterson, C.M., 1986, Rapid selection of viable transplantable human fetal pancreatic islets by trypan blue exclusion, Proc. of the Soc. For Exp. Bio. and Med. 182: 245-247.
16. Usadel, K.H., Schwedes, U., Bastert, G., Steinan, U., Klempa, I., Fassbinder, W., and Schoffling, K., 1980, Transplantation of human fetal pancreas: experience in thymusaplastic mice and rats and in a diabetic patient *Diabetes* 29: 74-75. 86.
17. Farkas, G., and Ferenc, J., 1984, Simple and reliable conditions for routine, long-term culturing of fetal human pancreatic tissue fragments,*Diabetes* 33: 1165-1168.
18. Mandel, T.E., and Georgiou, H.M., 1983, Insulin secretion by fetal human pancreatic islets of Langerhans in prolonged organ culture, *Diabetes* 32: 915-920.
19. Peterson, C.M., Jovanovic, L., Formby, B., Fuhrman, K., Walker,L., Brennan, M., and Rashbaum, W., 1986, Studies of human fetal pancreas. Proceedings of the Second International Conference on the Use of Human Tissues and Organs for Research and Transplant, National Diabetes Research Interchange Phila. PA. 220-222.
20. Jovanovic-Peterson, L., Williams, K., Brennan, M., Fuhrmann, K., Rashbaum, W., Walker, L., and Peterson, C.M., 1988, Studies of Transplantation of human fetal tissue in man. In Peterson, C.M., Jovanovic-Peterson, L., Formby, B., (eds) *Fetal Islet Transplantation,* Springer-Verlag New York. pp: 185-196.
21. Jovanovic-Peterson, L., Williams, K., Brennan, M., Rashbaum, W., and Peterson, C.M., 1989, Studies of human fetal pancreatic allografts in diabetic recipients without immunosuppression, *J. Diabetic Complications* 3. 1: 27-34.
22. The DCCT Research Group, 1985, "The informed consent: Is it truly informed?", *Controlled Clin. Trials.* 6:223.
23. Wells, S.A. Jr., Farndon, J.R., and Dale, D.K., 1980, Long term evaluation of patients with primary parathyroid hyperplasia managed by total parathyroidectomy and heterotopic autotransplantation, *Ann. Surg.* 192: 451-458.
24. Wells, S.A. Jr, Eltes, G.J., and Gunnells, J.C., 1976, Parathyroid autotransplantation in primary parathyroid hyperplasia, *N. Eng. J.* Med 295: 57-62.
25. Brennan, M.F., Marx, S.J., and Dappman, J.L., 1981, Results of reoperation for persistent and recurrent hyperthyroidism, *Ann. Surgery* 194: 671-676.
26. Pickup, J.C., Keen, H., Parsons, J.A., and Alberti, KGMM, 1978, Continuous subcutaneous insulin infusion: an approach to achieving normoglycemia. *Br. Med. J.*, 1:204-207.
27. Pavlovskii, M.P., and Boiko, N.I., 1990, *Imeni ii Grokova, 145:256-259.*

9

LONG-TERM STUDIES WITH CULTURED AND CRYOPRESERVED HUMAN FETAL ISLETS FOR ISLET TRANSPLANTATION IN HUNGARY

Gyula Farkas

Department of Surgery
Albert Szent-Györgyi Medical University
Szeged
P. O. Box 464, H-6701
Hungary

INTRODUCTION

The fetal pancreas has long been viewed as an attractive source of tissue for transplantation by virtue of its relative enrichment in endocrine tissue (or precursors) with respect to exocrine tissue (as compared to the adult organ), and its potentially lesser immunogenicity. However, the result of such transplantation depends on various factors: the quality, quantity and viability of the islets, and the possibility of immunomodulation. Isolated fetal islets basically have a great proliferative capacity in organ cultures, which can provide a large number of islets from one pancreas (36). Unfortunately, this quantity of islets is not sufficient for a complete cure of the diabetic condition in one recipient, but in combination with cryopreserved islet tissue (39), it may provide an opportunity for the treatment of diabetes mellitus and secondary diabetic complications. The fact that fetal islet cells can be maintained in organ cultures also leads to an opportunity for reduction of the immunogenicity of the islets of Langerhans (32, 33). In this article, we study the possibility of long-term cultivation, cryopreservation for the storage of fetal islets, the effect of these procedures in reducing immunogenicity and the role of these conditions in clinical transplantation.

MATERIALS AND METHODS

Organ cultures

A simple and reliable procedure for long-term culturing was developed earlier (11). Fetal pancreatic islets were isolated from 15 human embryos aged 16-24 weeks by means of a modified collagenase digestion technique. These isolated islets were cultured for 10

Fetal Islet Transplantation
Edited by C. M. Peterson, L. Jovanovic-Peterson, and B. Formby, Plenum Press, New York, 1995

weeks in Eagle's medium containing 20% human AB serum, L-glutamine (2 mM), and antibiotics (penicillin and streptomycin) in plastic Petri dishes (50 mm) at 37°C in an atmosphere of 5% CO_2 in air. The medium was changed three times per week and a measured aliquot from each sample was frozen for radioimmunoassay (RIA).

Cryopreservation

Tissue cultured for 7 weeks was removed and placed in 10% dimethyl sulfoxide (DMSO) in Eagle's medium containing 20% human AB serum. The tissue was equilibrated in this solution for 30 min at 4°C, and was then sealed in plastic ampoules in the same medium. The tissue was cooled to approximately -80°C at 1 degree/min. The ampoules were then plunged into liquid nitrogen and stored until further use. After 6 or 8 months, the frozen tissue was thawed in a 37°C water bath, removed from the ampoules and washed extensively in Eagle's medium until free of DMSO. These fetal islets were placed in cultures for an additional 2 weeks (12).

Glucose and Theophylline-Stimulated Release of Insulin from Fetal Islets

Fetal islet tissue (cultured or cryopreserved) was washed and resuspended in fresh medium containing either 5.5 mM or 22.0 mM glucose plus 5 mM theophylline. Samples for insulin assay were collected from the medium at the end of each 60-min challenge period.

Hormone Assay

The amount of insulin released into the medium during culturing and the glucose and theophylline-stimulation period was measured via an insulin RIA (IZINTA, Budapest, Hungary). Somatostatin release into the medium was determined by means of a somatostatin RIA (DRG Co., U.S.A.). The concentration of glucagon in the medium during culturing was measured by a glucagon RIA (NOVO, Copenhagen, Denmark).

Light and Electronmicroscopy

The islets or tissue fragments were fixed in Bouin's solution for light microscopy and embedded in paraffin embedding medium (Paraplast). The sections (5 μm) were stained with hematoxylin and eosin or immunocytochemically for insulin or glucagon or somatostatin by the peroxidase-antiperoxidase methods of Sternberg (34) with a light counterstain with hematoxylin. For electronmicroscopy, islets were fixed in an aldehyde solution of high osmolarity for 2 h. The further procedure was performed as described previously (11).

Immunostaining of Islets Following Long-Term Cultivation

Monoclonal antibody (Dianova, Hamburg, Germany) was used for the identification of class II MHC antigen-bearing cells in the islets. Immunostaining was accomplished on intact islets which were incubated with the antibody for 30 minutes, washed by centrifugation with phosphate-buffered saline in a microfuge, and incubated with fluorescein isothiocyanate (FITC)-conjugated goat anti-mouse IgG, followed by washing by centrifugation. The islets then were placed on a glass slide, covered with a coverslip and examined in a fluorescence microscope to determine the fluorescently labeled cells.

Transplant Patients and Procedures

Since 1982, 26 clinical transplantations of cultured islets have been performed. All recipients were suffering from IDDM with progressive retinopathy and 4 of them had nephropathy as well. The grafting was performed in 7 women and 19 men. The mean duration of IDDM was 20.5 years. No detectable C-peptide level was observed before transplantation. The fetal pancreatic islets were isolated from 42 embryos aged from 14 to 32 weeks by a modified technique (11). Fetal islet tissues were cultured at 37°C in 5% CO_2 for 10 weeks and 17 islet masses were also cryopreserved at -196°C for 6-10 months. After tissue typing (blood group; one, two or three HLA antigens were compatible), the transplantation was performed into the liver through the umbilical vein, with the exception of one patient, who had a simultaneous kidney and fetal islet transplantation. In this case, the cultured islet masses were grafted beneath the kidney capsule following revascularization of the kidney. Twelve patients were given only one compatible embryonic mass, while the other 14 subjects received two or three cryocultured tissue masses. Immunosuppression was carried out in all cases: temporary prednisolone and azathioprine in the first 3 patients, and cyclosporine-A in a reduced dose for 1 or 2 years in the other 22. In the case involving simultaneous kidney and islet transplantation, three immunosuppressive drugs (prednisolone, azathioprine and cyclosporine-A) were applied. Following transplantation, the plasma glucose, C-peptide, and glycosylated hemoglobin (HbA_{1C}) levels were monitored. The iv. glucose tolerance test (IVGTT) (1g/kg glucose) and iv. 1 mg glucagon were used as provocative tests of C-peptide and insulin secretion. The kidney functions were investigated by means of beta-2-microglobulin (B2M) and albumin RIA (Pharmacia, Sweden), while the alterations in the retinopathy were checked by means of color stereoopthalmography and fluorescence angiography.

Statistical Analysis

Results were expressed as means ± SD. Statistical significance was analyzed with the unpaired Student's *t* test.

RESULTS

Results of *in Vitro* Examinations

Fetal islet tissues were cultured for 10 weeks. The amount of insulin released into the medium during the 10-week culture period was measured by means of an insulin RIA. During this period, the insulin release was almost continuous (325±12 μU/ml). The somatostatin concentration was found to be slightly increased during the 10-week culturing period (from 47±5.1 to 92.5±6.5 pg/ml; $p<0.01$). In spite of the positive changes in the different hormone productions of the pancreatic islets, the glucagon production decreased continuously during the long-term culturing period (from 375±31 to 8.5±1.25 pg/ml; $p<0.001$). Figure 1 shows the changes in the release of different hormones into the medium during the long-term cultivation.

The results of the immunocytochemical examinations showed a close correlation with those of the laboratory measurements. As can be seen in Figs. 2-4, no glucagon positivity, but the strong insulin and strong somatostatin positivity of the cells were noted.

After the tenth week of culturing, the release of insulin from the fetal islets could be stimulated by glucose concentrations of 5.5 and 22.0 mM/l in the medium, the latter concentration resulting in a threefold elevation in insulin release over the lower concentration

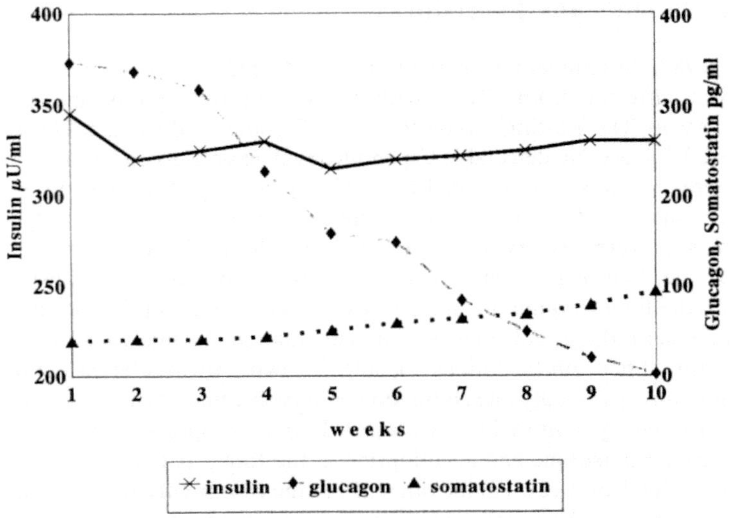

Figure 1. Mean insulin, glucagon and somatostatin concentrations during a 10-week culture period. (n=15). Values are means ± SD.

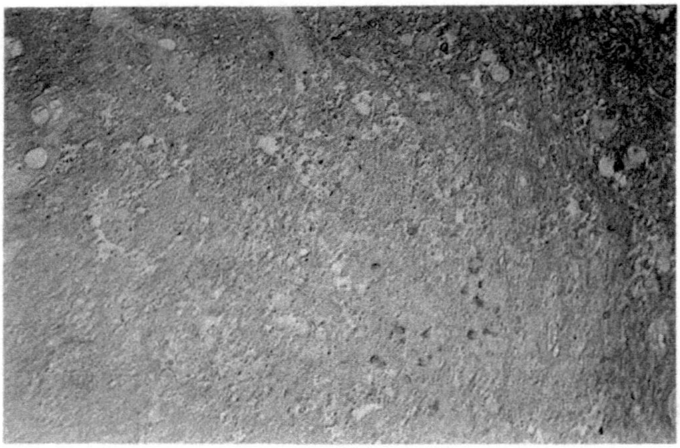

Figure 2. Ten-week cultured islet immunocytochemically stained for glucagon. Original magnification, x 460, reduced 66%.

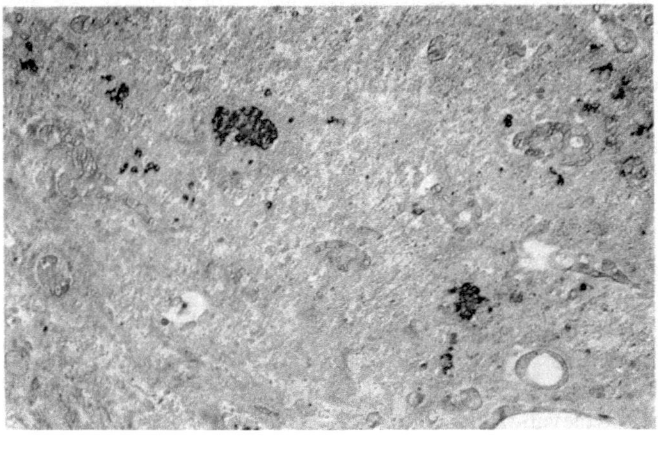

Figure 3. Ten-week cultured islet immunocytochemically stained for insulin. Original magnification, x 460, reduced 66%.

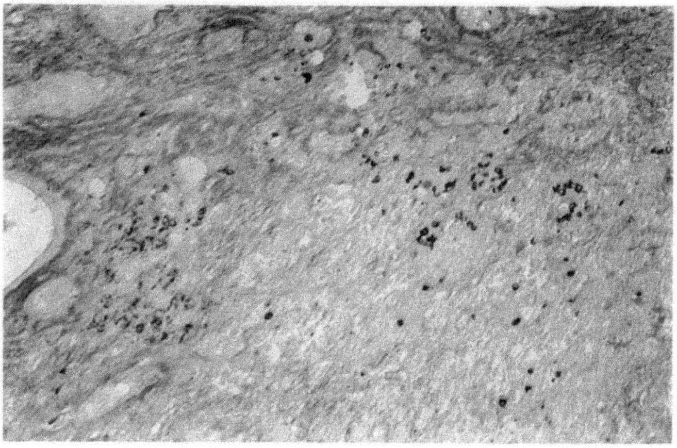

Figure 4. Ten-week cultured islet immunocytochemically stained for somatostatin. Original magnification, x 460, reduced 66%.

(52±2.5 and 150±4.5 μU/ml, respectively). After cryopreservation, the insulin production and viability of the thawed tissue were examined. During a 7-week cultivation, the insulin production was continuous, and after thawing the function remained at the same level (312±15 and 308±33 μU/ml, respectively). Functional analysis of cryopreserved islets was performed at different glucose concentrations (5.5 and 22.0 mM/l) and at 22.0 mM/l glucose plus 5 mM/l theophylline. The results demonstrated similar basal and stimulated insulin release in the medium as in the cases of only cultured islets (48±3, 152±3.5 and 248±6.5 μU/ml, respectively). Light microscopic examinations showed the normal morphological picture of the thawed islets after a one-week culturing. Immunohistochemical examination proved the strong insulin positivity of the cryopreserved islets and electronmicroscopy demonstated characteristic secretory granules too (12). In the first week of cultivation and following the 10-week culturing, the islet class II MHC expression was examined by immunostaining of the islets with monoclonal antibody. As shown in Fig. 5, a very strong class II MHC positivity was present connected with a large number of class II MHC-bearing lymphoid cells in the islets in the first week of cultivation. Figure 6 depicts the effect of a 10-week cultivation on the elimination of class II positive cells, *i.e.* minimal intraislet class II MHC positive cells were noted on immunostaining of the islets. These findings clearly indicated that long-term culturing almost completely eliminated lymphoid cells from the fetal islets.

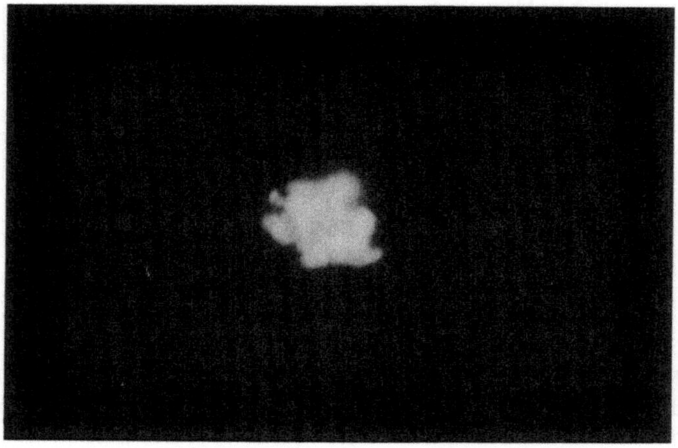

Figure 5. Immunofluorescent staining of uncultivated islet cells with monoclonal antibody for class II antigen expression. Original magnification, x160, reduced 66%.

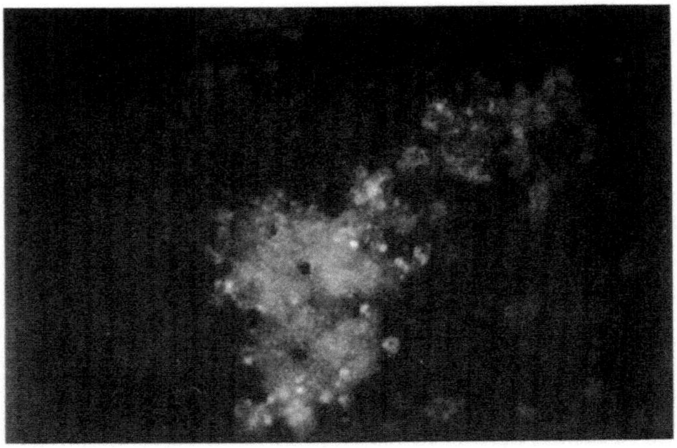

Figure 6. Immunofluorescent staining of islet cells with monoclonal antibody for class II antigen expression after a 10-week cultivation. Original magnification, x160, reduced 66%.

Clinical Results

The period that had elapsed following transplantation ranged from 1 to 8 years. Following transplantation, the mean concentration of serum C-peptide was 0.42 ng/ml (0.25-1.1 ng/ml), depending on the volume of the transplanted islet masses (one, two or three donor tissues), *i.e.* the number of grafted islets (between 10,000 and 40,000). The reduction in the insulin dose was 39.4% (mean for 24 patients). The HbA_{1C} level (6.0%) always revealed a normal carbohydrate metabolism. The graft function failed in 2 cases and in 3 cases before 1 and before 3 years following grafting, respectively, and the transplanted islet function ceased in another 7 patients after 5 or 6 years. In these cases, only one donor islet mass was grafted, and a decrease in the islet function was already noted 3 years after transplantation. As shown in Fig. 7, the insulin requirement was increased by 20%, correlating with the reduction in serum C-peptide level. In the other 14 patients (more than one

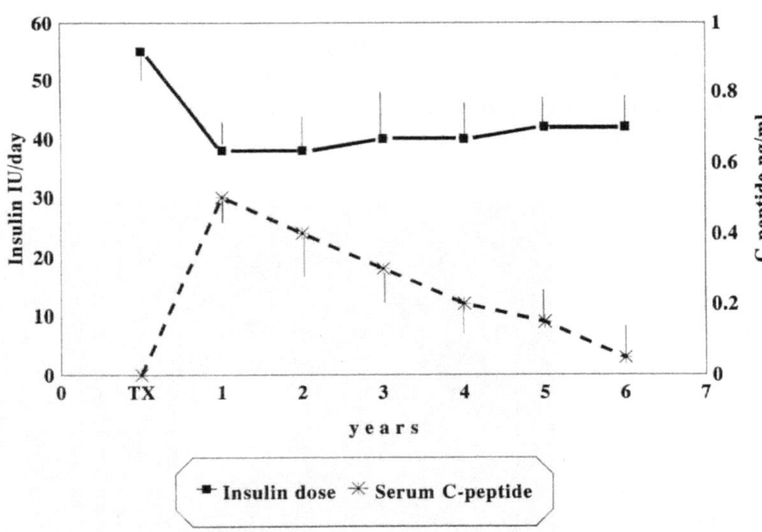

Figure 7. Islet function following grafting of one compatible islet mass. The circles and squares represent the daily insulin requirement and the serum C-peptide level respectively. Each point on the curve is the mean ± SD of the results on 7 transplanted patients.

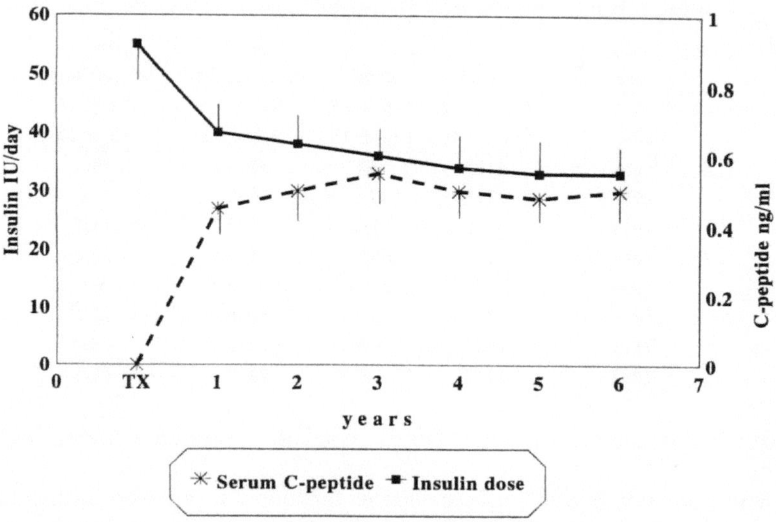

Figure 8. Islet function following transplantation of more than one compatible islet mass. The circles and squares represent the daily insulin requirement and the serum C-peptide level, respectively. Each point on the curve is the mean ± SD of the results on 14 transplanted patients.

islet mass was grafted), the graft function between 2 and 6 years posttransplantation was continuous supported, by a steadily reduced daily insulin dose and a higher C-peptide level; Fig. 8 presents these data. After grafting, glucose stimulation and serum C-peptide determination were performed in all patients at different times. In those cases which had more grafted islet masses, the stimulated C-peptide concentration was higher than in those with only one graft.

The alterations in the secondary complications were as follows in 24 patients (the exceptions were 2 cases with grafts functioning for less than one year). The background retinopathy was improved in 10 eyes, and was unchanged in 24 eyes, but in proliferative retinopathy 8 eyes were unchanged and in 6 eyes the condition had progressed. For checking of the kidney function, the B2M levels in the serum and urine and the protein excretion were determined. In 22 patients, diabetic nephropathy did not develop; both the serum and the urine levels of B2M remained in the normal range (serum B2M 1519-1528 μg/ml; urine B2M 106-116 μg/l) and only 3 patients exhibited microalbuminuria. In one of the transplanted nephropathic patients, the laboratory parameters displayed a temporary improvement, but after a one-year postgrafting period all the laboratory parameters demonstrated the progression of the nephropathy. In the other nephropathic patient, the grafting did not exert any beneficial effect on the renal function, because the patient had a preuremic condition at the time of transplantation. In contrast with these cases in one patient the kidney function showed a significant improvement, correlating with the successful transplantation performed before irreversible tissue damage (Table 1).

In the patient who underwent simultaneous kidney and fetal islet transplantation, the period that had elapsed following grafting was more than 2 years. The islet function was demonstrated by an immediately increased C-peptide level (0.25-0.39 ng/ml). At present, the fasting C-peptide level is in the range 0.30-0.90 ng/ml. The insulin requirement has fallen from 58 to 24 U/day, *i.e.* a reduction of 58%. The relation between the daily insulin requirement and the serum C-peptide level is shown in Fig. 9. The insulin dose reduction closely followed the increased C-peptide production. In spite of the significantly reduced

Table 1. Effects of Fetal Islet Transplantation on Kidney Function

Patient checking	time	B2M (μg/l) serum	urine	albumin excr.(mg/24h)	creatinin cir.(ml/min)
n=22	1988	1528 ± 32	106 ± 25	8.3 ± 1.3	91 ± 16
	1993	1519 ± 76	116 ± 18	9.1 ± 3.8	89 ± 22
L.B.	before tx	4253	658	3520.8	28.6
	1989	3723	411	2858.6	71.2
	1991	9750	5832	7500.2	15.3
A.B.	before tx	9618	6527	7105.0	20.4
	1990	11927	8485	8332.5	8.5
M.K.	before tx	5320	852	3640.8	22.3
	1991	2831	350	2640.2	65.4
	1993	2722	240	2410.2	66.1

insulin requirement, the HbA_{1C} level (5.6%) constantly revealed a normal carbohydrate metabolism.

Twenty-four months after grafting, the islet function was provoked with glucagon (Fig. 10), which led to a C-peptide elevation from 0.30 to 0.90 ng/ml and an insulin concentration increase from 14 to 25 μIU/ml. During IVGTT, an increased serum C-peptide level was noted, but the highest concentration appeared 90 min following glucose stimulation.

Improvements in retinopathy and peripheral microangiopathy were also noted, followed by a normoglycemic condition. During the 24-month posttransplantation period, laser treatment was not required at all and the peripheral pregangrenic lesions disappeared completely.

After grafting, three periods of kidney rejection were diagnosed, but these proved reversible on high-dose steroid treatment. The partially elevated serum and urine B2M and urine albumin levels displayed a good correlation with the rejection episodes and the recovery. More than 2 years postgrafting, the kidney function is acceptable: UN 7 mM/l, serum creatinine 92 μM/l, creatinine clearance 75 ml/min, serum B2M 2100 μg/l, urine B2M 117 μg/l, and urine albumin 9.1 mg/24 h.

DISCUSSION

It is known that approximately 100,000-200,000 islets have to be grafted into a human diabetic for successful reversal of the diabetic status. It is unlikely that such numbers

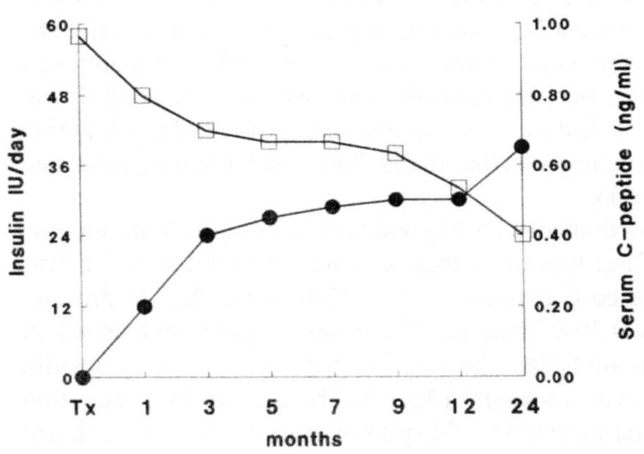

Figure 9. Islet function and relation between daily insulin requirement and serum C-peptide level during 24 months following transplantation. The squares and closed circles represent the daily insulin requirement and the serum C-peptide level, respectively.

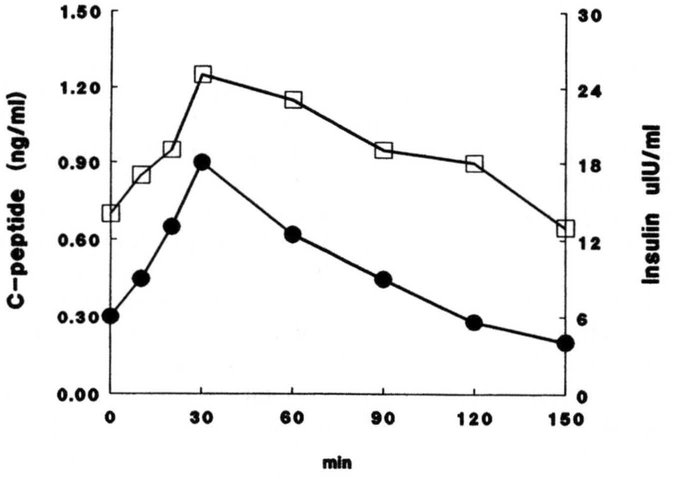

Figure 10. Serum insulin concentration and serum C-peptide level after stimulation with 1 mg glucagon iv. The squares and closed circles represent the daily insulin requirement and the serum C-peptide level, respectively.

of human fetal islets can be produced, but certain important factors that increase the number and function of islets for transplantation are well known.

Fetal pancreas transplantation requires a number of precautions before and after grafting. Perhaps the most important of the pretransplant factors is the gestational age of the grafting tissue used, which is usually 14-20 weeks. Hahn von Dorsche (9, 10) applied immunohistochemical, morphometric and ultrastructural examinations of the human fetal pancreas at different times of gestation and demonstrated that the β-cells formed larger clusters, this being the predominant type of islet cell at the 14th week of gestation. This result suggests that the fetal pancreas is useful for grafting only after the 14th gestational week. In our practice, therefore, the age of the human fetal tissue used in the *in vitro* and *in vivo* examinations was 14 weeks or older.

The yield of islet tissue for transplantation is a real problem, especially in the field of fetal pancreatic islets. Many authors have investigated the optimal culture conditions (1, 4, 6, 8, 24, 28). It is generally believed that culture maintenance requires rather special conditions: addition of hormones, the use of sophisticated culturing media (RPMI 1640 or TCM 199), and low concentrations of glucose. In contrast with these assumptions, we applied long-term culturing (10 weeks) in a relatively simple way, using 20% human serum, with glutamine in the culturing media instead of fetal calf serum. Additionally, the higher glucose concentration (400 mg/dl) used in this protocol might have supported the faster growth and differentiation. A high and constant insulin production was observed during the 10-week period, but the glucagon production into the media decreased steadily in spite of the increasing somatostatin secretion. The different hormone productions correlated with the results of immunocytochemical examinations on the islet: no glucagon positivity, an increased somatostatin positivity and the constant insulin positivity of the cells were noted. While some reports have described decreasing hormone productions during a short cultivation (30, 37), the increase in content was consistent with the increased insulin secretion by cultured fetal pancreas after several weeks in culture reported by Kover and Mandel (19, 23); no information was provided about the somatostatin production. Somatostatin is known to have beneficial humoral and metabolic effects in diabetes mellitus and is able to reverse some diabetic retinal vascular complications (14). Our results clearly demonstrated that the long-term cultivation (10 weeks) of fetal human islets did not impair the growth capacity of the islet tissue. The observed high chronic insulin secretion into the medium suggests that this organ culture may be useful in clinical work as a means of storage (organ bank) of human fetal islets. Further, the ability to maintain this fetal islet tissue *in vitro* with a relatively simple procedure for longer times provides an opportunity for the production of an increased and qualitatively different islet mass.

An opportunity for increasing the yield of islet tissue for transplantation is cryopreservation: the cryopreservation of isolated pancreatic islet grafts is an adequate technique for long-term storage prior to transplantation. This was also demonstrated by our results, as the cryopreservation permitted the storage of large numbers of human fetal pancreatic islets over long periods with high numerical recovery and maintenance of physiological functions. The islet tissue was stored for 6 or 8 months after a 7-week culturing. The post-thaw recovery of the islets was about 85%, as assayed via extractable insulin recovery after culturing for 2 weeks following thawing. On light and electronmicroscopy, the cryopreserved islets appeared to be histologically and ultrastructurally intact (12). Our experimental data indicate that long-term cultivation can ensure the growth capacity of fetal islet tissue, and that cryopreservation or methods combined with cryoculturing are useful for the storage of pancreatic islet tissue in order to establish an islet bank. Islet banking would also optimize the tissue matching of HLA before transplantation (18).

Graft rejection appears to be the major problem of transplantation, mainly in the field of fetal islet grafting. Fetal pancreatic tissue contains substantial quantities of primitive lymphoid tissue, which is highly immunogenic (31). This high immunogenicity is suggested by the presence of a large number of class II-positive lymphoid cells (26). These intraislet lymphoid cells are responsible for the destruction of islet cells in the immunological processes (21). There are several opportunities to solve the problem of graft immunogenicity: reduction of the antigen expression, selection of the best-matched donor-recipient combination, effective immunosuppression and choice of the site of transplantation. Our experimental work clearly demonstrated that a 10-week culturing resulted in an effective elimination of intraislet class II MHC positive cells and produced a reduction of the immunogenicity. On the other hand, cryopreservation could also reduce the immunogenicity of the fetal islets (5, 16, 25, 35) and combination with a long-term cultivation would allow optimized circumstances for transplantation: a significantly reduced antigenicity of the islets and time allowed for the best-matched donor-recipient combination (7). The cryoculturing method is likewise useful for the storage of fetal islet tissue in order to establish an islet bank and futher provides an opportunity for the accumulation of large numbers of samples of donor pancreatic tissue. The site of transplantation may have an important bearing on the effect of islet transplantation. In clinical applications, intrahepatic, intramuscular and intraperitoneal implantation are the favored methods. However, from a consideration of the experimental data, it could be suggested that the renal subcapsular space offers better growth conditions for islets than the liver, spleen or other sites (2, 20, 22). Further, the subcapsular space of the kidney could be an immunologically privileged space, where the islet graft could exhibit a significant acceleration of cell differentiation and maturation (38).

Transplantation of a whole pancreas or of isolated pancreatic islets prevents and reverses the development of secondary complications in diabetic animals (3, 27, 29, 40), and at present pancreas transplantation is currently the only treatment of type I diabetes that establishes an insulin-independent, constant normoglycemic state, because the success rate with clinical islet allotransplantation remains low (13, 15, 17). Successful transplantation produces long-term normoglycemia and provides a unique opportunity for evaluation of the impact of normalization of the blood glucose levels and the carbohydrate metabolism. Intensive insulin therapy can also exert a moderate effect in preventing of diabetic complications (41), whereas the multiple injection of human insulin is not able to ensure the same beneficial condition because exogenous insulin treatment cannot compensate the physiological function of the Langerhans islet. However, the grafting of long-term cultured and cryopreserved fetal pancreatic islets resulted in a partial cure of diabetes in our clinical practice. The transplanted islet mass was able to ensure a normoglycemic condition, as proved by the normal HbA_{1C} level. During the long-term follow-up, the graft function failed in 2 cases within the first year posttransplantation, while in 24 successful cases the long-term graft function depended on the volume of the transplanted islet mass. With the exception of 2 cases, the progression of the retinopathy stopped and the condition improved. Apart from the nephropathic cases, the renal function remained normal following transplantation. In nephropathy, the improvement was temporary in one case, whereas in another patient the kidney function showed a significant improvement correlated with the successful grafting performed before irreversible tissue damage.

In the case involving simultaneous kidney and long-term-cultured fetal pancreatic islet transplantation, the patient became normoglycemic during 24 months following grafting, and this condition provided a beneficial condition for the improvement or prevention of diabetic complications. It seems important to stress certain factors influencing successful transplantation in our case. The primary one is the use of matched long-term cultured fetal islets, grafted to the subcapsular site of the revascularized kidney. This region is an immunologically privileged one and provides an opportunity for the permanent growth of grafted islets. During the long-term posttransplantation period, the C-peptide secretion continuously increased and the reduction in daily insulin requirement showed an inverse correlation with this production, but the corticosteroid medication, as part of the immunosuppression, did not allow total elimination of the insulin dose. Following transplantation, kidney graft rejections were diagnosed on three occasions, but no rejection episode was noted for the islet grafts, which suggests that the kidney subcapsular area really is a suitable site for islet transplantation.

Our results suggest that the transplantation of long-term cultured and cryopreserved fetal islets is a hopeful method for curing diabetes mellitus, mainly at an early stage of diabetic complications, and if applied simultaneously with kidney grafting in end-stage nephropathy, the islet graft can additionally prevent diabetic complications in the transplanted kidney.

REFERENCES

1. Andersson, A., 1976, Tissue culture of isolated pancreatic islets, *Acta Endocrinol.* 83(Suppl. 205):283-293.
2. Andersson, A., Sandler, S., Groth, C.G., and Hellerström, C., 1988, Transplantation of fetal islet tissue. In: Groth, C.G., ed. *Pancreatic transplantation.* Philadelphia, Saunders Company, p. 391-406.
3. Ar'Rajab, A., Ahrén, B., Alumets, J., Lögdberg, L., and Bengmark, S., 1990, Islet transplantation to the renal subcapsular space improves late complications in streptozotocin-diabetic rats, *Eur. Surg. Res.* 22:270-278.
4. Bretzel, R.G., Flesch, B., Milde, K., Entenmann, H., and Federlin, K., 1989, Ia antigen-reducing effect of different cryopreservation programs on rat pancreatic islets, *Diabetes* 38(Suppl. 1):282-283.
5. Cottral, M.S., Warnock, G.L., Kneteman, N.M., Halloran P.P., and Rajotte, R.V., 1993, The effect of cryopreservation on the survival and MHC antigen expression of murine islet allografts, *Transplantation* 55:159-163.
6. Chick, W.L., and Boston, M.D., 1973, Beta cell replication in rat pancreatic monolayer cultures: Effect of glucose, tolbutamide, glucocorticoid, growth hormone and glucagon, *Diabetes* 22:687-693.
7. Clayton, H.A., Swift, S.M., James, R.F.L., Horsburgh, T., and London, N.J., 1994, Human islet transplantation - is blood group compatibility important? *Transplantation* 56:1538-1540.

8. Collier, S., Mandel, T.E., Hoffeman, L., and Caruso, G., 1981, Organ culture of fetal mouse pancreas: Effect of culture conditions on insulin and glucagon secretion, *Diabetes* 30:804-812.
9. von Dorsche, H.H., Fält, K., Titlbach, M, Reiher, H., Hahn, H-J., and Falmer, S., 1989, Immunohistochemical, morphometric, and ultrastructural investigations of the early development of insulin, somatostatin, glucagon, and pp cells in foetal human pancreas, *Diabetes Res.* 12:51-56.
10. von Dorsche, H.H., Fält, K., and Hahn, H.J., 1990, Ontogenesis of human fetal pancreas in use for transplantation. *Horm. Metab. Res.* Suppl. 25:227-233.
11. Farkas, G., and Joó, F., 1984, Simple and reliable conditions for routine, long-term culturing of fetal human pancreatic tissue fragments. *Diabetes* 33:1165-1168.
12. Farkas, G., Lázár, G., and Herczegh, J., 1990, The long-term cultivation and cryopreservation of human fetal pancreatic tissue. *Horm. Metab. Res.* Suppl. 25:64-68.
13. Farkas, G., 1993, Fetal islet cell transplants: promises and limits of the experience in the eastern countries. *Cell transplantation* 2:59-64.
14. Fassler, J.E., Hughes, J.H., and Titterington, L., 1988, Somatostatin analog: an inhibitor of angiogenesis? *Clin. Res.* 36:869A.
15. Fernandez-Cruz, L., Casanovas, D., and Lloveras, G., 1992, Pancreas transplantation: is islet transplantation the future? *Transplant. Proc.* 24:2379-2382.
16. Flesch, B.K., Entenmann, H., Milde, K., Bretzel, R.G., and Federlin, K., 1991, Islet transplantation in experimental diabetes of the rat. Cryopreservation reduces MHC class II but not class I antigens of rat pancreatic islets. *Horm. Metab. Res.* 23:1-6.
17. International islet transplant registry, 1994, 4:6-10.
18. Kneteman, N.M , Andersson, D., Scharp, D.W., and Lacy, P.E., 1989, Long-term cryogenic storage of purified adult human islets of Langerhans. *Diabetes* 38:386-396.
19. Kover, K., and Moore, W.V., 1989, Development of a method for isolation of islets from human fetal pancreas. *Diabetes* 38:917-924.
20. Korsgren, O., Andersson, A., Jansson, L., and Sundler, F., 1992, Reinnervation of syngeneic mouse pancreatic islets transplanted into renal subcapsular space. *Diabetes* 41:130-135.
21. Lacy, P.E., and Finke, E.H., 1991, Activation of intraislet lymphoid cells causes destruction of islet cells. *Am. J. Pathol.* 138:1183-1190.
22. Leow, C.K., Shimizu, S., Gray, D.W.R., and Morris, P.J., 1994, Successful pancreatic islet autotransplantation to the renal subcapsule in the cynomolgus monkey. *Transplantation* 57:161-164.
23. Mandel, T.E., and Georgiou, H.M., 1983, Insulin secretion by fetal human pancreatic islets of Langerhans in prolonged organ culture. *Diabetes* 32:15-20.
24. McEvoy, R.C., and Leung, P.E., 1982, Tissue culture of fetal rat islets comparison of serum supplemented and serum-free, defined medium on the maintenance, growth, and differentiation of A, B and D cells. *Endocrinology* 111:1568-1575.
25. Meloche, M., Ketchum, R.J., Serie, J.R., Sutherland, D.E.R., and Hegre, O.D., 1988, Elimination of Ia-bearing cells by in vitro isolation and culture of neonatal rat pancreatic islets. *Transplantation* 46:614-616.
26. Motojima, K., and Mullen, Y., 1987, IFN-gamma stimulates cryptic class II antigen expression in human and pig fetal pancreas. *Transplant. Proc.* 19:214-217.
27. Murray, F.T., Beyer-Mears, A., Johnson, R.D., Sima, A.A.F., Cameron, D.F., Sninsky, Ch.A., and Selawry, H., 1993, Assessment of proteinuria and neuropathy in the nonimmunossuppressed BB diabetic rat after abdominal intratesticular islet transplantation. *Transplantation* 56:680-686.
28. Milner, R.D.G., Cser, A., and Fennell, J.S., 1977, Effect of glucose on tissue culture of human endocrine pancreas. In: von Wasielewski, E., and Chick, W.L. eds., *Pancreatic beta cell culture.* Amsterdam, Excerpta medica, p. 143-147.
29. Orloff, M.J., Yamaka, N., Greenleaf, G.E., Huang, D.G., and Leng, X.S., 1986, Reversal of mesangial enlargement in rats with long-standing diabetes by whole pancreas transplantation. *Diabetes* 35:347-354.
30. Sandler, S., Andersson, A., Landström, A.S., Tollemar, J., Borg, H., Petersson, B., Groth, C-G., and Hellerström, C., 1987, Tissue culture of human fetal pancreas. *Diabetes* 36:1401-1407.
31. Simeonovic, C.J., Bowen, K.M., Kotlarski, I., and Lafferty, K.J., 1980 Modulation of tissue immunogenicity by organ culture. Comparison of adult islets and fetal pancreas. *Transplantation* 30:174-178.
32. Simeonivic, C.J., and Lafferty, K.J., 1982, The isolation and transplantation of fetal mouse proislets. *Aust. J. Exp. Biol. Med. Sci.* 60:383-390.
33. Simpson, A.M., Touch, B.E., and Vincent, P.C., 1991, Characterization of endocrine-rich monolayers of human fetal pancreas that display reduced immonogenecity. *Diabetes* 40:800-808.
34. Sternberger, L.A., 1986, *Immunocytochemistry* New York, Wiley, p. 90-209.

35. Taylor, M., Bank, H.L, and Benton, M.J., 1987, Selective killing of leucocytes by freezing: potential for reducing the immunogenicity of pancreatic islets. *Diabetes Res.* 5:99-103.
36. Tuch, B.E., Grigoriou, S., and Turtle, J.R., 1988, Long-term passage of human fetal pancreas in non-diabetic nude mice fails to allow maturation of the response to glucose. *Transplant. Proc.* 20:64-67.
37. Tuch, B.E., Jones, A., Ng, A.B.P., and Turtle, J.R., 1986, Characteristics of human fetal pancreas cultured in vitro. *Transplant. Proc.* 18:322-325.
38. Tuch, B.E., Osgerby, K.J., and Turtle, J.R., 1988, Human fetal pancreas grafted into non-diabetic nude mice normalizes blood glucose levels once diabetes is induced. *Transplantation* 46:608-610.
39. Vasir, B.S., Gray, D.W.R., and Morris, P.J., 1989, Normalization of hyperglycemia in diabetic rats by intraportal transplantation of cryopreserved islets from four donors. *Diabetes (Suppl. 1)* 38:185-188.
40. Woehrle, M., Spitzer, D., Linn, T., Federlin, K., and Bretzel, R.G., 1990, The effect of early islet transplantation on prevention of nephropathy in the spontaneously diabetic BB rat. *Transplant. Proc.* 22:819-820.
41. Zinmann, B., 1993, Insulin regiments and strategies for IDDM. *Diabetes care (Suppl. 3)* 16:24-28.

10

FETAL ISLET TRANSPLANTATION AND PREGNANCY

Charles M. Peterson,* Lois Jovanovic-Peterson, Hui-Min Chen, Wendy Bevier, Richard B. Pearce, Liberty Walker, Alison Okada Wollitzer, and Bent Formby

Sansum Medical Research Foundation
2219 Bath Street
Santa Barbara, CA 93105 USA

SUMMARY

Several animal models are now available for the study of pregnancy complicated by diabetes mellitus and thus studies of islet transplantation in these pregnant animals can also be performed. Animals may be made hyperglycemic by the use of alloxan or streptozotocin. Infusion protocols of glucose and/or insulin have been described in several species including rats and monkeys. Recently described genetic models include the BB Wistar rat, the NOD mouse, the C57/KsJdb+/+m mouse, and the chinese hamster with spontaneous diabetes (CHAD). The NOD mouse is particularly attractive for studies of transplantation since it has several features in common to the human autoimmune counterpart. Studies of subcutaneous fetal islet transplantation in this model as well as in humans during gestation suggest improved graft survival and insulin secretory capacity. The nature of the factors during pregnancy that lead to enhanced tissue vascularization, improved tissue growth and secretory capacity, and decreased immunological response in pregnant recipients are noteworthy and warrant further study.

INTRODUCTION

As a partial allograft, pregnancy has fascinated immunologists and transplantation biologists for decades. The protection of the fetus from immunologic rejection involves complex interactions at the fetal, placental, and maternal levels. In general, these interactions are yet to be completely defined.

The attempt to transplant viable insulin secreting fetal tissue into a pregnant diabetic woman introduces additional variables including that of an autoimmune disease on the part

*Tel: 805-682-7638; FAX: 805-682-3332.

of the recipient and multiple allogeneic determinants on the part of the grafted tissue since a single donor is unlikely to provide sufficient tissue under present protocols.

Little information is available on the interaction of pregnancy on the course of autoimmune diabetes. Studies of transplantation of fetal islets into pregnant recipients are few. Nevertheless, experiments performed to date suggest that pregnancy may provide an opportune time for transplantation of fetal islet tissue in autoimmune diabetes. This chapter reviews the animal models available for the study of diabetes, pregnancy and transplantation, animal studies to date, human studies, and the hormonal, vascular, growth factor, and immunologic responses during pregnancy that may warrant exploration in the development of protocols for the transplantation of fetal islet tissue into pregnant or nonpregnant recipients.

Animal Models for the Study of Diabetes and Pregnancy

The selection of an animal model for the study of problems related to human diabetes and pregnancy should ideally be based upon a close correlation between the pathology and pathophysiology of diabetes as displayed by the animal and the human condition. The etiology of diabetes complicating human pregnancy is multifactorial. Type I and type II diabetic women obviously have genetic differences leading to hyperglycemia and metabolic perturbations yet have similar pathologies associated with their condition (Table 1). The same problems occur in pregnancies complicated by gestational diabetes except that the malformations associated with first trimester hyperglycemia are not seen with a frequency above that observed in the normal population (1).

Our ability to quantify events during human gestation has increased markedly in the last decades. Nevertheless, there are still many aspects of genetic interactions, biochemical

Table 1. Problems Complicating Human Maternal Hyperglycemia by Trimester

First Trimester
Malformations
Growth Retardation
Fetal Wastage
Second Trimester
Hypertrophic Cardiomyopathy
Polyhydramnios
Erythremia
Placental Insufficiency
Preeclampsia/Eclampsia
Possible Fetal Loss
Third Trimester
Intrauterine Demise
Macrosomia
Neonatal Problems
Hypoglycemia
Hypocalcemia
Hyperbilirubinemia
Respiratory Distress
Hypomagnesemia
Developmental Problems
Metabolic
Mental

Table 2. Animal Models of Diabetic Pregnancy

Animals Made Hyperglycemic by Alloxan or Streptozotocin
Mice
Hamsters
Rats
Rabbits
Pigs
Sheep
Animals Made Hyperglycemic by Glucose Infusion
Rats
Animals Made Hyperinsulinemic by Insulin Infusion
Monkeys
Genetic Models of Hyperglycemia
BB Wistar Rat
NOD Mouse
C57/KsJdb+/+m Mouse
Chinese Hamsters with spontaneous diabetes (CHAD)

processes, and pathology which only can be studied in animal systems as has been noted by several authors (2-3). Given the complexity of human gestation, it is apparent that no one model will be able to speak to all of the questions surrounding diabetes and pregnancy. The numerous past advances and the use of embryo tissue culture systems is beyond the scope of the present chapter and is discussed elsewhere (2-8). While a number of animals including primates and domestic pets become diabetic spontaneously during gestation, the low frequency of these events makes these animals poor candidates for research.

CHEMICAL MODELS OF DIABETES APPLIED TO PREGNANCY

Table 2 summarizes the animal models of pregnancy complicated by diabetes currently being studied. Despite the confounding nature of administering chemical compounds which in and of themselves may have an effect on gestation, not to mention the immune system or transplanted tissue, the use of animals made diabetic by the administration of alloxan or streptozotocin remains popular.

The models are easy to produce and have the advantage that the timing of onset and the severity of diabetes can be strictly controlled. For example, to evaluate the effects of streptozotocin on maternal pancreatic beta-cell function, Dickinson and colleagues (9) administered the agent to 14 pregnant ewes at 85 to 90 days' gestation on two occasions, 4 days apart. Intravenous glucose tolerance tests were performed before the initial administration, before the second dose, and 4 weeks after the final dose of streptozotocin. There was a small but significant elevation in maternal fasting blood glucose (4.6 +/- 0.5 mmol/l before streptozotocin and 5.7 +/- 0.4 mmol/l after streptozotocin, p less than 0.05). Five late-gestation ewes were used as controls. The maternal insulin response to streptozotocin demonstrated a loss of the second-phase insulin response to the glucose load after one dose of streptozotocin and loss of the first phase after two doses. Comparison of fetal weights between the control and diabetic ewes showed a significant increase in fetal weight in the fetuses of diabetic ewes (3280 +/- 46 gm in control fetuses vs 3710 +/- 54 gm in diabetic fetuses, p less than 0.05). This study is consistent with the observation that the most common manifestation of pregnancy complicated by diabetes, macrosomia, results from even mild elevations in maternal glucose during the latter phases of pregnancy.

The use of larger animals such as sheep and pigs also allows the investigator to perform serial studies or studies in utero on the growing fetus. For example Lips et al. studied 25 female sheep of the Texel breed made hyperglycemic by administration of alloxan monohydrate in early pregnancy and 15 ewes served as controls (10). Average venous glucose levels (mean +/- standard deviation) increased from 3.5 +/- 0.2 to 14.0 +/- 1.8 mmol/l. All hyperglycemic sheep were treated with long-acting insulin in doses adjusted individually (0.2-1.0 U/kg per day) to keep glucose levels above 8 mmol/l. After a temporary significant increase, maternal venous concentrations of urea and creatinine returned to normal levels. One sheep died on day 6 after administration of alloxan. Another hyperglycemic sheep died at induction of anesthesia. Eight hyperglycemic ewes aborted between days 90 and 128 of gestation. Between days 103 and 135 of gestation the remaining hyperglycemic (n = 15) and control (n = 15) ewes were operated upon and the fetuses were provided with EEG, nuchal EMG and ECG electrodes and catheters in the trachea, amniotic fluid, jugular vein and carotid artery. Use of the chronic sheep preparation for the study of diabetes mellitus and fetal responses was successful in 10 out of 25 cases, as in the diabetic group postoperative intra-uterine fetal survival varied between 2 and 19 days and in 10 cases was at least 5 days. Postoperative intrauterine fetal survival in the controls was significantly longer and varied between 4 and 28 days, and in 13 cases was at least 5 days. While illustrating the potential utility of larger animal models, the difficulty in these types of catheterization studies with their concomitant expense are also made apparent from this study. The pig has received increasing attention as a potential source of transplant tissue (11) but little attention to date as a model of diabetes complicating gestation.

The use of rodents made diabetic by alloxan or streptozotocin is advantageous in that gestation is short and many offspring can be studied. In addition, studies involving multiple generations are relatively easy. Thus investigations of mice, hamsters, rats, and rabbits continue to be popular for metabolic, pathologic and behavioral studies (12-17). As noted below, the advent of genetic inbred strains of rodents with diabetes has in many cases provided a more useful model than the use of animals with drug induced diabetes.

Animals Made Hyperglycemic by Glucose Infusion

The advantages of these models is the ability to differentiate the effects of hyperglycemia per se from the autoimmune or insulin resistance factors that contribute to the complex syndrome known as diabetes. The technologies for maintaining animals with chronic catheters have progressed dramatically. Gauguier et al. took advantage of this technique in rats. Their study investigated whether a deterioration of glucose homeostasis and insulin secretion in adult female rats from hyperglycemic dams could be transmitted to the next generation independent of genetic interferences. Dams (F_0) were rendered hyperglycemic by continuous glucose infusion during the last week of pregnancy. Females born of these rats (F_1) exhibited glucose intolerance and impaired insulin secretion in vivo at adulthood. When they were 3 months old, they were matched with males born of control dams. During pregnancy, their glucose tolerance remained impaired compared with that of controls. Consequently, F_2 newborns of F_1 hyperglycemic dams showed the main features of newborns from diabetic mothers: they were hyperglycemic, hyperinsulinemic, and macrosomic. As adults, they displayed basal hyperglycemia and defective glucose tolerance and insulin secretion. These studies indicate that the long-range deteriorating effects on glucose homeostasis of late gestational hyperglycemia in the F_1 generation are transmitted to the F_2 generation and suggests that a perturbed fetal metabolic environment contributes to the inheritance of diabetes mellitus. These observations on transgenerational effects of hyperglycemia are consistent with the observations of others using chemical models of diabetes (18,19,20). These models then might provide a means for investigating the potential effect of implantation of islet cells on the metabolism and course of type II or noninsulin dependent diabetes mellitus (NIDDM).

ANIMALS MADE HYPERINSULINEMIC BY INSULIN INFUSION

These types of studies allow the differentiation of the effects of chronic hyperinsulinemia from those associated with other components of diabetes syndromes. Hyperinsulinemia is seen in most individuals with NIDDM and persons who inject insulin subcutaneously for diabetes management. Susa and colleagues have developed insulin infusion in the rhesus monkey as a model of hyperinsulinemia to isolate the effects of insulin from those of hyperglycemia (21-23). Recently, chronic in utero hyperinsulinemia was produced by the continuous subcutaneous delivery of 4.75 units of insulin per day for 18 +/- 1 days. After delivery, the insulin-containing pump was removed to allow neonatal insulin levels to drop to normal levels. By 6.5 +/- 1.0 hr after pump removal, plasma glucose, insulin, and C-peptide immunoreactivity were comparable in the control and experimental animals. At that point 300 micrograms of glucagon/kg body weight were given iv to stimulate insulin secretion. After 30 minutes, a significant elevation (expressed as the percentage of basal levels) in plasma glucose by 250%, insulin by 200%, and C-peptide by 200% was observed in the control animals. In contrast, no changes in plasma insulin or C-peptide concentrations occurred, with an attenuated glucose response that was only one-fifth of the control response, in the experimental animals. These results along with the observed lowered concentrations of C-peptide in the plasma and insulin in the pancreas at birth provides evidence that insulin is an inhibitor of its synthesis and secretion in utero and that this abnormal intrauterine environment causes changes that persist into extrauterine life. Whether these changes result in turn in gestational diabetes or affects the subsequent generation analogous to the findings noted above in rats remains to be determined.

GENETIC MODELS OF HYPERGLYCEMIA

One of the more exciting developments of the past decade has been the characterization of genetic models of hyperglycemia in rodents. The rapid evolution of genetic studies especially in the mouse and the rat have made these models especially attractive for the study of diabetes and pregnancy.

The BB Wistar rat is non-obese and displays hyperglycemia, hypoinsulinemia, ketosis, and glycosuria (24). The onset of diabetes is acute and usually occurs in animals 60 to 120 days of age. Pancreatic lesions consist of lymphocytic insulitis with rapid and complete destruction of beta cells. Daily insulin treatment is required for survival. Both genetic and immunological components are involved in the etiology of the disease and genetic susceptibility is linked *inter alia* to the major histocompatibility (RT1) locus. Hyperglycemic mothers treated with insulin have been shown to have intrauterine growth retarded fetuses, increased stillbirths, and numerous malformations including lumbosacral dysgenesis similar to that described in the caudal regression syndrome (25,26).

Kaufmann et al. (24) investigated the glucose metabolism of glucose intolerant BB female rats (study group) prior to pregnancy, during pregnancy, and postpartum using glucose tolerance tests (GTT). Control rats with normal GTT were studied and bred in a fashion similar to the study animals. Before becoming pregnant, the GTT levels of the chemically diabetic rats were significantly different from those of the controls (p less than 0.05). The GTT values of the study animals decreased during pregnancy to levels seen in pregnant controls. After pregnancy, the GTT values of the study animals returned to prepregnant levels. Based on these observations, it appears that pregnancy may block the autoimmune destruction of beta cells, causing an increase in insulin production and release, thereby improving glucose metabolism.

The other genetic model of diabetes that has been found useful for the study of pregnancy related questions is the glucose intolerant prediabetic NOD mouse (27). The NOD is a well accepted murine model of autoimmune diabetes. The females begin to evidence a cumulative incidence of diabetes following puberty which reaches up to 80% by 30 weeks of age. The autoimmune attack on the islets is characterized by islitis and has been linked to several genes including the major histocompatibility complex (MHC) (28). A MHC matched diabetes resistant strain has also been developed (29).

Our findings in mildly hyperglycemic animals include macrosomia, and hypoglycemia in the neonate, and increased peripheral and pancreatic insulin concentrations. The effect on intrauterine growth appears to be biphasic with animals with higher levels of glycemia showing a decrease in birthweight, and increased fetal loss similar to findings reported in humans (30,31).

As can be seen in Figure 1, pregnant NOD diabetic mice like their nondiabetic human counterparts show a drop in glucose levels by the second trimester if diabetes or glucose intolerance does not intervene. Mildly hyperglycemic mice gave birth to increasingly large pups with birthweights two standard deviations greater than the mean birthweight of pups born to normoglycemic mice. Macrosomic pups weighed at least 1.82g, had increased insulin content of their pancreas, and had large organs, similar to the pathology seen in human macrosomic infants.

We examined the relationship between birthweight and maternal blood glucose and glycosylated hemoglobin levels, litter size, maternal age, and parity (31). After observing 133 births we found that mean litter birthweight was significantly negatively correlated with the total number of pups in each litter ($r=-0.39$, $p \leq 0.001$) and significantly positively correlated with parity ($r=0.19$, $p \leq 0.05$) and maternal age ($r=0.22$, $p \leq 0.05$). The total number of pups was significantly negatively correlated with parity ($r=-0.33$, $p \leq 0.001$) and with parent age ($r=-0.21$, $p \leq 0.05$). Initial analysis showed no correlation between birthweight and antepartum or postpartum blood glucose or glycated hemoglobin (GHb). However, by

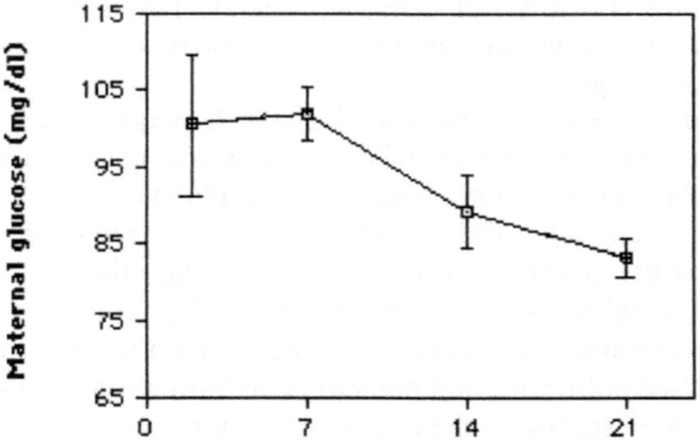

Figure 1. Maternal whole blood glucose obtained from the retro-orbital sinus of NOD mice (N = 7) during normal gestation. Day 0 is prior to mating and day 21 is one day following delivery. The error bars represent the Standard Deviation.

plotting birthweight versus GHb the reason for no correlation became clear. Below a GHb of 2.5% there was a great deal of variation. A significant positive correlation was found for birthweight and GHb when GHb was between 2.4% and 4.0% ($r=0.67$, $p\leq0.01$). Birthweight decreased when GHb was above 4.0%.

Our results show an initial increase in pup growth in response to rising maternal glucose followed by a decrease in growth with further increases in maternal glucose levels. The work of Schroeder et al. may in part explain the biphasic nature of the fetal growth response to maternal glycemia in NOD mice (32). They found that maternal glucose levels regulated placental glucose transporter gene expression. Gene expression increased linearly up to a maternal glucose of 12.7 mM but decreased at higher glucose levels.

During our study we noticed that many of the large pups died soon after birth. In 4 macrosomic pups that were sacrificed at birth, the average blood glucose was 0.1 mM. In 5 normal weight pups the average blood glucose was 2.77 mM. Thus, NOD pups clearly become severely hypoglycemic as may macrosomic infants of human diabetic mothers.

For all births we found that birthweight was significantly negatively correlated with the total number of pups in the litter but was positively correlated with parity and parent age, analogous to the situation in humans. However, the total number of pups in each litter decreased with increasing parity and age, contrary to the increase in twins seen with increasing age in humans. Thus as the animals became older they had fewer pups in each litter and birthweight appeared to increase (33-35).

Since birthweight is affected by the total number of pups, parity, and parent age, and appears to be affected by GHb, macrosomia in the Sansum Medical Research Foundation colony is now defined as a birthweight of 1.9g or greater (2 standard deviations above the normal mean) and a litter size of at least 6 pups. Macrosomia in the NOD mouse is also associated with an antepartum GHb of between 2.6 and 4.0%.

The C57/KsJdb+/+m mouse was evaluated by Kaufmann et al. as a model of gestational diabetes (35). This animal is frankly diabetic in the homozygous diabetic form. In the heterozygous form, it develops gestational diabetes, and in the homozygous normal form, it is normal. The pups of heterozygous males and females that were bred were weighed, classified by sex, and identified. At 4 weeks of age, the genetic makeup of the pups was determined. From 37 litters, 140 pups were born and raised to weaning age. Multiple regression analysis of the data revealed that the homozygous diabetic pups weighed most at birth; the heterozygous diabetic pups weighed less, and the homozygous normal pups weighed the least. All comparisons of these groups were statistically significant. Sex and interlitter variation also were found to be significant factors determining birthweight. Controlling for sex and interlitter variation did not change the significance of the effect of the genetic tendency for diabetes on birthweight. This study indicates that in this model of NIDDM, neonatal macrosomia in part may be determined by the genetic or congenital susceptibility to develop diabetes in the future.

Sasaki too studied the spontaneously diabetic hamster as a model of pregnancy complicated by diabetes (36). Females of Chinese hamsters with spontaneous diabetes (CHAD), which have been developed as a genetic strain of IDDM, were mated with males of non-diabetic Chinese hamsters (CHA). According to the grade of glucose intolerance, the females of CHAD were divided into four groups, i.e. normal, chemical and diabetic with mild and severe disease. In the diabetic groups, hyperglycemia in fetuses and a high incidence of fetal abnormalities were observed. Fetal lung lipid analysis revealed that the diabetic pregnancy in this animal model showed typical features of delayed fetal lung maturity. Therefore, this animal model may be useful for studying the mechanism of delayed fetal lung maturity as well as the development of respiratory distress syndrome in fetuses from dams with diabetes.

As can be seen, there are multiple animal models now available for the study of issues related to diabetes and pregnancy that can also be used for studies of transplantation. The two models that seem most applicable to the human condition of autoimmune diabetes would appear to be the BB rat and the NOD mouse. While transplantation studies are few, there is an increasing amount of information on the interaction of autoimmunity and pregnancy.

Studies of Pregnancy, Autoimmunity and Lymphokine Response

There is evidence that pregnant women undergo immunological changes consistent with weakening of cell-mediated immunity (Th1 responses) and strengthening of humoral immunity (Th2 responses) with increased production of the immunosuppressive cytokines IL-4 and IL-10. Immunosuppression during pregnancy may be critical for survival of the fetus, a partial allograft. These alterations in cytokine production associated with immunosuppression during pregnancy may in part account for the decreased ability of pregnant women to resist viral and bacterial infections. On the other hand, the immunological changes of pregnancy could be beneficial for individuals with increased Th1-like activities associated with autoimmunity. Cytokines may also play a role in the onset of normal labor, as well as in preterm labor induced by intrauterine infection. Cell-mediated and humoral immune responses are often mutually exclusive. Th1 and Th2 cells have provided a cellular basis for this observation (37,38).

Data reported by Dudley et al. (39) indicate that cytokine production by activated lymphocytes obtained from female mice during pregnancy is dramatically altered. As reflected by splenocyte cytokine production, systemic immune cytokine responses are marked by a progressive decline in the ability of activated T cells to produce IL-2, with a concomitant increase in IL-4 and IL-6 production. INF-g production by activated splenocytes was found to peak in the first days of pregnancy, but otherwise was unchanged. Decidual lymphocytes, representing local immune function in the uterus, were found to produce only modest amounts of IL-6, IL-3, and GM-CSF after activation. Because both IL-2 and INF-g have embryo-toxic properties (40), it is not surprising to find that decidual lymphocytes do not secrete IL-2 and INF-g after activation. Growth factor production is enhanced during pregnancy. IL-3 and GM-CSF production by decidual lymphocytes peaks early in pregnancy and declines as pregnancy progresses. IL-10 effectively suppresses secondary Th1 effector functions. It does so by strongly inhibiting the production of inflammatory cytokines such as INF-g, TNF-a and IL-1 (41).

Biologically active IL-10 is constitutively produced at the maternal-fetal interface and thus joins TGF-b2 and alpha-fetoprotein, among other substances, which have a potentially immunosuppressive role at the maternal-fetal interface (42). TGF-b2 inhibits IL-2 production at high concentrations and thus could be responsible for local immunosuppression.

Two striking features of the immunoregulation in pregnancy are the avoidance of cell-mediated immunity and the enhancement of antibody production. The continuous presence of locally secreted IL-10 offers a plausible explanation for this phenomenon because it is known for its ability to down-regulate Th1 cytokines (43). Most significantly, IL-10 inhibits the production of INF-g, a known abortifacient that may act either by activating NK cells that can damage the trophoblast (44) or by down-regulating the production of trophoblast growth-promoting GM-CSF by the uterine epithelium (45).

The relative excess of IL-10 and IL-4 throughout pregnancy also provides a potential mechanism for avoiding the harmful effects of various types of Th1-mediated immunity in the vicinity of the maternal-fetal unit. The significance of changes in cytokines produced by Th1 and Th2 cells during the course of normal murine pregnancy provide a possible cytokine basis for local avoidance of DTH and NK responses along with systemic enhancement of antibody-mediated immunity (46).

Similar types of studies in humans have not been reported in the literature. However, the significant changes in IL-2 and IL-4 production, along with other changes in cytokine production, suggest that activated lymphocytes during pregnancy produce cytokines that favor function of Th2 cells over Th1 cells. These changes in cytokine production parallel the increase in corticosterone levels during murine pregnancy and thus could be the result of increased circulating levels of corticosterone. Support for this possibility include previous findings (47) that glucocorticoids inhibit IL-2 production while enhancing IL-4. Also, these alterations in cytokine production that associate with immunosuppression as discussed above could partially account for the decreased ability of pregnant mice to resist infection with parasites (48). Additional substances that have been implicated in the reduced immune responsiveness of the mother during pregnancy include α-fetoprotein, placental proteins, early pregnancy factor, human chorionic gonadotropin (hCG), corticosteroids, estrogens, androgens and progresterone (49-52).

The feto-placental unit might secrete Th2 cytokines in order to divert the maternal immune response away from damaging Th1-mediated cellular immune responses. As mentioned above, Th1-type responses could lead to excessive uterine NK cell activation, which could, in turn, damage trophoblast tissue and compromise fetal survival. Experimental evidence for this hypothesis came from tissue culture experiments (52) where tissue from murine feto-placental unit (unstimulated decidual cells) as well as maternal lymphoid tissue (con A -stimulated spleen cells) from various stages were cultured from 1 to 24 hours. It was found that decidual cell cultures spontaneously released IL-4, IL-5 and IL-10 during all three trimesters of pregnancy with peak values occurring only 1 hour after establishing the cultures. INF-g was present in barely detectable levels only in the earliest phase of gestation. In general the ratio of Th2 to Th1 cytokines is dramatically increased compared to ConA-stimulated spleen cells. Thus the IL-4/INF-g ratio in unstimulated day 12 decidual cell supernatants was 614 which is 200-fold greater than the ratio of 3 found in supernatants of ConA-stimulated spleen cells. It remains to be determined whether a Th2 cytokine bias also occurs in normal human pregnancy. However, the important lesson from murine pregnancy is that the maternal immune state is most beneficial to reproductive fitness and is maintained by the local secretion of Th2 cytokines, particularly IL-4 and IL-10.

An intriguing question is which mechanisms are brought into play when the Th2 cytokine bias rapidly is reversed at the time of normal delivery and a post-partum maternal shift away from humoral immunity towards cell-mediated immunity occurs. Presently, one can speculate INF-g and TNF-a play a role. The effectiveness of the NK/INF-g/TNF response involved in terminating pregnancy is demonstrated by the ability of INF-g stimulated NK cells to assist in the separation of the placenta from the uterine wall during parturition and the ability of utero-placental TNF-a to initiate uterine contraction via stimulation of the prostaglandins associated with the induction of labor (53-). This scenario is indirectly supported by several observations. In normal human pregnancy and labor, Opsjoen et al. (57) investigated the cytokines TNF-a, IL-1 and IL-6 (cytokines produced by Th2 cell) in extraembryonic coelomic fluid, amniotic fluid, placenta, and maternal and cord serum. Little or no TNF-a, IL-1, or IL-6 was found in coelomic fluid or amniotic fluid in the first trimester. IL-6 appeared in second-trimester fluid. At term TNF-a was present (median 17 pg/ml) and increased with the onset of labor (median 58 pg/ml), as did IL-1 (median 188 to 680 pg/ml) and IL-6 (median 399 to 4800 pg/ml). Maternal serum IL-6 increased during pregnancy with a further increment with the onset of labor. Cord IL-6 also increased with labor but at a lower level. The study suggests all three cytokines may play a role in the onset of normal labor, albeit at a lower level than that seen in preterm labor with infections.

Appreciable numbers of pregnancies that culminate in preterm labor are complicated by infectious processes that involve intrauterine tissues, i.e. extraembryonic fetal membranes and/or decidua (58). Although the association of infection and preterm labor is unfortunate, it may constitute a model system to evaluate key biomolecular processes involved in spontaneous parturition at term. Results from *in vitro* culture studies (62) suggest increased formation of cytokines are involved in the pathogenesis of infection-associated preterm labor. Thus TNF-a was synthesized and secreted into the culture medium by human decidual cells and explants in response to treatment with the bacterial toxin LPS. LPS treatment also caused an increase in PGF2a production by decidual cells and explants. The prostaglandins (principally PGE2a) serve as mediators (uterotonins) of the myometrial contractions that are characteristic of labor. In amnion cells in monolayer culture, TNF-a stimulated PGE2a formation, and TNF-a were cytostatic but not cytolytic in amnion cells. It is likely, therefore, that cytokine formation in macrophage-like decidua may serve a fundamental role in the pathogenesis of preterm labor, including increased prostaglandin formation and premature rupture of the membranes. In a recent study (62) it was found that *in vitro* the production of PGE2 by human decidual cells was inhibited by two cytokines, namely IL-4 and TGF-b1. Because labor is associated with enhanced prostaglandin production, suppression of prostaglandin production may serve to prevent untimely labor.

Thus pregnancy produces immunological changes consistent with a weakening of cell-mediated immunity (Th1 responses) and strengthening of humoral immunity (Th2 responses) with increased production of the immunosuppressive cytokines IL-4 and IL-10 (although only demonstrated in a murine model). The above discussion emphasizes the need for clarification of the Th1/Th2 interactions and their significance for normal pregnancy, autoimmune diseases, and transplantation.

AUTOIMMUNE DISORDERS AND HUMAN PREGNANCY

Based on our understanding of pregnancy related immune changes, pregnancy might be expected to exacerbate or ameliorate a given autoimmune response depending on the humoral or cellular nature of the pathophysiologic process. As noted below, the clinical response of the pregnant individual with an autoimmune syndrome provides testimony to our inadequate understanding of the physiological response of both autoimmunity and pregnancy.

RHEUMATOID ARTHRITIS

Approximately 77% of women with rheumatoid arthritis (a Th1-mediated autoimmune disorder) experience a temporary remission of their symptoms during gestation (63-66). Symptomatic relief is apparent from the first trimester in the majority of cases reported and tends to become more pronounced as pregnancy progresses. Unfortunately the remission is not long lasting: most of the patients experiencing partial or complete remission during pregnancy relapse in the post-partum period. Of 168 individuals involved in 6 studies 81% had relapsed 3 months after delivery. Over 60% of the patients had relapsed within 8 weeks of delivery and almost all before the sixth month. As a consequence patients will need to return to medication and the level of disease activity is similar to the one that preceded pregnancy.

What are the mechanisms involved in the remission relapse phenomena? A recent provocative finding has been the observation that significantly more maternal-fetal disparity in HLA-DR and DQ antigens is found in pregnancies characterized by the remission or improvement of rheumatoid arthritis than in pregnancies characterized by active disease. In 76% of pregnancies characterized by remission or improvement, maternal-fetal disparity occurred in alleles of HLA-DRB1, DQA, and DQB, suggesting that the maternal immunosuppressive response to paternally inherited fetal HLA antigens may play a role in the pregnancy-induced remission of rheumatoid arthritis. The mechanism is likely to be complex and multifactorial, although activation of HLA-DQ restricted immune suppressor mechanisms might be involved (67). For example, HLA class II molecules, in addition to presenting foreign antigens, are also known to present self peptides. In a recent study in which peptides were eluted from mouse MHC class II molecules and sequenced, one of the peptides eluted from the mouse I-A molecule (analogous to human DQ) was a self peptide derived from the I-Ea molecule (analogous to human DRa) (68). Thus peptides derived from HLA class II molecules of the fetus might compete with or displace maternal self peptides therefore creating a shift away from autoimmunity.

MULTIPLE SCLEROSIS

Pregnancy has been reported to have a favorable effect on the course of multiple sclerosis on both a short-and a long-term basis (69,70). Multiple sclerosis (MS) is a chronic, immune-mediated neurologic disease generally acquired during young adulthood. At highest risk for the development of MS are young women in the reproductive age group. They are often faced with difficult decisions regarding childbearing and parenthood following diagnosis. Retrospective studies have reported reduced exacerbation rates and disability during pregnancy. During pregnancy, exacerbation rates are reduced to about half that expected in nonpregnant patients with MS. Of all adverse events surrounding pregnancy and the puerperium, two thirds occur in the postpartum period. The actual risk or worsening post partum for individuals with MS has been estimated at 20% to 40% (71).

Birk et al. (70) reported a prospective study of eight pregnant women with MS. These investigators measured T cell subsets and pregnancy-associated proteins with immunosuppressive properties twice during the pregnancy and twice during the first postpartum year to seek correlation with MS activity through pregnancy. The MS relapse rate during pregnancy was less than half that expected, but 75% of the women experienced a flare in their MS post partum. The calculated annualized relapse rate for the initial 6 months post partum was 10 times the rate observed in the same women during gestation. No differences were found between pregnant patients with MS and pregnant control women for levels of AFP, a2-pregnancy-associated glycoprotein, or pregnancy-associated plasma protein A. There were differences in T cell subsets between patients with MS and controls throughout pregnancy. The number of CD4 T cells in patients with MS at 35 weeks' gestation had increased to a percentage that was not statistically different from pregnant controls (34%±4.6 vs 41%±7.6 n=8, p=NS). The percentage of CD8 T cells was decreased in pregnant patients with MS, although this difference did not reach statistical significance. The CD4/CD8 T cell ratio was higher in the pregnant patients with MS compared with pregnant control women throughout pregnancy and the first six months Clues to effective and safe treatment to control MS may lie in the natural protection that pregnancy provides. The responsible mechanisms therefore need to be clarified in animal and *in vitro* studies.

SYSTEMIC LUPUS ERYTHEMATOSIS

Systemic lupus erythematosis (SLE) is a connective tissue disorder more prevalent in women, especially in those of childbearing age. The female to male ratio is 15:1 during childbearing years. SLE is characterized by the overproduction of autoantibodies, mainly IgG, that are directed against various endogenous antigens. These antibodies are most commonly directed toward nucleic acid (anti-dsDNA), nucleoproteins (ANA, anti-SSA, anti-SSB, anti-Ro), and cell surface antigens. It is likely that Th2 cells are important in amplifying this autoantibody response (72). A suggested model for the initiation and expansion of autoimmune T cell responses to lupus autoantigens involve a model of molecular mimicry whereby autoantigen-presenting B cells are generated by foreign cross-reactive determinants than can, in turn, elicit an autoimmune T cell response with the subsequent induction of Th2 cytokines that sustain autoantibody responses typical of SLE (75). Additional evidence for the involvement of Th2 cytokines in the immunopathogenesis of SLE came from studies reported by Al-Janadi et al. (74), who investigated T cell function and role of IL-4 and IL-6 in B cell induced Ig synthesis from SLE patients. Expression of activation antigens on T cells and monocytes (i.e. CD25, CD38 and CD71) were increased in the circulation of patients with SLE. Patients with prominent clinical presentation like lymphadenopathy had a higher percentage of T cells in blood. Of note was the observation that $CD4^{+}CD29^{+}$ T cell subsets, the major T cells secreting IL-6, were increased in the circulation. These cells provide effective helper function to B cells in their enhanced *in vitro* Ig synthesis in SLE, hence suggesting that overproduction of the Th2 cytokine IL-6 may contribute to the B cell hyperactivity and enhanced antibody synthesis characteristic of this autoimmune disease. Whether pregnancy places the patient with SLE at an increased risk of exacerbation remains debated (75).

AUTOIMMUNE THYROID DISEASES

Graves' disease (hyperthyroidism) to Hashimoto's thyroiditis encompass a disease spectrum because both diseases are associated with cellular and humoral immune system abnormalities and have associations with other autoimmune disorders. It has often been stated that clinical thyroid disease may worsen or present during early pregnancy but tends to ameliorate during late gestation.

The complexity of autoimmune thyroid diseases is clearly demonstrated by a study reported by Grubeck-Loebenstein et al (76). These investigators studied cytokine production in 63 thyroid-derived $CD4^{+}$ T cell clones from four patients with Graves' disease, one with Hashimoto's thyroiditis, and one with non-toxic goiter in order to define whether $CD4^{+}$ T cells from autoimmune and non-autoimmune thyroid tissue could be classified according to their mediator production. No cytokine production assessed at the mRNA level was found in unstimulated clones, whereas 56% of the clones produced IL-2, INF-g, TNF-a, lymphotoxin, IL-6 and TGF-b simultaneously after activation with anti-CD3 plus IL-2. In the remaining 44% usually not more than one cytokine was missing from the complete panel. Cytokine mRNA concentrations varied between different clones and different patients, but not between the diseases from which the clones were originated. There was a significant correlation between IL-6, lymphotoxin, and IL-2 mRNA levels and Th function, which was estimated by the stimulation of thyroid microsomal autoantibody production using autologous peripheral B cells. Thus, intrathyroid T cells from autoimmune and non-autoimmune thyroid disorders cannot be classified according to their cytokine production, unlike *in vitro*-induced mouse T cell clones, where two populations, Th1 and Th2, have been described (76). In patients with autoimmune thyroid diseases it therefore should be noted that single T cells are capable of producing a whole panel of cytokines and thus capable of triggering a multitude of different processes.

MYASTHENIA GRAVIS

Myasthenia gravis is a chronic autoimmune neuromuscular disorder characterized by weakness of the voluntary muscles following repetitive activity. The pathologic mechanism of myasthenia gravis is interference of the conduction of nerve impulses across the myoneuronal junction caused by autoantibodies against the nicotinic acetylcholine receptors (anti-AChR Ab) in skeletal muscle (77-79). The disease prevalence is between 1 in 10,000 to 50,000, with 65% to 70% of affected individuals being women. Myasthenia gravis may coexist with other autoimmune or suspected autoimmune diseases, including Hashimoto thyroiditis, SLE, polymyositis, and sarcoidosis.

The immunopathogenesis of MG involves production of anti-AChR autoantibodies, which have a high affinity and requires AChR specific $CD4^+$ (Th) cells. These Th cells are present in the blood and thymus of MG patients and can be propagated *in vitro* from such tissues by stimulation with AChR antigens which are recognized as specific AChR epitopes presented by MHC class II antigens (DR-restricted). Since anti-AChR Th cells of a particular epitope specificity are involved in the development of MG symptoms, due to their preferential pairing with B cells secreting highly pathogenic antibodies, suggests the involvement of different subpopulations of Th cells. In a recent study Yi et al. (78) investigated Th subsets in T cells isolated from peripheral blood from MG patients. Autoantigen-stimulated IL-4 secretion was found in 55% of the patients. INF-g secretion was found in 86% and IL-2 secretion in 72%. T cells from all patients who responded with increased IL-2 secretion also showed increased INF-g secretion. Stimulated IL-4 secretion was detected both in the presence and absence of stimulated INF-g secretion. Furthermore, a positive correlation was found between the numbers of INF-g- and IL-2 secreting T cells and the numbers of B cells secreting antibodies against AChR. Taken together, the results indicate that AChR stimulated T cells secrete IL-4, INF-g and/or IL-2 in a MHC class II restricted response which is monocyte/macrophage-dependent and hence indicate both Th1/Th2 or Th0 subsets of the T cells are involved in the autoimmune response in MG.

Although an uncommon autoimmune disorder of neuromuscular transmission, myasthenia gravis occurs frequently enough in women of childbearing years to warrant awareness of the disease. The clinical course of myasthenia gravis in pregnancy is unpredictable. Recent studies have demonstrated the following: (1) approximately one-third of patients remain the same symptomatically, one-third improve, and the remaining one-third worsen; (2) the clinical course of one pregnancy does not predict that in subsequent pregnancies; (3) exacerbations occur equally in all three trimesters; and (4) therapeutic termination does not demonstrate consistent benefit in cases of first-trimester exacerbation (79).

AUTOIMMUNE DIABETES

No studies are available regarding the role of pregnancy in exacerbating or ameliorating autoimmune diabetes (IDDM) in humans or animals.

THE NOD PREGNANT MOUSE AS A MODEL OF ISLET TRANSPLANTATION

Since, as noted above, the non-obese diabetic mouse has been shown to be a useful model of pregnancy complicated by diabetes with macrosomia the most common fetal complication, we performed a study of neonatal subcutaneous pancreatic isograft implants into

Table 3. Histological Analysis of Subcutaneous Neonatal Pancreatic Implants

	Control	Pregnant
N	13	11
Score: range	4.5-5	1-4
mean	4.9	2.9
S.D.	0.2	1.2

p-value; $p < 0.0001$.

NOD females primarily to determine *inter ali*a the effect on pup birthweight (80). Outcome variables included graft histology, maternal glycemic status, and birth weight of the offspring. One hundred and thirteen twelve-week-old NOD female mice were randomized into four groups as follows: 1) non-pregnant NOD mice received a sham operation, 2) non-pregnant NOD mice received neonatal pancreatic transplants, 3) pregnant NOD mice received a sham operation and 4) pregnant NOD mice received neonatal pancreatic transplants. Pancreas transplants from 3 neonatal one day old NOD mice were placed via an incision 1-2 mm distal to the ear-skull junction of the recipient. Maternal blood glucose and glycated hemoglobin were determined between day 18 to 20 after the surgery. Histology was graded by two observers using a standardized grading scale. Pups were weighed within 4-6 hours after delivery.

Histological review of the implanted tissue showed that pregnancy was associated with less rejection. The mean rejection score was lower (Table 3) and the pattern of infiltration of lymphoytes was qualitatively and quantitatively different. Whereas nonpregnant animals showed lymphocytic infiltration throughout the grafted tissue, pregnant animals had grafts characterized by less lymphocytic infiltrate that was confined to the perivascular areas.

Pregnant NOD that received transplants (N=29) had significantly lower glucose and glycated hemoglobin (GHb) than sham operated pregnant controls (N=26) (88 ± 18 vs. 162 ± 138 mg/dL, $p<0.01$ for glucose and 2.0 ± 0.4 vs. $3.0 \pm 2.4\%$, $p<0.01$ for GHb) at 18-20 days of gestation.

Controlling for litter size of 8-10 pups (see discussion above on pup birthweight) showed a decrease in birth weight for offspring of transplant recipients versus pregnant controls (1.5 ± 0.1 vs. 1.6 ± 0.1 gm, $p< 0.01$). The prevalence of macrosomic pups as defined above was significantly lower in the offspring of recipients of transplants (Table 4).

These observations reaffirm that glucose influences birth weight in NOD mice. More important for transplantation studies, these findings document that transplantation during gestation is feasible and provides three differential means of quantifying efficacy and toxicity: 1) glycemia as quantified by glucose levels and glycated proteins, 2) graft histology, and 3) outcome of pregnancy with birthweight being an especially sensitive variable to changes in glycemia. The subcutaneous site of transplantation is advantageous because of its ease of access, the benign nature of the procedure, and the comparability to our human protocols.

Table 4. Effect of Subcutaneous Neonatal Pancreatic Transplantation on the Prevalence of Macrosomia (Birth Weight > 1.9 g, Litter Size of 8-10 Pups)

	Pregnant + Sham	Pregnant + Transplant
Total # Pups	117	123
% Macrosomic	10	3
# Macrosomic*	12	4

*p-Value≤0.03.

While it has been known for some time that fetal pancreatic transplants can reverse diabetes (81,82) and fetal rat islets transplanted at day 15 of gestation normalize maternal and pup blood glucose levels in STZ-induced diabetic rats (83,84). There have been few studies of pancreatic transplantation in NOD mice and none to our knowledge during gestation.

Others have examined the effect of a single STZ administration on subsequent islet isograft and allograft survival in NOD mice (85,86). Young prediabetic NOD mice were rendered diabetic by STZ administration and transplanted with islet isografts 8-11 days later. The earliest loss of islet function occurred on postgraft day 49. In sharp contrast, 15 of 16 isografts in spontaneously diabetic mice were destroyed within 17 days postgrafting (not unlike our results above). A comparison of the age of islet isograft destruction in STZ-induced diabetic NOD mice with the course of diabetes development in the NOD mouse colony clearly showed that STZ administration at the prediabetic stage led to a significant delay of diabetes onset in isografts. However, the degree of prolongation induced by STZ was much smaller compared with that induced by anti-lymphocyte serum (ALS). In vitro mixed lymphocyte culture experiments showed that spleen cells of mice given STZ exhibited time-dependent reduction of their alloantigen reactivities. These results demonstrate the feasibility of transplantation in the NOD in an immunomodulated environment.

The above investigations also attest to the rapid rejection of transplanted tissue into the NOD without immunomodulation. We found, for example (Walker CL, Peterson CM, unpublished observations), that the T1/2 histological rejection of an allograft (C57) placed under the kidney capsule of NOD mice to be 7-9 days. Kai et al. using isografted adult pancreatic tissue placed under the kidney capsule found rapid rejection that could be prevented with FK506 (86). Purcell and colleagues have studied segmental pancreas iso- and allografts using a vascular anastomosis technique in NOD mice (87,88). They also confirmed the rapid rejection of isografts (9.5 days) in this model. Nomura and colleagues have used the NOD mouse to document that syngeneic islets transplanted into the thymus of newborn mice have enhanced survival (89). Weber et al. showed that ultraviolet-B irradiation plus encapsulation can enhance survival of donor islets (90). These studies confirm the need for immunomodulation protocols to enhance graft survival in NOD mice and place our findings in pregnant animals in striking perspective.

Wang and colleagues used an isograft protocol in NOD mice to determine whether CD4+ cells are the helper cells for the activation of cytotoxic CD8+ cells that directly destroy islet beta cells in type I diabetes (91). Their data challenged this interpretation because of two observations: (1) Destruction of syngeneic islet grafts by spontaneously diabetic NOD mice (disease recurrence) was CD4+ and not CD8+ T-cell dependent. (2) Disease recurrence in islet tissue grafted to diabetic NOD mice was not restricted by islet major histocompatibility complex antigens. From these observations they propose that islet destruction depends on CD4+ effector T cells that are restricted by major histocompatibility complex antigens expressed on NOD antigen-presenting cells. Both of these findings argue against the CD8+ T cell as a mediator of direct islet damage. They therefore postulate that islet damage in the NOD mouse results from a CD4+ T-cell-dependent inflammatory response. Thus their data would attest to the importance of Th1/Th2 mechanisms as a potential means of ameliorating autoimmunity or graft rejection and support the utility of transplantation studies during gestation in NOD mice.

STUDIES OF FETAL ISLET TRANSPLANT IN HUMANS

During our studies of subcutaneous fetal islet transplantation in humans three women have become pregnant. These three women's C-peptide responses have had the most dramatic response following the procedure described in detail elsewhere in this volume. The mean C-peptide value (± standard deviation) at baseline was 0.02±0.035 ng/ml and rose to 0.32±0.028 ng/ml, $p = 0.04$. This represents a mean delta increase in C-peptide peak response in the fasting state of 0.3 ng/ml at the three month time point. The full Sustacal challenge test was not given to the pregnant participants because of the fear of hyperglycemia and potential harm to the infant. When these women's C-peptide levels were expressed as a linear regression line over the first three months of gestation the rise was also significant : $p < 0.001$, $r = 0.878$.

The insulin requirements of these three women were half of the requirement expected for the gestational week. The insulin requirement for 12 weeks of gestation is 0.6-0.8 units per kilogram per day (92). All three transplanted women had insulin requirement of 0.34 to 0.41 units per kilogram per day.

The above responses on the part of women who became pregnant during our studies of fetal islet cell transplantation provide several important pieces of information. The transplantation of fetal islet tissue did not appear to inhibit the ability to conceive. The fetal islet transplant procedure thus continues to be viewed as benign. The C-peptide response of the pregnant women indicates that the graft hormonal response may benefit from the pregnant milieu. Thus pregnancy may provide a model for the enhancement of graft protocols in the nonpregnant individual as well. Whether and how pregnancy might enhance graft success via vascular, hormonal, growth factor, and/or immunologic responses warrants further consideration and study.

HORMONES OF PREGNANCY THAT MAY FACILITATE FETAL ISLET CELL TRANSPLANTATION

With (and perhaps antecedent to) implantation of the trophoblast, the production of pregnancy related hormones begins. These hormones immediately alter the metabolism of nutrients to shift the priority of metabolic products towards the growing fetus. A buffering mechanism must be initiated early in pregnancy to prevent the mother from suffering deleterious hypoglycemia between feedings as her reserves continue to flow to the fetal placental unit. Maternal glucose homeostasis is sustained by an intricate interplay of maternal hormones designed *inter alia* to increase fat storage, decrease energy expenditure and delay glucose clearance. In addition, fetal needs are met through the fetal control of nutrients mediated via a variety of placental and fetal hormones. Hormonal messages from the conceptus not only affect metabolic processes but also uteroplacental and whole body blood flow, cellular differentiation, and immune response.

Immediately after ovulation, the corpus luteum is converted to make 17OH- progesterone. Luteinizing hormone from the pituitary is necessary to keep the corpus luteum functioning. Once conception and subsequent implantation occurs, human chorionic gonadotropin (hCG) stimulates the corpus luteum's production of 17OH- progesterone until the placental production of steroids is adequate. Thus, hCG is needed only for the first 12 weeks of gestation as the corpus luteum is needed only during these early phases of placental growth (93). HCG does not seem to have any effect on glucose homeostasis. Other hormones which do promote production of glucose are therefore urgently needed early in pregnancy.

The adult ovary is capable of making steroids directly from acetate, but this capability is not true of the placenta. Estrogen formation by the placenta is dependent on precursors which reach it from both the fetal and maternal compartments. To form estrogens, the placenta aromatizes androgens coming primarily from the fetus. The fetal adrenal gland provides dihydro-epiandrosterone (DHEA) which proceeds through a series of hydroxyla-

Table 5. Sequential Rise and Potency of the Diabetogenic Hormones of Pregnancy

Hormone	Onset of Elevation (Days)	Peak Elevation (Weeks)	Relative Diabetogenic Potency on a Scale of 1=Weak to 5=Strong
Estradiol	32	26*	1
Prolactin	36	10	2
Human Chorionic Somatomammotropin	45	26*	3
Cortisol	50	26*	5
Progesterone	65	32†	4

*Optimal time to screen for gestational diabetes.
†Optimal time to re-screen for gestational diabetes in those women who screen negative at 26 weeks.

tions and then double bond formation or aromatization into estrone and 17-beta estradiol. In addition, some of the fetal DHEA undergoes 16-alpha hydroxylation in the fetal liver and/or fetal adrenal gland to become 16 alpha hydroxy-dihydro-epiandrosterone (HDHEA) sulfate that is cleaved in the placenta to 16-alpha OH HDHEA and aromatized to estriol (94). The time course of the appearance of estrogens during pregnancy are listed in Table 5. As can be seen, estrogens rise within 35 days of conception.

Estrogens have weak anti-insulin properties. Table 5 also ascribes relative diabetogenic properties to hormones of interest and Table 6 their less understood immunologic activity. In each table, estrogen has a relative potency of 1 on a scale of 1 to 5. Their major gluconeogenic property is derived from their stimulating effect on liver production of cortisol binding globulin (CBG). As CBG is increased, the maternal adrenal gland secretes more cortisol to compensate for the elevated CBG and will produce in addition, enough cortisol to increase the level of free cortisol. Hypercortisolemia causes insulin resistance, delayed glucose clearance, and thus more available glucose for fetal use. In Table 2, the appearance of cortisol is timed to contribute to the rising demand for glucose and presents with the strongest diabetogenic property.

In contrast to estrogen, progesterone production by the placenta is independent of the quantity of precursor available, uteroplacental perfusion, fetal well being or even the presence of a live fetus. Thus, progesterone is not useful as a marker of impending abortion (95). The majority of placental progesterone is derived from cholesterol which is readily available. The placenta does not make 17OH- progesterone until the 32nd week when it starts to metabolize progesterone. Once the corpus luteum deteriorates, progesterone is the major form of the hormone. Progesterone has a direct effect on glucose metabolism (96). When

Table 6. Hormones of Pregnancy

	Vascular Effect	Growth Promoting Effect	Relative Immunologic Potency on a scale of 1=Weak to 5=Strong
Estradiol	+	?	1
Androgens	?	?	1-2
Prolactin	?	?	2-5
Human Chorionic Somatomammotropin	?	++	1
Cortisol	+	?	5
Progesterone	+	?3	
Transforming Growth Factor ß	+	+	5
Early Pregnancy Factor	?	?	4

progesterone is administered to normal fasting women, the serum insulin concentration rises while glucose remains unchanged. In monkeys, progesterone increases both the early and total insulin secretory responses to glucose (97). Progesterone does not peak until the 32nd week of gestation. Those women who screen negative on a glucose screening test for gestational diabetes at 26 weeks may not pass the test at 32 weeks due to the diabetogenic properties of progesterone (a 4 on the scale of 1-5) (Table 5). Many workers feel that progesterone is the main element responsible for immunosuppression in early gestation (Table 6) and that the serial evaluation in the luteal phase of this steroid may be used as a marker of achieved implantation (97,98). Estrogen and progesterone appear synergistic in their immunomodulatory properties. Falling levels of progesterone might lead to a loss of the pregnancy through either immunologic or metabolic mechanisms (99).

Two other pregnancy related hormones warrant discussion: prolactin (hPRL) and human chorionic somatomammotropin (hCS). Barberia and Associates(100) showed that the initial rise in hPRL in pregnancy occurs within a few days after the estradiol levels start to increase above nonpregnant levels (30 to 33 days after the LH peak), whereas the rise in hPRL levels above the nonpregnancy luteal phase levels occurs 32 to 36 days after the LH peak (Table 6). The estrogen level seems to initiate the "turning on" of prolactin. Without a rise in estrogen with a resultant rise in prolactin levels, spontaneous abortion seems imminent (95).

WHAT IS THE FUNCTION OF PROLACTIN SO EARLY IN PREGNANCY?

Prolactin is so named because it is necessary for lactation, a third trimester event. What is a lactation promoting hormone doing in the first few days of pregnancy? Some researchers feel that prolactin is "luteotropic" and works in concert with hCG to nourish the corpus luteum (101). Others (102) have suggested that prolactin enhances cell-to-cell communication among the beta-cells in pancreatic islets. These investigators have shown a ten-fold increase in beta cell coupling, independent of glucose stimulation. Thus, prolactin may be necessary early in pregnancy to stimulate both maternal and fetal beta cell hypertrophy. Others hypothesize that prolactin increases insulin resistance and thus potentiates glucose transfer to the fetus. In Table 5, prolactin has a diabetogenic potency of 2 on the scale of 1-5.

As shown in Table 6, prolactin also has profound effects on the immune system (103). Both humoral and cell-mediated immunity are compromised in hypophysectomized rats. The reintroduction of prolactin to these animals restores their immune function. Prolactin receptors have been identified on the membranes of white blood cells, and lymphocytes have been shown to secrete prolactin. Cyclosporin A directly competes with prolactin for binding to these receptors. This may be one mechanism of the immunosuppressive action of cyclosporin A. In addition to diminished levels, prolactin excess may also result in immunocompromise. This has been demonstrated in lactating female and prolactin-treated male rats, as well as hyperprolactinemic humans. Prolactin abnormalities have also been described in a number of immunologic disorders, including systemic lupus erythematosus, adjuvant arthritis, experimental allergic encephalomyelitis, and autoimmune uveitis and thyroid disease. Dopaminergic agents that suppress serum prolactin are now being used in clinical trials to treat a number of autoimmune diseases and to prevent rejection in organ transplant recipients.

Human chorionic somatomammotropin (hCS) is a protein hormone with immunologic epitopes and biologic and growth factor properties similar to pituitary growth hormone (hGH). The original name, human placental lactogen, was so named because of its lactogenic properties in animals, however such properties in women have not been confirmed. Josimovich et al (104,105) found that hCS has luteotropic properties which would explain the rise of this hormone so early in pregnancy. Similar to prolactin, hCS has an effect on glucose metabolism. HCS rates a potency of 3 in the diabetogenic property scale (Table 5).

HCS does have growth hormone-like effects on tibial epiphysial growth, body weight gain, and sulfate uptake by costal cartilage in the hypophysectomized rat, although the effective dose required is 100 to 200 times that of growth hormone (104). As noted elsewhere in this volume, this hormone may be an important component of the maternal serum used for the culture of human fetal islets.

The effects of hCS on fat and carbohydrate metabolism are similar to those following treatment with growth hormone. There is inhibition of peripheral glucose uptake and stimulation of insulin release. A comparable maximal increase in plasma free fatty acids occurs following administration of hCS or hGH in hypopituitarism. In addition, infusion of hCS into an hypophysectomized, diabetic man caused the blood glucose to rise four-fold above baseline (105-108).

The final class of hormone that warrants discussion comprises androgens (109). As noted above, androgens are increased during gestation. As for a number of autoimmune syndromes, the penetrance of autoimmune diabetes in NOD mice is greater among females than males. A role for androgens is suggested in that diabetes can be prevented by dihydrotestosterone (DHT) implants. Since diabetes is T-cell mediated, we examined whether or not DHT could affect T-cells directly (R. B. Pearce, K. Healey, B. Formby, and C. M. Peterson unpublished observations). We found that cytokines released by Con A activated NOD splenocytes were differentially altered in vitro by physiological levels of DHT. Following a 60-minute exposure to 10^{-7} M DHT and 24-hr culture in the presence of 4 μg/ml Con A, the levels of immunoreactive and bioactive IL-2 rose 22% while the level of immunoreactive IL-4 fell 39% ($P<0.0001$). DHT, over a wide range of concentrations, had no effect on the level of high-affinity IL-2R. Another unusual feature of the NOD strain is an elevation of the percentage of CD4+ peripheral blood lymphocytes (PBL). The mean percent CD4+ for NOD is 48.6 ± 7.7% compared to 26.8 ± 3.2% for C57BL/6 and 30.3 ± 9.3% for the non-obese, non-diabetic (NON) strain. Within the NOD strain, female levels are higher than males (50.2 ± 5.2 vs. 44.0 ± 6.6; $P = 0.008$). Amongst [NOD X (NON X NOD)F1]BC1 segregants we observed that only females showing high levels of CD4+ T cells at an early age (4 weeks) went on to develop diabetes later in life (>12 weeks). Thus this T-cell phenotype, like diabetes, is sexually dimorphic and links with diabetic gene(s) and/or is necessary for the diabetic process. In vivo, DHT lowered the percentage of CD4+ PBL to male-like levels. Thus DHT may exert some of its effects on the immune system by modulating Th1 and Th2 pathways as well as a T cell frequency (Tlf) locus in the NOD mouse. The effect of pregnancy on T cell frequency has not been evaluated.

In summary, the hormonal changes in pregnancy are classically viewed as a serial rise in hormones intended to maintain a constant glucose supply to the fetus. These hormones also have immunologic, vascular, and growth promoting consequences. As the fetal metabolic requirements increase, the gluconeogenic properties and concentration of hormones rise. The order of hormonal presentation in pregnancy does appear to be inverse to their relative gluconeogenic property which in turn tends to parallel systemic immune effects (Tables 5 and 6). The first hormone, human chorionic gonadotropin has no gluconeogenic and minimal if any immunologic effect. Cortisol, a relatively late appearing hormone, has the most potent gluconeogenic effect as well as potent immunosuppressive effects.

CONCLUSION

Studies in the NOD mouse and humans provide evidence that pregnancy may provide a fortuitous environment for the transplantation of fetal islet cells into an insulin dependent diabetic recipient. The availability of numerous animal models of diabetes and pregnancy makes this hypothesis amenable to rigorous scientific inquiry. While still rudimentary, our understanding of the immunological, vascular, hormonal, and growth factor changes of pregnancy give promise that further studies of these factors will be rewarded with improved approaches to fetal islet transplantation. Studies of pregnancy may provide not only improved methods of handling tissue prior to implantation to improve growth and secretory capacity but also an improved understanding of the optimum recipient milieu.

REFERENCES

1. Neufeld, N.D., 1986, Gestational diabetes and congenital anomalies. IN: Jovanovic, L., Peterson, C.M., Fuhrmann, K., eds. *Diabetes and Pregnancy* New York, Prager 37-50.
2. Baird, J.D., Aerts, L., 1987, Research priorities in diabetic pregnancy today: the role of animal models, *Biology of the Neonate* 51:119-127.
3. Freinkel, N., 1980, Of pregnancy and progeny, *Diabetes* 29:1023-1035.
4. Eriksson, U.J., 1988, Importance of genetic predisposition and maternal environment for the occurrence of congenital malformations in offspring of diabetic rats, *Teratology* 37:365-374.
5. Eriksson, U.J., Karlsson, M.G., Styrud, J., 1987, Mechanisms of congenital malformations in diabetic pregnancy, *Biology of the Neonate* 51:113-118.
6. Eriksson, U.J., Borg, L.A., Forsberg, H., Styrud, J., 1991, Diabetic embryopathy. Studies with animal and in vitro models, *Diabetes* 40 Suppl 2:94-98.
7. Sadler, T.W., Horton, W.E., Hunter, E.S., 1986. Mechanisms of diabetes-induced congenital malformations in infants of diabetic mothers as studied in mammalian embryo culture. In: Jovanovic, L., Peterson, C.M., Fuhrmann, K. eds. *Diabetes and Pregnancy*. New York: Prager, 51-71.
8. Freinkel, N., 1988. Diabetic embryopathy and fuel-mediated organ teratogenesis: lessons from animal models, *Hormone and Metabolic Research* . 20:463-475.
9. Dickinson, J.E., Meyer, B.A., Chmielowiec, S., and Palmer, S.M., 1991, Streptozocin-induced diabetes mellitus in the pregnant ewe, *American Journal of Obstetrics and Gynecology* 165:1673-1677.
10. Lips, J.P., Jongsma, H.W., and Eskes, T.K., 1988, Alloxan-induced diabetes mellitus in pregnant sheep and chronic fetal catheterization, *Laboratory Animals* 22:16-22.
11. Thompson, S.C., and Mandel, T.E., 1990, Fetal pig pancreas. Preparation and assessment of tissue for transplantation, and its in vivo development and function in athymic (nude) mice, *Transplantation*, 49:571-581.
12. Levy, J., Gavin, J.R. 3rd, Scott, M.J., and Avioli, L.V., 1987, Mineral homeostasis in neonates of streptozotocin-induced noninsulin-dependent diabetic rats and in their mothers during pregnancy and lactation. *Bone* 8:1-6.
13. Johansson, B., Meyerson, B., and Eriksson, U.J., 1991, Behavioral effects of an intrauterine or neonatal diabetic environment in the rat, *Biology of the Neonate* 59:226-235.
14. Thomas, C.R., Eriksson, G.L., and Eriksson, U.J.,1990, Effects of maternal diabetes on placental transfer of glucose in rats, *Diabetes* 39:276-282.
15. Neufeld, N.D., Corbo, L., Stoddard, A., Klein, A.H. and Tadokoro, N., 1989, Oxygen consumption and guanosine diphosphate binding by fetal brown adipose tissue in diabetic pregnancy, *Metabolism: Clinical and Experimental,* 38:831-836.
16. Canavan, J.P., Holt, J., and Goldspink, D.F., 1991, Growth of the rat foetal liver in gestational diabetes. Comparative Biochemistry and Physiology. a: Comparative Physiology, 99:473-476.
17. McDowell, E.M., Coleman, W.P., De Santi, A.M., Newkirk, C., and Strum, J.M., 1990, Development of the conducting airway epithelium in fetal Syrian golden hamsters during normal and diabetic pregnancies, *Anatomical Record*, 227:111-123.
18. Gauguier, D., Bihoreau, M.T., Ktorza, A., Berthault, M.F., and Picon, L., 1990, Inheritance of diabetes mellitus as consequence of gestational hyperglycemia in rats. *Diabetes*, 39:734-739.

19. Van Assche, F.A., Aerts, L., and Verhaeghe, J., 1988, Fetal consequences of maternal diabetes. IN: Weiss, P.A.M., Coustan, D.R., Eds. *Gestational Diabetes*. Vienna: Springer-Verlag, 153-160.
20. Aerts, L., Sodoyez-Goffaux, F., Sodoyez, J.C., Malaisse W.J., and Van Assche, F.A., 1988, The diabetic intrauterine milieu has a long-lasting effect on insulin secretion by B cells and on insulin uptake by target tissues. Am. J. Obstet. Gynecol. 159:1287-1292.
21. Susa, J.B., Boylan, J.M., Sehgal, P., and Schwartz, R., 1990, Impaired insulin secretion in the neonatal rhesus monkey after chronic hyperinsulinemia in utero. *Proc. of the Society for Exper.Biol.and Med.*, 194:209-15.
22. Susa, J.B., McCormick, K.L., Widness, J.A., Singer, D.B., Oh, W., Adamsons, R., and Schwartz, R., 1979, Chronic hyperinsulinemia in the fetal rhesus monkey. *Diabetes* 18: 1058-1063.
23. Susa, J.B., Gruppuso, P.A., Widness, J.A., Domenech, M., Sehgal, P., and Schwartz R.,1984. Chronic hyperinsulinemia in the fetal rhesus monkey: Effects of physiologic hyperinsulinemia on fetal substrates, hormones, and hepatic enzymes. *Am .J. Obstet. Gynecol.* 150:415-420.
24. Kaufmann, R.C., Khosho, F.K., Verhulst, S.J., and Amankwah, K.S. 1991.Effect of pregnancy on glucose metabolism in glucose intolerant 'BB' Wistar rats. *American Journal of Perinatology*, 8:11-14.
25. Brownscheidle, C.M., 1986, The BB rat: Type I diabetes and congenital malformations. IN: Jovanovic, L., Peterson, C.M., Fuhrmann, K. eds. *Diabetes and Pregnancy*. New York: Prager, 15-36.
26. Brownscheidle, C.M., Wootten, B., Mathieu, M.H., Davis, D.L., and Hofmann, I.A. 1983, The effects of maternal diabetes on fetal maturation and neonatal health. Metabolism 32 (Suppl 1):148-155.
27. Formby, B., Schmid-Formby, F., Jovanovic, L., and Peterson, C.M. 1987, The offspring of the female diabetic "nonobese diabetic" (NOD) mouse are large for gestational age and have elevated pancreatic insulin content: a new animal model of human diabetic pregnancy. *Proc. of the Society for Exper. Biol. and Med.* 184:291-4.
28. Todd, J.A., Altman, T.J., Cornall, R.J., Ghosh, S., Hall, J.R.S., Hearne, C.M., Knight, A.M., Love, J.M., McAleer, M.A., Prinws, J-B., Rodrigues, N., Lathrop, M., Pressey, A., DeLarato, N.Y.H., Peterson, L.B., and Wicker LS. 1991, Genetic analysis of autoimmune type 1 diabetes mellitus in mice. *Nature* 351:542-47.
29. Prochazka, M., Serreze, D.V., Frankel, W.N., Leiter, E.H. 1992, NOR/Lt mice: MHC matched diabetes-resistant control strain for NOD mice. *Diabetes* 41:98-106.
30. Siddiqi, T.A., Miodovnik, M., Mimouni, F., Clark, E.A., Khoury, J.C., and Tsang, R.C. 1989, Biphasic intrauterine growth in insulin-dependent diabetic pregnancies. *J. of the Am. Coll. of Nutri.* 8:225-234.
31. Bevier, W.C., Jovanovic-Peterson, L., Formby, B., and Peterson, C.M., 1994, Maternal hyperglycemia is not the only cause of macrosomia: Lessons learned from the non-obese diabetic mouse. *Am. J. Perinatol.* 11:51-56.
32. Schroeder, R., Devaskar, U., Holtzclaw, L., deMello, D., and Devaskar, S., 1990 Maternal diabetes regulates placental glucose transporter (GT) gene expression. *Clinical Resrch.* 38:804A.
33. Hrubec, Z., Robinette, C.D., 1984, The study of human twins in medical research. *N. Engl. J. Med.* 310:435.
34. Kramer, M.S.,1987, Determinants of low birth weight: methodological assessment and meta-analysis. *Bull. W.H.O.* 65:683-737.
35. Kaufmann, R.C., Amankwah, K.S., Colliver, J.A., and Arbuthnot, J., 1987, Diabetic pregnancy. The effect of genetic susceptibility for diabetes on fetal weight. A*m. J. of Perinatol.* 4:72-74.
36. Sasaki, K., 1987, Studies of fetal lung maturity of maternal spontaneous diabetes in the Chinese hamster. Nippon Sanka Fujinka Gakkai Zasshi. *Acta Obstetrica et Gynaecologica Japonica*, 39:1607-14 .
37. Mosman, T.R., and Coffman, R.L., 1989, Th1 and Th2 cells: Different pattern of cytokine secretion leads to different functional properties. *Ann. Rev. Immunol.* 7:145.
38. Mosman, T.R., and Coffman, R.L., 1987, Two types of mouse helper T-cell clone. *Immunol. Today* 8:223
39. Dudley, D.J., Chen, C-L., Mitchell, M.D., Dajres, R.A., Araneo B.A., 1993, Adaptive immune responses during murine pregnancy: Pregnancy-induced regulation of lymphokine production by activated T lymphocytes. *Am. J. Obstet. Gynecol.* 168:1155.
40. Clark, D.A., Falbo, M., Rowley, R.B., Banwatt, D., and Stedronska-Clark, J., 1988, Active suppression of host-vs-graft reaction in pregnant mice. IX. Soluble suppressor activity obtained from allopregnant mouse decidua that blocks the cytolytic effector response to IL-2 is related to transforming growth factor-b. *J Immunol.* 141:3833.
41. Fiorentino, D.F., Bond, M.W., and Mosman, T.R., 1989, Two types of mouse T helper cell. IV. Th2 clones secret a factor that inhibits cytokine production by Th1 clones. *J. Exp. Med.* 170:2081.
42. Lin, H., Mosmann, T.R., Guilbert, L., Tuntipapitat, S., and Wegmann, T.G.,1993, et al: Synthesis of T helper 2-type cytokines at the maternal-fetal interface. *J. Immunol.* 151:4562.

43. Chaouat, G.E., Menu, E., Clark, D.A., Dy, M., Minkowsk, M., and Wegmann, T.G., 1990, Control of fetal survival in CBAxDBA/2 mice by lymphokine therapy. *J. Reprod. Fertil.* 89:447.
44. Drake, B.L., and Head, J.R., 1989, Murine trophoblast can be killed by lymphokine-activated killer cells. *J. Immunol.* 143:9.
45. Robertson, S.A., Mayrhofer, G., and Seamark, R.F. 1992, Uterine epithelial cells synthesize granulocyte-macrophage-stimulating factor (GM-CSF) and interleukin-6 (IL-6) in pregnant and non-pregnant mice. *Biol. Reprod.* 46:1069.
46. Holland, D., Bretscher, P., and Russell, A.S., 1984, Immunologic and inflammatory responses during pregnancy. *Clin. Lab. Immunol.* 14:177.
47. Boumpas, D., 1993, Glucocortoid therapy for immune-mediated diseases: Basic and clinical correlates. *Ann. Intern. Med.* 119:198.
48. Luft, B.J., and Remington, J.S., 1984. Effect of pregnancy on augmentation of natural killer activity by corynebacterium parvum and toxoplasma gondii. *J. Immunol.* 132:2375.
49. Madden, J.D., Siiteri, P.K., and MacDonald, P.C., 1976, The pattern and rates of metabolism of maternal plasma dehydroepiandrosterone sulfate in human pregnancy. *Am. J. Obstet. Gynecol.* 125:915.
50. Asibey-Berko, E., Thomas, J., and Stricker, R.C., 1986, 3b-Hydroxy-steroid dehydrogenase in human placental microsomes and mitochondria: co-solubilization of androstene and pregnene activities. *Steroids* 47:351.
51. Szekeres-Bartho, J., Varga, P., Kinsky, R., and Chaou, A.T., 1990, Progesterone mediated immunosuppression and the maintenance of pregnancy. *Rsrch. in Immunology.* 175-181.
52. Wegmann, T.G., Lin, H., Guilbert, L., and Mesnamm, T.R., 1993, Bidirectional cytokine interactions in the maternal-fetal relationship: Is successful pregnancy a Th2 phenomen? *Immunol. Today.*14:353.
53. Chen, H.L., Yang, Y.P., HU, X.L., Velavarthi, K.K., Fishbach, and Hunt, J.S., 1991, Tumor necrosis factor alpha mRNA and protein are present in human placental and uterine cells at early and late stages of gestation. *Am. J. Pathol.* 139:327.
54. Austgulen, R., Liabakk, N.B., Brockhaus, M., and Espevik, T., 1992, Soluble TNF receptors in amnionic fluid and urine from pregnant women. *J. Reprod. Immunol.* 22:105.
55. Austgulen, R., Espevik, T., and Mescei, R., 1992, Expression of receptors for tumor necrosis factor in human placenta at term. *Acta. Obstet. Gynecol. Scand.* 71:417.
56. Austgulen, R., Johnsen, H., Kjollesdal, A.M., Liabakk, N.P., and Espevik, T., 1993, Soluble receptors for tumor necrosis factor: occurrence in association with normal delivery at term. *Obstet. Gynecol.* 82:343.
57. Opsjin, S.L., Wathen, N.C., Tingulstad, S., Wiedswang, G., Sundan, A., Waage, A., and Austgulen, R., 1993, Tumor necrosis factor, interleukin-1, and interleukin-6 in normal human pregnancy. *Am. J. Obstet. Gynecol.* 169:397.
58. Wahbeh, C.J., Hill, G.B., Eden, R.D., and Gall, S.A., 1984, Intra-amniotic bacterial colonization in premature labor. *Am. J. Obstet. and Gynecol.* 148:739.
59. Chamberlain, G.,1984, Epidermiology and etiology of the preterm baby. *Clin. Obstet. Gynecol.* 11:297.
60. Casey, M.L., Cox, S., Beutler, B., Ward, R.A., Mand MacDonald, P.L. 1990, Cytokines and infection induced preterm labor. *Fertility and Develop.* 2:499.
61. Novy, M.J., and Liggens, G.C. 1980, Role of prostaglandins, prostacyclin, and thomboxanes in the physiological control of the uterus in parturition. *Sem. Perinatol.* 4:45.
62. Bry, K., and Lappalainen, U., 1994, Interleukin-4 and transforming growth factor-b1 modulate the production of interleukin-1 receptor antagonist and prostaglandin E2 by ducidual cells. *Am. J. Obstet. Gynecol.* 170:1194.
63. Da Silva, J.A., and Spector, T.D.,1992, The role of pregnancy in the course and aetiology of rheumatoid arthritis. *Clin. Rheumatol.* 11:189.
64. Oka, M., and Vainio, U., 1966, Effect of pregnancy on the prognosis and serology of rheumatoid arthritis. *Acta. Rheum. Scand.* 12:47.
65. Ostensen, M., Aune, B., Husby, G., 1983, Effect of pregnancy and hormonal changes on the activity of rheumatoid arthritis. *Scand. J. Rheumatol.* 12:69.
66. Nelson, J.L., Hughes, K.A., Smith, A.G., Nisperoc, B.B., Branchand, A.M., and Hansen, J.A., 1993, Meternal-fetal disparity in HLA class II alloantigens and the pregnancy-induced amelioration of rheumatoid arthritis. *N. Engl. J. Med.* 329:466.
67. Salgame, P., Convit, J., and Bloom, B.R., 1991, Immunological suppression by human CD8 T cells is receptor dependent and HLA-DQ restricted. *Proc. Natl. Acad. Sci.* USA 88:2598.
68. Rudensky, A.Y., Preston-Hurlburt, P., Hong, S.C., Barlow, A., and jareway, C.A., 1991, Sequence analysis of peptides bound to MHC class II molecules. *Nature* 353:622.
69. Duquette, P., Girard, M., 1993, Hormonal factors in susceptibility to multiple sclerosis. *Opinion Neurol. Neurosurg.* 6:195.

70. Birk, K., and Rudick, R., 1986, Pregnancy and multiple sclerosis. *Acta. Neurol.* 43:719.
71. Korn-Lubetzki, I., Kahana, E., and Cooler, G., 1984, Activity of multiple sclerosis during pregnancy and puerperium. *Ann. Neurol.* 16:229.
72. Mamula, M.J., Fatenejad, S., and Craft, J., 1994, B cells process and present lupus autoantigens that initiate autoimmune T cell responses. *J. Immunol.* 152:1453.
73. Mao, C., Osman, G.E., Adams, S., Datta, S.K., 1994, T cell receptor alpha-chain repertoire of pathogenic autoantibody-inducing T cells in lupus mice. *J. Immunol.* 152(3):1462-1470.
74. Al-Janadi, M., and Raziuddin, S., 1993, B cell hyperactivity is a function of T cell derived cytokines in systemic lupus erythematosus. *J. Rheumatol.* 20:1885.
75. Varner, M.W., 1991, Autoimmune disorders and pregnancy. *Sem. Perinatol.* 15:238.
76. Grubeck-Loebenstein, B., Turner, M., Pirich, K., Kassal, H., Londei, M., Waldhausl, W., 1990, CD4+ T-cell clones from autoimmune thyroid tissue cannot be classified according to their lymphokine production. *Scand. J. Immunol.* 32(5):433-440.
77. Protti, M.P., Manfredi, A.A., and Horton, R.M., 1993, Myastenia gravis: recognition of a human autoantigen at the molecular level. *Immunol Today* 14:363.
78. Yi, Q., Ahlberg, R., Pirskanen, R. Lefvert, A.K., 1994, Acetylcholine receptor-reactive T cells in myasthenia gravis: evidence for the involvement of different subpopulations of T helper cells. *J. Neuroimmunol.* 50(2):177-186.
79. Mitchell, P.J., and Bebbington, M., 1992, Myasthenia Gravis in pregnancy. *Obstet. Gynecol.* 80:178.
80. Chen, H-M., Jovanovic-Peterson, L., Desai, T.A., and Peterson, C.M., 1994, Leasons learned from the NOD mouse: Studies of subcutaneous neonatal/fetal islet transplantation. Submitted.
81. Brown, J., Clark, W.R., Molnar, I.G., and Mullen, Y.S., 1976. Fetal pancreas transplantation for reversal of streprozotocin-induced diabetes in rats. *Diabetes*, 25:56-64.
82. Brown, J., Molnar, I.G., Clark, W.R., and Mullen, Y.S., 1974, Control of experimental diabetes mellitus in rats by transplantation of fetal pancreas. *Science* 184:1377-1379.
83. Aerts, L., and Assche, F.A., 1992, Islet transplantation in diabetic pregnant rats normalizes glucose hormeostasis in their offsprings. *J.of Develop. Phys.iol,* 17(6):283-287.
84. Ryan, E.A., Tobin, B.W., Tang, J. and Finegood, D.T., 1993, A new model for the study of mild diabetes during pregnancy. Syngeneic islet-transplanted STZ-induced diabetic rats. *Diabetes*, 42(2):316-323.
85. Takayama, Y., Ichikawa, T., and Maki, T., 1993, Effect of STZ administration on islet isograft and allograft survival in NOD mice. *Diabetes,* 42:324-329.
86. Kai, N., Motojima, K., Shiogama, T., Terada, M., Tamaki, S., Tsunoda, T., and Kanematsu, T., 1992, A study on the timing of immunologic priming in autoimmune insulitis in NOD mice. *Transplan. Proc.*, 24:1040-1041.
87. Purcell, L.J., Mottram, P.L., and Mandel, T.E., 1992, The transplantation of segmental pancreas isografts in onoobese diabetic mice. *Transplant. Proc.* 245:2299.
88. Purcell, L.J., Mottram, P.L., Green, M.K., and Mandel, T.E., 1992, Transplantation of the segmental pancreas in STZ-treated diabetic mice. *Transplant. Proc.* 24;236-237.
89. Nomura, Y., Mullen, Y., and Stein E., 1993, Syngeneic islets transplanted into the thymus of newborn mice prevent diabetes and reduce insulitis in the NOD mouse. *Transplant. Proc.* 25:963-964.
90. Weber, C., Krekun, S., Koschitzky, T., Zabinski, S., D'Agati, V., Hardy, M., and Reemtsma, K., 1991, Prolonged functional survival of rat-to-NOD mouse islet xenografts by ultraviolet-B (UV-B) irradiation plus microencapsulation of donor islets. *Transplant. Proc.* 23:764-766.
91. Wang, Y., Pontesilli, O., Gill, R.G., La Rosa, F.G., and Lafferty, K.J., 1991, The role of CD4+ and CD8+ T cells in the destruction of islet grafts by spontaneously diabetic mice. *Proc. National Acad. of Sci. of the USA*, 88(2):527-531.
92. Jovanovic, L., Druzin, M., and Peterson, C.M., 1981, The effect of euglycemia on the outcome of pregnancy in insulin-dependent diabetics as compared to normal controls. *Am. J. Med.* 71:921-927.
93. Csapo, A.L., Pulkkinen, M.O., and Wiest, W.G., 1973, Effects of luteectomy and progesterone replacement in early pregnant patients. *Am. J. Obstet. Gynecol.* 115:759.
94. Jaffe, R.B., 1978, The Endocrinology of Pregnancy. In: Yen, S.S.C., Jaffee, R.B., eds. *Reproductive Endocrinology: Physiology, Pathophysiology, and Clinical Management.* Philadelphia: WB Saunders, 521-536.
95. Jovanovic, L., Dawood, M.Y., Landesman, R., and Saxena, B.B., 1978, Hormonal profile as a prognostic index of early threatened abortion. *Am. J. Obstet. Gynecol.* 130:274-276.
96. Hiriis-Nielsen, J., Nielsen, V., Molsted-Pedersen, L., and Deckert, T., 1986, Effects of pregnancy hormones on pancreatic islets in organ culture. *Acta-Endocrinol.* (Copenh);lll:336-341.
97. Kalkhoff, R.K., Jacobson, M., and Lemper, D. 1970, Progesterone, pregnancy and the augmented plasma insulin response. *J. Clin. Endocrinol. Metab.,* 31:24.

98. Scarpellini, F., Scarpellini, L., Dino, N., and Benvenuto P., 1993, Progesterone immunosuppressive levels and luteal steroid profiles in the cycles induced with clomiphene citrate. *Clin. and Exper. Obstet. and Gynecol.*, 20:182-188.
99. Kalo-Klein, A., and Witkin, S.S., 1991, Regulation of the immune response to Candida albicans by monocytes and progesterone. Am. J. Obstet.and Gynecol.,164:1351-1354.
100. Barberia, Jr., Whu-Fadil, S., Kletzky, O.A., Nakamura, R.M. and Mishell, D.R., 1975, Serum prolactin patterns in early human gestation. *Am. J. Obstet. Gynecol.*, 121:1107.
101. Ho Yuen, B., Cannon, W., Lewis, J., Sy, L., and Woolley, S., 1980, A possible role for prolactin in the control of human chorionic gonadotropin and estrogen secretion by the fetoplacental unit. *Am. J. Obstet. Gynecol.*, 136:286.
102. Michaels, R.L., Sorenson, R.L., Parsons, J.A., and Sheridan, J.D., 1987, Prolactin enhances cell-to-cell communication among beta-cells in pancreatic islets. *Diabetes*, 36:1098-1103.
103. Reber, P.M., 1993., Prolactin and immunomodulation. Am. J. of Med., 95(6):637-644.
104. Josimovich, J.B. 1971, Placental lactogenic hormone. In: *Endocrinology of Pregnancy*, New York: Harper & Row, 184-196.
105. Josmovich, J.B., and MacLaren, J.A., 1962, Presence in the human placenta and term serum of a highly lactogenic substance immunologically related to pituitary growth hormone. *Endocrinology*, 71:209.
106. Spellacy, W.N., Buhi, W.C., Schram, J.C., Birk, S.A., and McCreary, S.A., 1971, Control of human chorionic somatomammotropin levels during pregnancy. *Obstet. Gynecol.*, 37:567.
107. Kim, Y.J., and Felig, P. 1971, Plasma chorionic somatomammotropin levels during starvation in mid-pregnancy. *J. Clin. Endocrin. Metab.*, 32:864.
108. Gaspard, V.J., Sandront, H.M., Luyckx, A.S., and Lefebvre, P.J. 1975, The control of human placental lactogen (HPL) secretion and its interrelation with glucose and lipid metabolism in late pregnancy. In: Camerini-Davalos, R.H., Coles, H.S., eds. *Early Diabetes in Early Life*, New York:Academic Press 273-278.
109. Medina, K.L., and Kincade, P.W., 1994, Pregnancy-related steroids are potential negative relators of B lymphopoiasis. *Proc. Natl. Acad. Sci.* 91:5382-5386.

11

ENCAPSULATED HUMAN ISLET TRANSPLANT TRIALS IN TYPE I DIABETIC PATIENTS

Patrick Soon-Shiong

Islet Transplant Center
St. Vincents Medical Center
Los Angeles, CA

BACKGROUND

Conventional insulin therapy has not prevented the devastating secondary complications of insulin-dependent diabetes. Diabetes results in significant morbidity and mortality in this country. It is the fifth leading cause of death and is the leading cause of blindness in individuals between 20 and 74 years old, and results in a significantly higher incidence of amputation, stroke, coronary artery disease and renal failure. It is estimated that the direct and indirect cost to the country as a result of diabetes is approximately $18 to 20 billion annually.

The findings of the Diabetes Control and Complication Trial, a landmark multicenter trial designed to examine the hypothesis that secondary complications of diabetes are related to poorly controlled blood sugar, have now convincingly established that maintenance of tight glycemic control (by intensive insulin therapy) prevents secondary complications of diabetes. Tight glycemic control reduced the risk of developing clinically meaningful retinopathy by 34 % to 76%, reduced the progression of diabetic nephropathy and reduced the development of neuropathy.

The levels of glucose control which achieved these benefits were a mean blood glucose of 155mg/dl and HbAlc of 7.2%. Unfortunately, a significant complication of this intensive insulin management was a 2 to 3 fold increased risk of severe hypoglycemic attacks.

The challenge scientists now face is to identify a therapy which will match the outcomes of the DCCT trial but without the dangers of hypoglycemic events, without the risks of a major surgical procedure, and without the morbidity of life-long immunosuppression. Islet transplantation, first reported by Ballinger and Lacy (1), has not lived up to its promise of reversing diabetes. Clinical results have been extremely disappointing. Despite the use of high dose immunosuppression, rejection and graft failure is the usual outcome. It is reasonable to believe that the drugs used for immunosuppressive therapy, which include Cyclosporine and Prednisone, are damaging to allografts, since Prednisone has been shown

Fetal Islet Transplantation
Edited by C. M. Peterson, L. Jovanovic-Peterson, and B. Formby, Plenum Press, New York, 1995

to cause insulin resistence and Cyclosporine toxicity to islets (2,3). While there have been sporadic incidences of normoglycemia and insulin independence in patients receiving islet allografts (4-9), the overall results of intraportal islet allografts have been extremely disappointing. It appears that the major obstacles facing islet transplantation are a combination of failure of cell engraftment, inadequate protection of engrafted islets from damage by the patient's immune system, toxic effects of the drugs used for immunsuppression, and graft rejection.

In view of these formidable obstacles, it is apparent that alternative methods of protecting the islets from the patients' immune system must be found for islet transplantation ever to be relatively successful. Encapsulation of islets in an alginate-based immunoprotective membrane may be such a method, and the preliminary findings of our first patient to have received such a transplant offers a glimpse into the potential of this technology.

The ultimate goal of our research is to establish that intraperitoneal transplanted encapsulated human islets may reverse diabetes in patients with early-onset disease and without the need for life-long immunosuppression. To achieve this goal, several issues need to be addressed including the safety and efficacy of encapsulated human islets, the dose of islets required and the immunoprotectivity of the capsule in non-immunosuppressed patients. These questions are being explored in a step-wise fashion by first examining the safety and efficacy of encapsulated islets transplanted in a dose escalation schedule in Type I diabetic patients with functioning kidney allografts. Once the efficacy of this therapy in this patient population has been established and insight has been gained into the optimal islet dose required, trials will be progressed into early-onset diabetic patients on no immunosuppression.

An objective end-point of the encapsulated islet transplant trials is the demonstration of tight glycemic control achieved by intensive insulin therapy as reported in the DCCT trial (mean blood glucose of 155 mg/dl and HbAlc $\leq$ 7.2%), without the attendant risks of severe hypoglycemic attacks. If encapsulated islet transplantation can result in long-term glycemic control, even with insulin supplementation, but avoid the risks of severe hypoglycemia, then the potential exists that long-term secondary complications of diabetes may be averted, as has been conclusively demonstrated by the DCCT Trial.

PRECLINICAL DATA

The preclinical data leading up to the initiation of the human clinical trials will be described in detail in the overall research plan. Over the course of the past 8 years, the following key issues have been addressed leading our group ultimately to the first human clinical trials of intraperitoneally transplanted encapsulated islets:

- Optimizing methods for organ preservation, islet isolation and islet function.
- Identifying fundamental factors preventing successful reversal of diabetes using the alginate-polyamino acid membrane as it relates to:
  - (i) Underlying cause of fibrosis associated with test failures of microcapsule technology.
  - (ii) Kinetics of insulin release and diffusion characteristics.
  - (iii) Immunoprotectivity characteristics
- Demonstrating the safety and efficacy of encapsulated islets in the large animal model.

Optimizing Methods for Organ Preservation, Islet Isolation and Islet Function

Purity and viability of islets is critical to the success of our clinical trials, and especially so when combined with a biocompatible immunoprotective membrane. We have explored numerous methods for improving islet purity, including the possible utilization of anti-acinar monoclonal antibodies. We identified and partially characterized two blood group-reactive monoclonal antibodies (mAb), CACl and CAC2, with specific binding activity to acinar cells but not islets (10). These are of the IgM subclass, and were found on immunocytochemical analysis to possess broad interspecies cross reactivity, binding to antigens expressed in the acinar tissue of rats, dogs, and man. The antigens that these mAb recognize were glycolipid in nature and thus were not denatured by collagenase digestion of the pancreas. We reported (11) a rapid reproducible method of rat islet purification utilizing magnetic microspheres coated with these antiacinar monoclonal antibodies, and demonstrated excellent islet yields, purity, and function both in vitro and in vivo. Unfortunately, when we applied this technique to human islet isolation, we discovered that islets with residual coatings of acinar cell tissue were contaminated by magnetic beads attached to such tissue, thus rendering the islets inappropriate for clinical application.

We then identified and characterized two monoclonal antibodies, CBL3 and TT62, with specific binding activity to human islets allowing islet identification by fluorescein isothiocyanate-labeled CBL3 and TT62 (12). Again, we found this method not practical with regard to clinical application because of the limitations of cell sorters. Thereafter, we turned our attention to a non-ficoll based purification solution, consisting of an overlayer of RPMI/2% FCS and an underlayer of a benzoic acid derivative, TRIS/HCl, and hydroxyethyl starch, and described the purification of canine and human islets by a simple two-phase aqueous separation method (13). Using this method, we were able to achieve consistent islet purity with excellent function, both in vitro and in vivo. We have subsequently used this method for islet purification in all canine and human clinical trials to date.

Identifying factors which optimize islet yield, purity and function is critical to successful clinical islet transplantation. Our laboratory retrieved and processed fifty-four human pancreata from multicenter donor sources to establish optimal methods for islet isolation. The data base generated from this experience with 54 consecutive islet isolations by the standard method of automated collagenase digestion provided an opportunity to examine the effect of donor age and cold ischemia time (CIT) on islet yield, purity and function. The pancreata ranged widely in donor age (13 to 60, 33.2 ± 1.9 yrs (x ± SE), weight (32 to 96, 60.7 ± 1.9 gms) and CIT (1.5 to 26, 10.1 ± 0.6 hrs), resulting in islet yields ranging from 140 to 6550 islet equivalents/gm with a mean purity of 76%. Good islet function was defined as insulin release >3X basal in response to in vitro glucose stimulation (Stimulation Index). Analysis of the effect of CIT in donor pancreata stratified into three age groups demonstrated no significant difference in islet yield, purity and function from pancreata with CIT ≤ 10 hrs compared to pancreata with CIT hrs (but less than 20 hrs). The effect of donor age in donor pancreata stratified into two CIT groups (≤ 10 hrs. and ≥ 10 hrs.) and analysis of islet yield, purity and function from donors within the three age groups are shown below in Table 1.

From this study we concluded that (1) donor age is an important factor affecting islet yield and function, (2) islet function is significantly better from pancreata from younger (≤ 40 yrs) than from older donors (≥ 40 yrs), islet yields are significantly higher from older (≥ 40 yrs) than from younger donors, and (4) CIT is less critical in affecting islet yield, purity and function if the isolation is performed within 20 hrs of cold storage in UW solution.

Table 1.

	<20 yrs. (n=14)	21-40yrs. (n=21)	40-60 yrs. (n=19)	P
Yield (Islet Eq/gm):	801 ± 132	1586 ± 318	2114 + 35	<0.05*
Purity (%):	79 ± 13.9	76 ± 19.8	73 ± 22.4	>0.05
Stim. Index >3 (% of donors):	82%	67%	45%	<0.05*

IDENTIFYING FUNDAMENTAL FACTORS PREVENTING SUCCESSFUL APPLICATION OF THE ALGINATE POLYAMINO ACID MICROCAPSULE

Biocompatibility

The alginate poly-L-lysine microencapsulation system was invented by Franklin Lim in the late 1970's, and the first report of its application in reversing diabetes was reported in Science in 1980. Further progress in the application of this technology has failed to occur, mainly due to the issue of fibrous overgrowth associated with implanted microcapsules. The underlying cause of this fibrosis has remained a mystery to investigators for the past two decades.

In 1990, we identified an immunologic basis for the fibrotic reaction to implanted microcapsules and discovered that a specific monomer within the alginate polysaccharide (mannuronic acid) was responsible for cytokine stimulation (IL-l and TNF), and thereby fibroblast proliferation. (14,15)

With this insight, we were able to devise a capsule formulation which did not evoke this inflammatory response, and led us to the first proof of principle of this technology in large animal models.

KINETICS OF INSULIN RELEASE

To explore the question of in vivo insulin release, an external jugular catheter model in diabetic rats was established, allowing the study of insulin release from transplanted encapsulated islets in response to a systemic glucose challenge.

We demonstrated that a bioartificial pancreas without any vascular access can respond appropriately to an increase in blood glucose concentration (a systemic glucose challenge), without overshoot hypoglycemia and within a lag lapse compatible with normal physiologic insulin delivery(16).

We further demonstrated the ability of encapsulated human islets in a highly discordant xenograft model to normalize a systemic glucose challenge, and were the first to demonstrate the in vivo correlation of human C-peptide release in rats from intraperitoneally placed encapsulated human islets, coincident with the reduction of serum glucose levels in response to an IV glucose challenge, (17) as shown in Table 2 (8). STZ-induced diabetic Lewis rats were transplanted intraperitoneally with either free (n=5) or encapsulated (n=5) human islets, followed by a ten-day course of oral cyclosporine. In the free islet controls, euglycemia was maintained for only two days.

Table 2. Twelve Days Post-encapsulated Islet Transplant, an IVGTT Showed the Following Glucose and Human C-peptide Levels in the Recipients

Time post-glucose challenge (min)	Glucose (mg %)	Human C-peptide (ng/ml)
0	90 ± 6	1.1 ± 0.4
1	444 ± 54	7.3 ± 7.9
5	256 ± 17	3.9 ± 1.8
10	209 ± 20	4.2 ± 4.4
20	161 ± 22	5.0 ± 4.6
30	141 ± 25	8.9 ± 8.3
60	121 ± 26	3.2 ± 4.1
90	105 ± 31	4.0 ± 5.7

M-values in these recipients were normalized (3.5 ± 0.7) in comparison to normal control rats (3.9 ± 0.4) and in contrast to control untreated diabetic rats (0.4 ± 0.1).

In contrast, the five rats receiving encapsulated islets remained euglycemic (off insulin) for a median of 45 days.

Twelve days post-encapsulated islet transplant, an IVGTT showed the following glucose and human C-peptide levels in the recipients:

K-values in these recipients were normalized (3.5 ± 0.7) in comparison to normal control rats (3.9 ± 0.4) and in contrast to control untreated diabetic rats (0.4 ± 0.1).

To our knowledge, this is the first report that demonstrated the in vivo correlation of human C-peptide released intraperitoneally placed encapsulated human islets, coincident with the reduction of serum glucose levels in response to a glycemic challenge. These data provided important insight to the potential of encapsulated islets transplanted intraperitoneally in our proposed human clinical trials.

IMMUNOPROTECTIVITY

We developed in vitro methods for assessing immunoprotectivity - (18).

It became apparent that the immunoprotective characteristics of a capsule for successful xenograft transplantation required a mechanically stable membrane with very tight porosity. To develop such a membrane, fundamental insights into the properties of alginate as well as that of hydrogels were required.

DEMONSTRATION OF SAFETY AND EFFICACY IN THE CANINE MODEL

Human clinical trials could not proceed until encapsulated islets could be successfully applied in the large animal model.

In 1991, we reported the successful reversal of diabetes in the spontaneous diabetic dog following IP injection of encapsulated islets.

Ten insulin-dependent, spontaneous diabetic dogs (insulin requirement; 1 to 4 units/kg/day; absence of circulating C-peptide; and diabetic K-values of 0.6 ± 0.4) were studied. Islets from mongrel donor pancreata were isolated and transplanted intraperitoneally either as free islet controls (n=3) or microencapsulated islet allografts (n=7). In all seven encapsulated islet recipients, euglycemia was achieved within 24 hrs (serum glucose falling from 304 ± 117 to 116 ± 72 mg/dl). IVGTT performed 14 days post islet transplant demonstrated normalization of K-values changing from a pre-transplant level of 0.6 ± 0.4 to 2.6 ± 0.6. These animals remained euglycemic, without exogenous insulin, for a period of 63 to 172 days, with a median insulin-independence for 105 days. In contrast, recipients receiving free islets rejected their graft within 7 days of implantation. (19)

To assess the safety and efficacy of multiple (IP) retransplants of encapsulated islets in maintaining nomoglycemia in this model, and to evaluate long-term graft function and metabolic control, five dogs were followed for two years, four of which received retransplants. In these retransplant studies, the recipients received a subtherapeutic dose of CsA (30-50 ng/ml HPLC blood level) for 30 days, after which all CsA was discontinued. Euglycemia, independent of any exogenous insulin requirement, was noted for 56, 95, 115, 119 and 172 days following the first transplant in the five recipients. With still ongoing islet function, four recipients were retransplanted to determine if insulin-independence could be safely reestablished. All four became euglycemic within 12 to 48 hours following the second transplant, and maintained this state for 83, 95, 98 and 130 days. There was no statistical difference between the duration of insulin-independence following the first transplant and that of the second. One recipient received a third transplant, and maintained euglycemia for 138 days thereafter. Graft survival was determined in each recipient, by evidence of positive fasting and stimulated C-peptide, as well as significantly improved K-values and HbAlc levels. Based on the last data point of positive C-peptide data at the time of this report, duration of graft survival in these recipients are 228, 269, 550, 641 and 726 days to date. Further evidence of long-term survival was provided by histological evidence of viable islets (positive insulin stain) retrieved from the peritoneal cavity six months post-transplant. (20)

We conclude that encapsulated islets transplanted IP can result in long-term reversal of diabetes in the spontaneous diabetic dog model, even after discontinuation of all immunosuppression and that multiple retransplants are both safe and efficacious. These findings formed the preclinical basis for the human clinical trials, which we initiated in 1993.

INITIATION OF THE FIRST HUMAN CLINICAL TRIALS OF ENCAPSULATED ISLETS

Patient #1

Following FDA and IRB approvals, the first transplant was performed at St. Vincent Medical Center in a 38-year old Type I diabetic male who received an intraperitoneal injection of 10,000 islets per kg. In the six months following this procedure, he demonstrated tight glycemic control with significant improvements in metabolic parameters including HbAlc, glycosylated albumin and values with a significant (≥ 70%) reduction in his insulin requirements. In addition, the patient demonstrated both subjective (loss of pain) and objective evidence of improvement in peripheral neuropathy (improvement of axonal function demonstrated by nerve conduction studies).

In the face of this ongoing islet function, we were granted permission to transplant a further dose of 5,000 islets/kg in this patient to explore the possibility that this supplemental islet dose may render the patient fully insulin independent. Following the transplantation of this second dose, the patient demonstrated a period of euglycemia without the need for any exogenous insulin therapy(21). Details of the fourteen month follow-up of this patient are shown in Table 4.

Patient #2

Our second recipient, a 35-year old female with Type I diabetes for 22 years, received 10,000 islets per kg, injected intraperitoneally. The procedure was successfully accomplished under local anesthetic without any complications, and, like our first patient, we have demonstrated efficacy without any evidence of adverse effects from the encapsulated islet transplant.

OUTCOME: SAFETY

In both patients, no adverse effects have been reported to date. In the case of the first patient, almost fourteen months since the procedure, he reports weight gain and remarkably, has noted only five recordings out of a total of 1833 blood glucose observations since his initial procedure of blood glucose levels below 50 mg/dl.

OUTCOME: EFFICACY

Islet Function

Our first patient, now over fourteen months since his initial transplant, demonstrates ongoing insulin secretion from the intraperitoneally transplanted encapsulated islets.

Following the injection of the sub-clinical dose of 10,000 islets/kg, insulin secretion from the transplanted cells was noted within 24 hours of transplantation. On the second post-operative day, all exogenous insulin was discontinued. The patient maintained normoglycemia and tolerated breakfast and lunch without requiring any insulin therapy. Occasional hyperglycemic episodes were noted post-prandially and the patient was placed on a minimal dose of insulin to maintain normoglycemia. He maintained a stable daily mean blood glucose levels ranging from 125 ± 4 to 153 ± 5mg/dl, with less lability relative to his pre-transplant levels while on a significantly ($p < 0.001$) reduced dose of insulin of approximately 0.2 units/kg/day for a period of six months.

Following the dose escalation of a further 5,000 islets per kg in the seventh month, the patient's insulin requirements dropped even further to .07 units per kg per day, and he achieved insulin independence in the ninth month (Figure 1).

The patient maintained insulin-independence for the entire 30-day period, with a daily mean blood glucose of 134 ± 4.2 mg% (114 observations) and M-value of 1.16. During this period of insulin independence, he demonstrated no evidence of ketosis, and maintained his body weight (67.3 kg.) (Fig. 1).

Fasting proinsulin levels were high (1.24 ng/ml), suggesting stress from the sub-clinical dose of islets and it was decided to supplement the patient with NPH insulin on a daily basis. He was thus returned to exogenous insulin therapy (Fig. 2), and to date, demonstrates ongoing islet function with tight glycemic control.

In the fourteenth month, his daily mean blood sugar is 108 ± 3.5 mg% (111 observations), with a normal M-value of minus 3.97 (Table 4). During this month, the patient has found that he had to remove himself from exogenous insulin in order to maintain

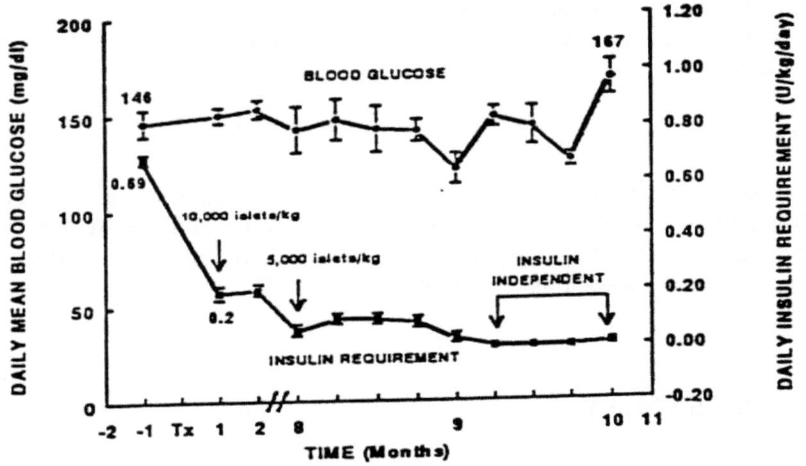

Figure 1.

nomoglycemia. For example, on days 416 and 417, the patient's blood glucose levels are shown below Table 3 in the face of zero exogenous insulin:

C-PEPTIDE AND PRO-INSULIN SECRETION

Basal C-peptide secretion increased, concomitant with the drop in insulin requirement, from a pretransplant level of < 0.1 ng/ml to a post-transplant fasting level of 1.0 ng/ml at the 8th month (Table 4), confirming sustained insulin secretion from the encapsulated islets. C-peptide levels have subsequently fallen as shown in Table 4, with a concomitant increase in proinsulin levels from <.04 ng/ml pre-transplant to 1.24 ng/ml in the ninth month, to 2.3 ng/ml in the 14th month (Fig. 3), suggesting stress on the subclinical dose of islets

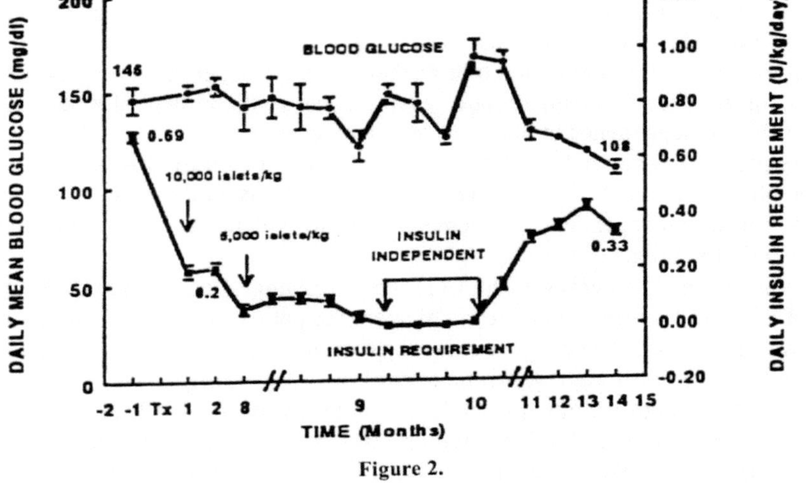

Figure 2.

Table 3.

Time	Day 415	Insulin	Day 416	Insulin	Day 417	Insulin
0700	65 mg%	6 units	49 mg%	0 units	83 mg%	0 units
1300	76 mg%	—	72 mg%	—	120 mg%	—
1900	53 mg%	4 units	90 mg%	—	122 mg%	—
2300	69 mg%	—	102 mg%	—	100 mg%	—
	X = 66 mg%	10 units	X = 79 mg%	0 units	X = 106 mg%	0 units

and overstimulation of the beta cells regulated secretory pathway, resulting in defective proinsulin conversion.

GLYCEMIC CONTROL

The M-value provides an index of glycemic control and is a measure of how far a given glucose level deviates from (above or below) a given standard. Using a standard blood glucose level of 120 mg/dl, the patient demonstrated a >100 fold improvement in M value at 6 months (0.20) compared to the pretransplant level of 4.35, indicating significantly less glycemic lability over 24-hour periods since the transplant. Over the fourteen month period, M-values have continued to improve with a normal minus 3.97 level noted in the fourteenth month (Fig. 4).

These improvements of glycemic control over an extended time period were corroborated by improvements in both glycosylated serum albumin and glycosylated hemoglobin levels. Glycosylated serum albumin decreased from 10.6% pre-transplant to 5.1% at 6 months and 5.1% at 14 months, while glycosylated hemoglobin fell from 9.3% to 7.9%.

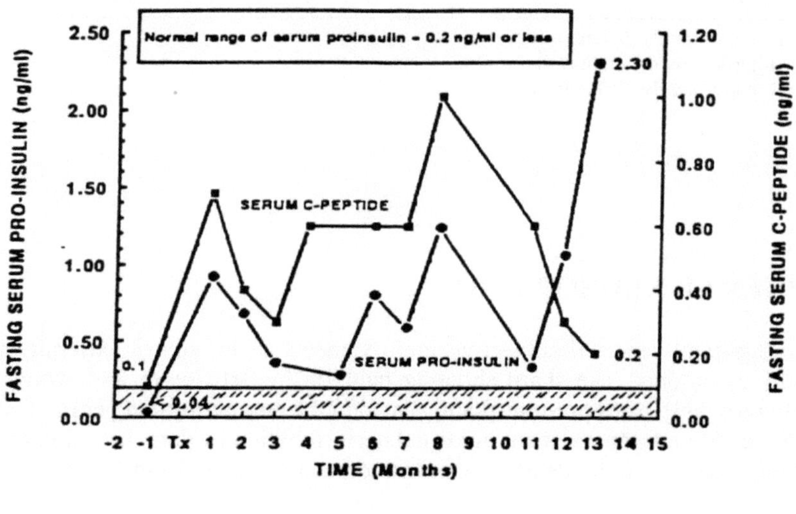

Figure 3.

Table 4. Indices Demonstrating Improved Glycemic Control and Insulin Requirement Post Encapsulated Islet Transplantation Post Tx

	Pre-Tx	2 mo.	4 mo.	6 mo
Blood Glucose Evaluation				
# of observations	60	182	114	117
Daily Mean±SE (mg/dl)	146±7.1	150±4.01*	150±4.95*	129±2.61*
<50 mg/dl episodes (%)	0.00	0.00	0.00	0.00
>200 mg/dl episodes (%)	11.7	16.48	15.79	1.71
M-Value (Standard-120 mg/dl)	4.35	4.83	3.60	0.20
Body Weight (Kg)	68.1	68.1	67.7	67.3
Daily Insulin Requirement				
Daily Mean± SE (Units/kg/day)	0.69±0.01	0.21±0.01***	0.27±0.00***	0.25±0.01***
Metabolic Parameters				
Fasting Pro-Insulin (ng/ml)	<0.04	—	0.36	0.28
Fasting C-Peptide (ng/ml)	0.1	0.40	0.60	0.6
Hemoglobin A1c (%TL HB)	9.3	8.20	7.60	7.8
Glycosylated Albumin (%TL ALB)	10.6	4.40	4.30	5.1
Renal Function				
Creatinine	1.1	—	—	1.3
BUN	19	—	—	25

	8 mo.	10 mo.	12 mo.	14 mo.
Blood Glucose Evaluation				
# of observations	120	116	120	111
Daily Mean±SE (mg/dl)	144±4.52	164±5.6*	124±1.69**	108±3.50**
<50 mg/dl episodes (%)	0.83	0.00	0.00	1.8
>200 mg/dl episodes (%)	10.00	22.41	0.00	0.00
M-Value (Standard-120 mg/dl)	3.04	6.18	-0.22	-3.97
Body Weight (Kg)	66.4	68.1	68.2	69.1
Daily Mean± SE (Units/kg/day)	0.07±0.01***	0.14±0.00***	0.35±0.00	0.35±0.00
Fasting Pro-Insulin (ng/ml)	0.59	—	1.06	2.30
Fasting C-Peptide (ng/ml)	1.0	—	0.3	—
Hemoglobin A1c (%TL HB)	7.8	—	7.9	—
Glycosylated Albumin (%TL ALB)	5.1	—	5.6	—
Renal Function				
Creatinine	1.1	—	1.0	—
BUN	22.1	—	19.8	—

*P>0.05, not significantly different from Pre-Tx.
**P<0.05, significantly different from Pre-Tx.
***P<0.001, significantly different from Pre-Tx.

PERIPHERAL NEUROPATHY

The patient reported subjective improvements in his lower extremity peripheral neuropathy symptoms. The sharp shooting pains in his left lower foot, which occurred constantly on a daily basis pre-transplant, abated in the post-transplant period. EMG studies (Figure 5) confirmed improvement in axonal nerve function by demonstration of continued bilateral increases of amplitude of peroneal motor latencies at 3, 6 and 11 months post-transplant (from 45 m.v. to 194 m.v. at 11 months on the left, and from 200 m.v. to 444 m.v. at 11 months on the right).

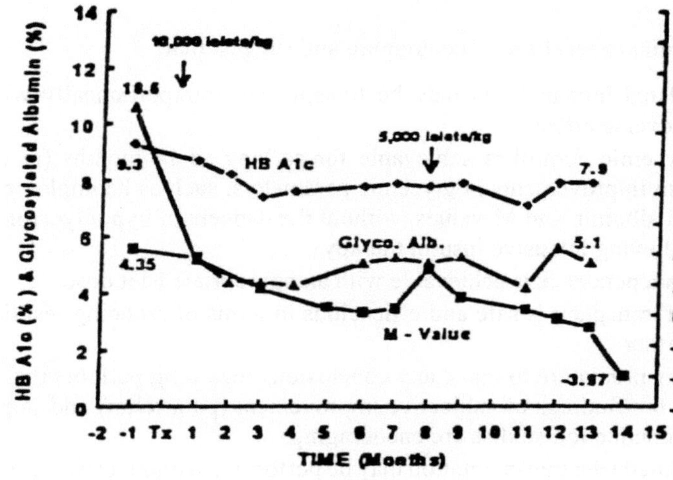

Figure 4.

RENAL FUNCTION

Throughout the 14-month period, the patient's renal function has remained stable with serum creatine levels ranging from 0.7 to 1.3 mg/dl.

Quality of Life

A quality of life questionnaire was completed by the patient pre-transplant, and again at 3 and 6 months post-transplant. The patient reported significant improvement in various aspects of quality of life including an increased energy level, an ability to walk further and a general feeling of improved health. He has recently secured full-time employment, an accomplishment he was not able to achieve due to his diabetes for almost a decade prior to his transplant.

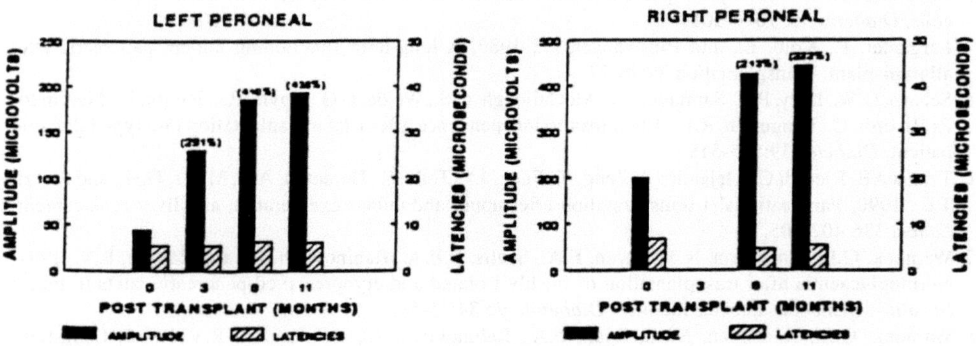

Figure 5. Peroneal proximal motor latencies and amplitude.

PRELIMINARY CONCLUSIONS

These preliminary results are encouraging and suggest that:

1. Encapsulated human islets may be transplanted intraperitoneally without any serious adverse affects.
2. Tight glycemic control is achievable for as long as 14 months (to date) with significant improvements in glycemic parameters, such as hemoglobin Alc, glycosylated albumin and M-values, without the dangers of hypoglycemic episodes noted following intensive insulin therapy.
3. Insulin independence is achievable with an appropriate islet dose.
4. A second transplant is safe and efficacious in terms of reducing insulin requirements further.
5. While it is premature to make any conclusions regarding peripheral neuropathic changes, the findings of subjective improvement (pain relief) and improvement in nerve conduction studies are encouraging.
6. Encapsulated islet transplantation may be performed without complications under local anesthesia.

SUMMARY

The DCCT Trial has incontrovertably demonstrated that tight glycemic control prevents secondary complications of diabetes. Our challenge remains to identify a therapy which can achieve these results without the dangers of hypoglycemia. The preliminary findings of encapsulated islets intraperitoneally injected into insulin dependent diabetic patients is encouraging. We have demonstrated the feasibilty of the encapsulated islet technology. Our challenge to identify sufficient sources of insulin producing cells remains. Once this is met, the potential exists that a therapeutic, minimally invasive procedure may be available for the millions of diabetic patients who may benefit from such a procedure.

REFERENCES

1. Ballinger, W.F., and Lacy, P.E., 1972, Transplantation of intact pancreatic islets in rats. *Surgery* 72:175-86.
2. Yale, J.F., Roy, R.D., Grose, M., Seemayer, T.A., Murphy, G.F., and Marliss, E.B., 1985, Effects of cyclosporine on glucose tolerance inthe rat. *Diabetes* 34:1309-1313.
3. Robertson, R.P., 1986, Cyclorsporin-induced inhibition of insulin secretion in isolated rat islets and HIT cells. *Diabetes* 35: 1016-1019.
4. Largiader, F., Kolb, E., and Binswanger, U., 1980, A long-term functioning human pancreatic islet allotransplant. Transplantation 29:76-77.
5. Scharp, D.W., Lacy, P.E., Santiago, J.V., McCullough, C.S., Weide, L.G., Boyle, P.J., Falqui, L., Marchetti, P., Ricordi, C., Gingerich, R.L., 1990, Insulin independence after islet transplantation into type I diabetic patient. *Diabetes* 39:515-518.
6. Tzakis AB, Ricordi C, Alejandro R, Zeng, Y., Fung, J.J., Todo, S., Demetris, A.J., Mintz, D.H., and Starzl, T.E., 1990, Pancreatic islet transplantation after upper abdominar exenteration and liver replacement. *Lancet* 336:402-405.
7. Warnock, G.L., Kneteman, N.M., Ryan, E.A., Seelis, R.E.A., Rabinovitch, A., and Rajotte, R.V., 1991, Normoglycaemia after trasnplantation of freshly isolated and cryopreserved pancreatic islets in type I (insulin-dependent) diabetes mellitus. *Diabetologia* 34:55-58.
8. Warnock, G.L., Kneteman, N.M., Ryan, E.A., Rabinovitch, A., and Rajotte, R.V., 1992, Long-term follow-up after trasnplantation of insulin-producing pancreatic islets into patients with type I (insulin-dependent) diabetes mellitus. *Diabetologia* 35:89-95.

9. Gores, P.F., Najarian, J.S., Stephanian, E., Lloveras, J.J., Kelley, S.L., and Sutherland, D.E.R., 1993, Insulin independence in type I diabetes after transplantation of unpurified islets from single donor with 15-deoxyspergualin. *Lancet* 341:19-21.
10. Soon-Shiong, P., Terasaki, P.I., Lanza, R.P., 1991, Immunocytochemical identification of monoclonal antibodies with binding activity to acinar cells but not islets. *Pancreas* 6:318-323.
11. Fujioka, T., Terasaki, P.I., Heintz, R., Merideth, N., Lanza, R.P., Zheng, T.L., and Soon-Shiong, P., 1990, Rapid purification of islets using magnetic microspheres coated with anti-acinar cell monoclonal antibodies. *Transplantation* 49:(2)404-407.
12. Soon-Shiong, P., and Grewal, I.S., 1988, Enhancement of lectin-induced cap formation in human neutrophils by cyclosporin A. (M)*Biochem. Biophys. Res. Commun.* 151:435-440.
13. Lanza, R.P., Heintz, R., Meredith, N., Yao, Z., Yao, Q., Zavitz, D., Chen, C., and Soon-Shiong, P., 1990, Large scale canine and human islet isolation using a physiological islet purification solution. *Diabetes* 39(suppl 1):309A.
14. Soon-Shiong, P., Otterlie, M., Skjak-Braek, G., Smidsrod, O., Heinta, R., Lanza, R.P., and Espevik, T., 1991, An immunologic basis for the fibrotic reaction to implanted microcapsules. *Trans. Proc.* 23(1pt 1):758-759.
15. Otterlei, M., Ostgaard, K., Skjak-Braek, G., Smidsrod, O., Soon-Shiong, P., and Espevik, T., 1991, Induction of cytokine production from human monocytes stimulated with alginate. *J. of Immunotherpy*, 10:286-291.
16. Soon-Shiong, P., Heintz, R., Yao, Q., Sanford, P., Lanza, R.P., and Meredith, N., 1992, Glucose-insulin kinetics of the extravascular bioartificial pancreas. *Asaio J.* 38(4):851-854.
17. Yao, Z., Heintz, R., Yao, Q., Sandford, P., and Soon-Shiong, P., 1992, Human c-peptide response in xenotransplanted diabetic Lewis rats. *Trans. Proc.* 24:2948-2949.
18. Soon-Shiong, P., Lu, Z.N., Grewal, I., Lanza, R.P., and Clark, W., 1990, An in vitro method of assessing the immunoprotective properties of microcapsule membranes using pancreatic and tumor cell targets. *Trans. Proc.*22:754-755.
19. Soon-Shiong, P., Feldman, E., Nelson, R., Komtebedde, J., Smidsrod, O., Skjak-Braek, G., Espevik, T., Heintz, R., and Lee, M.,1992, Successful reversal of spontaneous diabetes in dogs by intraperitoneal microencapsulated islets. *Transplantation*, 54:769-774.
20. Soon-Shiong, P., Feldman, E., Nelson, R., Heintz, R., Yao, Q., Yao, Z., Zheng, T., Merideth, N., Skjak-Braek, G., Espevik, T., et al. (1993, Long term reversal of diabetes by the injection of imunoprotected islets. *Proc. NAS* 90:5843-5847.
21. Soon-Shiong, P., Heintz, R.E., Meridith, N., Yao, Q., Yao, Z., Zheng, T., Murphy, M., Moloney, M.K., Schmehl, M., Harris, M., et al., 1994, Insulin independence in a type I diabetic patient after encapsulated islet transplantation. *Lancet* 343:950-951.

12

OPTIMAL SURVEILLANCE OF DIABETIC EYE DISEASE

Barbara E. K. Klein,* Ronald Klein, and Scot E. Moss

Department of Ophthalmology and Visual Sciences
University of Wisconsin Medical School
Madison, Wisconsin 53792-3220

INTRODUCTION

Although the sequelae of diabetes mellitus occur in many tissues and organs in humans, direct observation of these effects can be most easily done by examining the eye. Retinopathy of diabetes has importance because of the potential for compromising the vision of the patient, and also because it can serve as an indicator of systemic involvement of other organs. Thus, this chapter is devoted to description of the stages of diabetic retinopathy, to describing its course as based on epidemiologic data, to methods of documentation, and to grading for systematic classification of the severity of this outcome. The reason to include this piece in the current volume is because of the major impact of retinopathy itself, and because monitoring it provides a useful surrogate for estimating effects of treatments of diabetes in clinical studies.

CLINICAL DESCRIPTION OF DIABETIC RETINOPATHY

Generally, the features appearing in the fundus of the eyes of people with diabetes are hemorrhages and various vascular abnormalities. Although these lesions are not pathognomonic of diabetic retinopathy, their orderly appearance and progression in people with known diabetes is a nearly universal observation.

Retinopathy is usually first manifest as microaneurysms, which appear as discrete red dots, and deep punctate retinal hemorrhages.[1] They commonly occur just temporal to the macula. With the progression of retinopathy, these lesions may become more numerous, although specific microaneurysms and hemorrhages may come and go.

The next lesion to appear is usually the "soft exudate" or "cotton wool patch". These areas are generally larger than the microaneurysms and than most retinal hemorrhages, are

*Correspondence: Barbara E.K. Klein, Dept. of Ophthalmology and Visual Sciences, University of Wisconsin-Madison, 610 North Walnut Street, 487 WARF, Madison, WI 53705-2397. (608) 263-0276; FAX (608) 263-0279.

Fetal Islet Transplantation
Edited by C. M. Peterson, L. Jovanovic-Peterson, and B. Formby, Plenum Press, New York, 1995

white and may be near microaneurysms and hemorrhages. Their name is meant as a morphologic description of these lesions which are probably due to nerve swelling from microinfarcts in the nerve fiber layer of the retina. These tend to disappear as retinopathy progresses.

Hard exudates may begin to develop contemporaneous with soft exudates. They probably result from exudation from permeable retinal vessels. These appear to be firm, yellowish deposits in the retina.

Early in the course of retinopathy, arterioles generally appear to be normal, but later opacification of the vessel wall may occur. This may occur in the presence of intraretinal microvascular abnormalities that are dilated precapillary vessels.

Neovascularization or proliferative retinopathy is a later stage in the process. Proliferative changes usually begin on the optic disc or along one or more of the major retinal veins. The vessels may be accompanied by transparent glial tissue. These new and fragile blood vessels may bleed and the resulting preretinal or vitreous hemorrhage may cause temporary or permanent abrupt decrease in vision. Timely laser photocoagulation reduces the risk of such hemorrhage and the resultant decrease in visual acuity.

Macular edema (thickening of the retina in the macular area) may occur with or without proliferative retinopathy. It, too, may be responsible for a significant decrease in visual acuity.[2,3]

EPIDEMIOLOGY

Much of the information presented is derived from the Wisconsin Epidemiology Study of Diabetic Retinopathy. This is a population-based cohort study of persons who received care for their diabetes in an 11-county area of southern Wisconsin. The baseline evaluations were performed in 1979-1980. This cohort is still under surveillance. Although people with younger onset (insulin-taking with diabetes diagnosed prior to 30 years of age) and older onset (diabetes diagnosed at 30 years of age or older) diabetes are included in that study, only data from the first group is included in this chapter.[4]

It is virtually a universal finding that no retinopathy is apparent at the onset of insulin-dependent diabetes. However, the frequency and severity of retinopathy increase with increasing duration of diabetes.[4] In prevalence data from the Wisconsin Epidemiologic Study of Diabetic Retinopathy in the younger onset group, the prevalence of retinopathy varied from 17% in those with diabetes for less than five years to 98% in those with diabetes for 15 or more years (Figure 1). Proliferative retinopathy was absent in those with less than five years of diabetes but was found in 48% of those with 15 or more years of diabetes. About 6% of persons had macular edema.

Because duration is such an important factor to consider when evaluating retinopathy, it is necessary to take account of this when evaluating other risk factors. Figure 2 demonstrates the association of glycosylated hemoglobin with the severity of retinopathy.[5] The severity of retinopathy in those with glycosylated hemoglobin levels in the lowest quartile are contrasted with those whose glycosylated hemoglobin is in the highest quartile in each interval of duration. Although there was no association in the first five years of diabetes, thereafter persons with higher glycosylated hemoglobin had more severe retinopathy. Figure 3 is similarly constructed to describe the association of severity of retinopathy to diastolic blood pressure by category of duration.[5] For this characteristic, there is also a relationship to severity of retinopathy although the relationship is not as strong as the previous one. There are other characteristics besides duration of diabetes, glycosylated hemoglobin, and blood pressure which may influence severity, but these appear to be the most important.

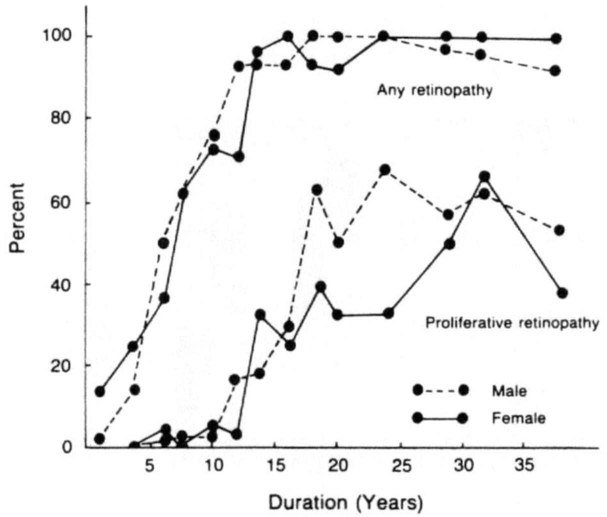

Figure 1. Prevalence of any or proliferative diabetic retinopathy, by sex and duration, in 995 insulin-taking persons diagnosed as having diabetes prior to 30 years of age examined in the Wisconsin Epidemiologic Study of Diabetic Retinopathy (Wisconsin HSA-1, 1980-82). SOURCE: Klein R, Klein BEK: Vision Disorders in Diabetes. In: Diabetes in America, Diabetes Data Compiled 1984. Hammon R, Harris MWH (eds). US Public Health Service, Bethesda. NIH Publication No. 85-1468. Chapter XIII, pp 1-36, August 1985.

For prognostic purposes, longitudinal data are most important. One can then compare the incidence of retinopathy or frequency progression of its severity in the population under surveillance taking account of the characteristics or treatments being evaluated. In incidence data, as in prevalence data, it is essential to account for those characteristics already known to influence progression before evaluating the treatment effect. Overall, in the Wisconsin Epidemiology Study of Diabetic Retinopathy incidence of retinopathy after a four year

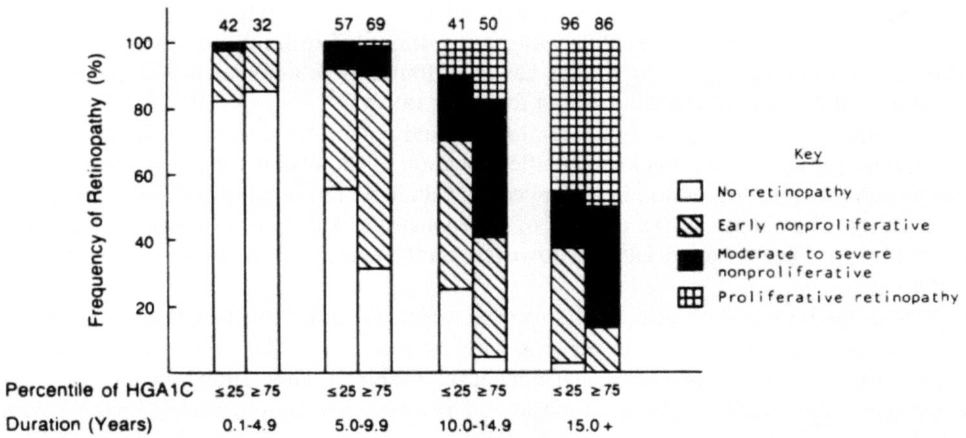

Figure 2. The relationship of the frequency and severity of diabetic retinopathy to glycosylated hemoglobin level, by duration of diabetes, in 995 insulin-taking persons diagnosed as having diabetes prior to 30 years of age in the Wisconsin Epidemiology Study of Diabetic Retinopathy (Wisconsin HSA-1, 1980-82). SOURCE: Klein R, Klein BEK: Vision Disorders in Diabetes. In: Diabetes in America, Diabetes Data Compiled 1984. Hammon R, Harris MWH (eds). US Public Health Service, Bethesda. NIH Publication No. 85-1468. Chapter XIII, pp 1-36, August 1985.

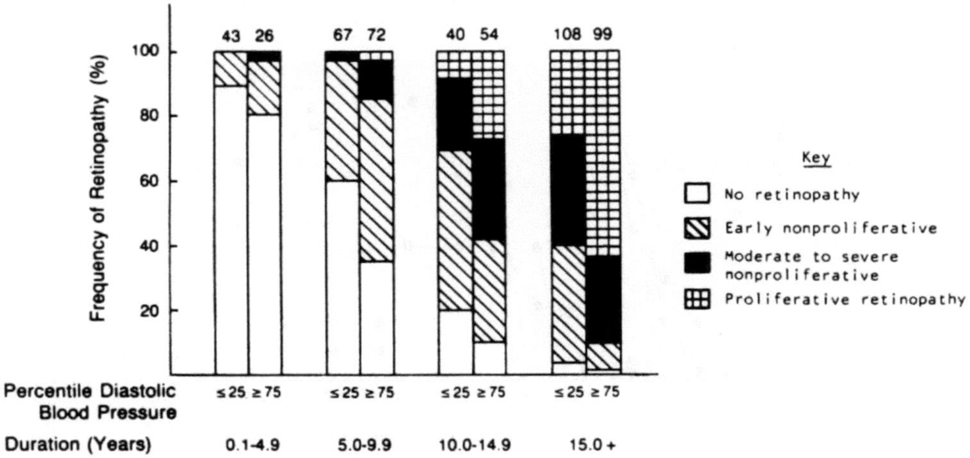

Figure 3. The relationship of the frequency and severity of diabetic retinopathy to diastolic blood pressure level, by duration of diabetes, in 995 persons diagnosed as having diabetes prior to 30 years of age participating in the Wisconsin Epidemiology Study of Diabetic Retinopathy (Wisconsin HSA-1, 1980-82). SOURCE: Klein R, Klein BEK: Vision Disorders in Diabetes. In: Diabetes in America, Diabetes Data Compiled 1984. Hammon R, Harris MWH (eds). US Public Health Service, Bethesda. NIH Publication No. 85-1468. Chapter XIII, pp 1-36, August 1985.

interval was 59%, progression of severity of retinopathy was 41% and the new development of proliferative retinopathy was 11% in those with younger onset diabetes.[6] Glycosylated hemoglobin at the baseline examination was a consistent predictor of all three retinopathy endpoints (Table 1).[7] Diastolic blood pressure at baseline also had a significant effect, especially for progression to proliferative retinopathy[6] (Table 2).

In studies involving those persons with relatively short duration of diabetes, evaluating retinopathy status in a more subtle way may be desired. The number of microaneurysms within a well-defined area of the fundus has been found to be associated with subsequent progression of diabetic retinopathy over a four year interval.[8]

In data from the Wisconsin Epidemiology Study of Diabetic Retinopathy, tripling of the number of microaneurysms in a specified location of the ocular fundus was associated with the subsequent progression in the severity of diabetic retinopathy and with decreased visual acuity. The change in the number of microaneurysms has been used in at least two clinical trials.[9,10] This measure has not, however, gained acceptance as a clinically meaningful endpoint.

The development of macular edema is an important endpoint because of its relationship to decreased visual acuity in persons with diabetes.[2,11-13] The incidence of macular edema was 8% over a four year interval in our study[14] (Table 3). This lesion is not consistently present with other signs of diabetic retinopathy. Its incidence is associated (Table 4) with the severity of retinopathy four years earlier.[14]

Visual impairment is the functionally important result of retinopathy.[12,13] Thus, in studies in which ocular sequelae of diabetes are the endpoints of interest, rather than the surrogate for other systemic complications of diabetes, visual acuity measurement is paramount. In our prevalence study of younger onset persons, 1% had moderate visual impairment (visual acuity of 20/80 to 20/160 equivalent on Snellen charts) and 4% were legally

Table 1. Four-Year Incidence and Progression Rates by Quartile of Glycosylated Hemoglobin for Persons With Nonproliferative Retinopathy at the Baseline Examination

	Incidence of Any Retinopathy				Progression of Retinopathy				Progression to Proliferative		
Glycosylated Hemoglobin	No. at Risk	%	RR*	95% CI*	No. at Risk	%	RR	95% CI	%	RR	95% CI
Younger onset											
1st quartile	80	45.0	1.0	—	177	17.0	1.0	—	1.1	1.0	—
2nd quartile	68	50.0	1.1	0.8-1.6	164	32.9	1.9	1.3-2.9	3.0	2.7	0.5-14.1
3rd quartile	50	66.0	1.5	1.1-2.0	172	49.4	2.9	2.0-4.2	16.3	14.8	3.5-62.4
4th quartile	59	84.8	1.9	1.4-2.5	167	68.3	4.0	2.0-5.7	24.0	21.8	5.3-90.5

* RR indicates relative risk; CI, confidence interval

SOURCE: Klein R, Klein BEK, Moss SE, Davis MD, DeMets DL: Glycosylated hemoglobin predicts the incidence and progression of diabetic retinopathy. JAMA 260:2864-2871, 1988.

blind (visual acuity of 20/200 or worse in the better eye).[12] Incidence of visual impairment was 5% and of legal blindness was 1% over a four year interval in these younger onset persons.[13]

METHODS OF DOCUMENTATION

Perhaps the most thorough evaluation of the eye is one done by a retinal specialist using ophthalmoscopy and slit lamp biomicroscopy through a dilated pupil. However, such evaluations are time consuming and do not provide a permanent nor objective recording of the findings. Therefore, for purposes of clinical studies, alternative techniques must be employed. The procedures that have been adopted by most studies was to obtain photographs of the ocular fundus with a 30° camera. Seven standard photographic fields as described by the protocol for the Diabetic Retinopathy Study are taken of each eye[15] (Figure 4). This requires dilation of the pupil and a well-trained photographer. It might improve compliance and reduce cost to take fewer photographs. However, the frequency of agreement in assigning a level of severity of retinopathy was 80% when only two photographic fields were used and 91% when four fields were used, compared to the levels assigned when the complete seven standard photographic fields were used. The frequency of agreement was dependent upon the specific severity of retinopathy. The agreement was poorest when proliferative reti-

Table 2. Four-Year Incidence and Progression Rates by Quartile of Diastolic Blood Pressure in the Younger Onset Group

		Incidence of Any Retinopathy				Progression of Retinopathy				Progression to PDR		
Quartile	Range (mmHg)	No. at Risk	%	RR*	95% CI*	No. at Risk	%	RR	95% CI	%	RR	95% CI
1st	42-71	105	58.1	1.0	—	207	35.3	1.0	—	2.9	1.0	—
4th	86-117	35	71.4	1.2	0.9,1.6	140	46.4	1.3	1.0,1.7	20.0	6.9	2.9,16.2

* RR indicates relative risk; CI, confidence interval

† PDR = proliferative diabetic retinopathy

SOURCE: Klein R, Klein BEK, Moss SE, Davis MD, DeMets DL: Is blood pressure a predictor of the incidence or progression of diabetic retinopathy? Arch Intern Med 149:2427-2432, 1989.

Table 3. Four-Year Incidence of Macular Edema by Duration of Diabetes at the Baseline Examination

Duration of Diabetes (yrs)	Younger Onset	
	No. at Risk	Incidence (%)
0-2	69	0
3-4	79	2.5
5-6	95	6.3
7-8	72	8.3
9-10	68	8.8
11-12	42	7.1
13-14	34	11.8
15-19	66	18.2
20-24	37	16.2
25-29	25	12.0
30+	23	8.7
Total	610	8.2
Test of trend	P<0.001	

SOURCE: Klein R, Moss SE, Klein BEK, Davis MD, DeMets DL: The Wisconsin Epidemiologic Study of Diabetic Retinopathy. XI. The incidence of macular edema. Ophthalmology 96:1501-1510, 1989.

nopathy was present. This can be particularly unfortunate for the individuals involved and may be scientifically important in studies involving subjects with longer duration of diabetes. Overall, this study shows that there is a reduction in the sensitivity to detect and accurately classify the severity of retinopathy when using fewer photographic fields.[16] When designing a study, this may lead to an increase in the necessary number of subjects and thereby increase the time and/or cost of the study. Similar concerns apply when considering the use of a 45° camera which has the advantage of not having to pharmacologically dilate the pupil.[17]

There are measures of retinal vascular and neurologic function that have been obtained in some studies of diabetic ocular changes. Fluorescein angiograms have been obtained in the Early Treatment of Diabetic Retinopathy Study.[18] The angiograms disclose details of retinal blood flow, capillary closure and leakage of fluorescein. However, angiography has been associated with allergic side effects. In addition, it is more difficult to obtain consistent quality between photographers, subjects, and visits, than is true for fundus photography. Moreover, it appears that fluorescein angiography offers no advantage over

Table 4. Four-Year Incidence of Macular Edema by Retinopathy Severity at the Baseline Examination of the Wisconsin Epidemiologic Study of Diabetic Retinopathy, 1979-198

	Younger Onset		Older Onset	
	No. at Risk	Incidence (%)	No. at Risk	Incidence (%)
Proliferative				
none	286	1.0	450	1.1
minimal	150	10.0	100	6.0
mild	88	14.8	64	20.3
Non-proliferative				
moderate to severe	70	22.9	34	23.5
test of trend	P<0.0001		P<0.0001	

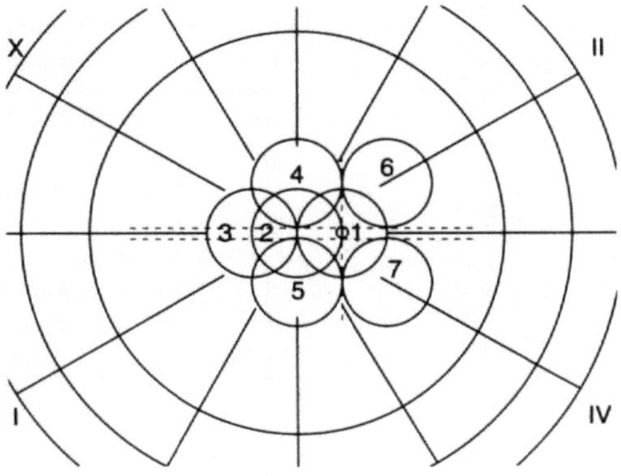

Figure 4. Schematic diagram of the 7 standard photographic fields of the right eye. Field 1 is centered on the optic disc. Fields 2-5 are temporal to Field 1 and Fields 6 and 7 are nasal to Field 1.

color fundus photography in predicting progression of retinopathy.[18] For all those reasons, and the additional costs involved, fluorescein angiography is not used often in studies designed to follow incidence or progression of retinopathy.

Other measures include vitreous fluorophotometry,[19,20] laser doppler velocimetry,[21] electroretinography,[22] visually evoked responses,[22] color vision testing,[23] and perimetry[24]. These tests have not been used routinely in epidemiologic observational studies of diabetes, nor in clinical trials of treatment of diabetes mellitus, nor, specifically, in studies of retinopathy.

CLASSIFICATION SYSTEMS

The progressive lesions characterizing diabetic retinopathy have been categorized into stages or steps on a scale of increasing severity. The system in current use is a refinement of that developed for the Diabetic Retinopathy Study.[15] It has been shown to be useful for describing the subsequent progression of retinopathy.[25] The system has been expanded to reflect finer description of the morphology of the progressive lesions as seen in Table 5).[26]

GRADING PHOTOGRAPHS

Training of graders entails instruction about the appearance and progression of diabetic retinopathy. Graders are trained to recognize characteristic lesions and to estimate their extent and severity by comparing them to standard photographs. They assign scores based on the standard photographs.[27] They grade test eyes on a regular basis and feedback is given to maintain consistency in grading. Initial training takes about six months and quality assurance is monitored throughout the studies. Graders are masked as to subject characteristics to minimize the opportunity for biasing the graders.

The photographic slides are mounted in plastic holders and viewed on a lightbox with a stereoscopic viewer. For most studies, slides of each eye and from each visit are graded independently (at different times, often by different graders) from each other. Thus, grading of the lesions in each eye is not biased by the appearance of the other eye, nor by the appearance of the fundus at previous or subsequent visits.

Table 5. Severity Scale for Diabetic Retinopathy in Each Eye

Level	Description of Severity of Retinopathy
10	None
20	Microaneurysms only
35	Mild non-proliferative
43	Moderate
53	Severe non-proliferative
61	Mild proliferative
>61-90	Moderate to advanced proliferative

ASSIGNING A SEVERITY SCORE

Grading procedures result in a severity score for the given eye at each encounter (Table 5). This is computer generated, based on the graders' indication of the lesions present in the eye. Many studies are concerned with systemic factors that may affect both eyes. The two eyes may be asymmetric in the initial severity of retinopathy and they may progress asymmetrically. One way to deal with this has been to adopt a convention that summarizes the severity of retinopathy for the individual at each study visit. Usually the worse eye is emphasized, but weight is also given to the less involved eye. This is usually expressed as a concatenated score, with the first number indicating severity in the worse eye and the second number reflecting the dichotomy of either an equal severity level in the second eye, or a less severe level.[25] Examples of the grades resulting from this scoring scheme are: 20/<20, which indicates that the individual had definite microaneurysms in one eye only; 61/61 which indicates mild proliferative retinopathy of the same severity in each eye. When estimating changes in the severity of retinopathy for an individual between two visits, many studies use a change of more than one step on the concatenated scale to be meaningful (and less prone to error in classification).

STUDY DESIGN

The nature of the study question will determine the specific design. For example, for therapeutic modalities which aim to prevent retinopathy, and, one might hope by analogy, would prevent other complications of diabetes, the study cohort would be free of retinopathy at inception. For maximum study efficiency and to minimize cost, one might prefer to limit enrollment to persons of a similar duration of diabetes and perhaps of similar blood pressure. However, restricting the study population will either increase the time necessary for recruitment or the geographic area one must recruit from in order to obtain a sufficient number of subjects.

The size of the study will also be dictated by the expected effect of treatment. One must take into account the anticipated frequency of events (e.g., incidence or rate of progression) in the control group and that in the treatment group, and the desired degree of certainty that the differences in observed rates between the groups is not due to chance. With these bits of information, one can then calculate a sample size estimate.

CONCLUSIONS

Diabetic retinopathy is an important event to monitor during the course of diabetes, both because of its intrinsic importance to visual function and because it reflects other complications of diabetes. Retinopathy can be documented by photography, a non-invasive procedure, and serial photographs can be monitored for a change in severity. Thus, this endpoint may be useful to follow in preventive and therapeutic trials for diabetes mellitus.

REFERENCES

1. Symposium on the Treatment of Diabetic Retinopathy, 1968, Goldberg MF, Fine S (eds). U.S. Department HEW, Public Health Service, Neurological and Sensory Disease Control Program, Diabetes and Arthritis Control Program. Clinical Observations Concerning the Pathogenesis of Diabetic Retinopathy. Arlington, VA, Chapter 4.
2. Patz, A., Schatz, H., Berkow, J.W., et al., 1973, Macular edema - an overlooked complication of diabetic retinopathy. *Trans Am Acad Ophthal Otolaryngology* 77:OP34-42.
3. Early Treatment Diabetic Retinopathy Study Research Group, 1985, Photocoagulation for diabetic macular edema. Early Treatment Diabetic Retinopathy Study Report No. 1. *Arch Ophthalmol* 103:1796-806.
4. Klein, R., Klein, B.E.K., Moss, S.E., Davis, M.D., DeMets, D.L., 1984, The Wisconsin Epidemiologic Study of Diabetic Retinopathy. II. Prevalence and risk of diabetic retinopathy when age at diagnosis is less than 30 years. *Arch Ophthalmol* 102:520-526.
5. Diabetes in America. Diabetes Data Compiled 1984. Harris MI, Hammon RF (eds). NIH Publication No. 85-1468, August 1985. U.S. Department of Health and Human Services, Public Health Service, National Institutes of Health, National Institute of Arthritis, Diabetes and Digestive and Kidney Diseases. Chapter XIII, p 16.
6. Klein, R., Klein, B.E.K., Moss, S.E., Davis, M.D,, DeMets, D.L., 1989, Is blood pressure a predictor of the incidence or progression of diabetic retinopathy? *Arch Intern Med* 149:2427-2432.
7. Klein, R., Klein, B.E.K., Moss, S.E., Davis, M.D., DeMets, D.L., 1988, Glycosylated hemoglobin predicts the incidence and progression of diabetic retinopathy. *JAMA* 260:2864-2871.
8. Klein, R., Meuer, S.M., Moss, S.E., Klein, B.E.K., 1989, The relationship of retinal microaneurysm counts to the 4-year progression of diabetic retinopathy. *Arch Ophthalmol* 107:1780-1785.
9. The DAMAD Study Group, 1989, Effect of aspirin alone and aspirin plus dipyridamole in early diabetic retinopathy: A multicenter randomized controlled clinical trial. *Diabetes* 38;491-498.
10. TIMAD Study Group, 1990, Ticlopidine treatment reduces the progression of non-proliferative retinopathy. *Arch Ophthalmol* 108;1577-1583.
11. Aiello, L.M., Rand, L.I., Briones, J.C., et al., 1981, Diabetic retinopathy in Joslin Clinic patients with adult-onset diabetes. *Ophthalmology* 88:619-23.
12. Klein, R., Klein, B.E.K., Moss, S.E., 1984, Visual impairment in diabetes. *Ophthalmology* 91:1-9.
13. Moss, S.E., Klein, R., Klein, B.E.K., 1988, The incidence of vision loss in a diabetic population. *Ophthalmology* 95:1340-1348.
14. Klein, R., Moss, S.E., Klein, B.E.K., Davis, M.D., DeMets, D.L., 1989, The Wisconsin Epidemiologic Study of Diabetic Retinopathy. XI. The incidence of macular edema. *Ophthalmology* 96:1501-1510.
15. Diabetic Retinopathy Study Research Group, 1981, A modification of the Airlie House classification of diabetic retinopathy. Report No. 7. *Invest Ophthalmol Vis Sci* 21:210-226.
16. Moss, S.E., Meuer, S.M., Klein, R., Hubbard, L.D., Brothers, R.J., Klein, B.E.K., 1989, Are seven standard photographic fields necessary for classification of diabetic retinopathy? *Invest Ophthalmol Vis Sci* 30:823-828.
17. Klein, R., Klein, B.E.K., Neider, M.W., Hubbard, L.D., Meuer, S.M., Brothers, R.J., 1985, Diabetic retinopathy as detected using ophthalmoscopy, a nonmydriatic camera and a standard Fundus camera. *Ophthalmology* 92:485-491.
18. Early Treatment Diabetic Retinopathy Study Research Group, 1991, Fluorescein angiographic risk factors for progression of diabetic retinopathy. Early Treatment Diabetic Retinopathy Study Report No. 13. *Arch Ophthalmol* 98(Suppl):834-840.
19. Waltman, S.R., 1983, Vitreous fluorophotometry. In: Little HL, Jack RL, Patz A et al. (eds). Diabetic retinopathy. New York: Thieme-Stratton Inc. pp 72-81.
20. Engler, C., Krogsaa, B., Lund-Anderson, H., 1991, Blood-retina barrier permeability and its relation to the progression of diabetic retinopathy in Type 1 diabetes. An 8-year follow-up study. *Graefe Arch Clinic Exp* 229:442-446.
21. Grunwald, J.E., Riva, C.E., Sinclair, S.H., et al., 1986, Laser doppler velocimetry study of retinal circulation in diabetes mellitus. *Arch Ophthalmol* 104:991-996.

22. Bresnick, G.H., Palta, M., 1987, Predicting progression to severe proliferative diabetic retinopathy. *Arch Ophthalmol* 105:810-814.
23. Birch, J., Chisholm, I.A., Kinnear, P., Marre, M., Pinckers, A.J.L.G., Pokorny, J., Smith, V.C., Verriest, G.P., 1979, Acquired color vision defects. Pokorny J, Smith VC, Verriest G, Pinckers AJLG (eds). In: Congenital and Acquired Color Vision Defects. Grune and Stratton, New York, pp 243-348.
24. Klein, B.E.K., Meuer, S.M., Klein, R., Dalton, D.S., 1991, A pilot study of glaucoma visual field screening in diabetes. *Europ J Ophthalmol* 1:111-114.
25. Klein, B.E.K., Davis, M.D., Segal, P., Long, J.A., Harris, W.A., Haug, G.A., Magli, Y., Syrjala, S., 1984, Diabetic retinopathy: Assessment of severity and progression. *Ophthalmology* 91:10-17.
26. Early Treatment Diabetic Retinopathy Study Research Group, 1991, Fundus photographic risk factors for progression of diabetic retinopathy. Early Treatment Diabetic Retinopathy Study Report No. 12. *Ophthalmology* 98(Suppl.):823-833.
27. Early Treatment Diabetic Retinopathy Study Research Group, 1991, Grading diabetic retinopathy from stereoscopic color fundus photographs- an extension of the modified Airlie House classification. Early Treatment Diabetic Retinopathy Study Report No. 10. *Ophthalmology* 98(Suppl.):786-806.

13

DETECTION OF PANCREATIC ISLET TRANSPLANT REJECTION

Barbara Brooks-Worrell[2] and Jerry Palmer[1,2]

[1] Veterans Affairs Medical Center
[2] University of Washington
Veterans Affairs Medical Center
Endocrinology (111)
1660 S. Columbian Way
Seattle WA 98108

INTRODUCTION

The immune system in multicellular organisms evolved with the major function to discriminate self from non-self. Thus, the immune system of each individual is able to recognize and respond to many foreign antigens, but is normally unresponsive to the individual's own "self" proteins. The integrity of the individual resides in the immune system carrying out this basic role. Abnormalities in the induction or maintenance of this major function lead to overwhelming infection by common organisms or to immune responses against "self" proteins resulting in autoimmune disease. When an organ or tissue is diseased or damaged, this basic function of the immune system must be circumvented when attempting to replace the damaged or diseased tissues through organ transplantation. In recent years, the understanding of the mechanisms involved in "self" recognition, organ/tissue rejection, and the development of autoimmune disease, have played a major role in improving the success of transplants and treatments for autoimmune diseases.

TRANSPLANT REJECTION

There are three general categories of organ/tissue rejection categorized primarily on histopathology rather than on immune effector mechanisms: hyperacute; acute; and chronic. Hyperacute rejection is a rapid process occurring immediately following transplantation whereas acute and chronic rejection can occur at almost any time after transplantation. Often times, acute and chronic rejection coexist in the same transplanted tissue or organ. Hyperacute rejection is mediated primarily by preexisting ABO blood group antibodies that bind to ABO antigens expressed on the endothelium of the transplant and activate complement with resulting vasculitis and ischemia. In the early years of transplantation, hyperacute

Fetal Islet Transplantation
Edited by C. M. Peterson, L. Jovanovic-Peterson, and B. Formby, Plenum Press, New York, 1995

rejection was common (1). In recent years, hyperacute rejection of allografts has become infrequent due to blood and tissue typing and matching of donor and recipient.

Acute vascular rejection can be mediated by IgG antibodies against endothelial cell alloantigens and activation of complement. With this form of rejection, lymphocytes may also be involved and contribute by responding to alloantigens present on the vascular endothelial cells, leading to direct lysis of these cells. The lymphocytes may also produce cytokines that activate inflammatory cells, causing endothelial necrosis. Another form of acute rejection termed acute cellular rejection involves several different effector mechanisms including cytotoxic T cell mediated lysis, activated macrophage-mediated lysis, and natural killer cell-mediated lysis. Several lines of evidence suggest that recognition and lysis of foreign cells by alloreactive T cells is probably the most important mechanism in acute cellular rejection (1).

Lastly, chronic rejection is characterized by fibrosis with loss of normal organ structures and function. Chronic rejection may represent a form of chronic delayed-type hypersensitivity reaction; however, the pathogenesis of chronic rejection is less well understood. In many cases, chronic rejection occurs without evidence that acute rejection ever occurred. Although antibodies are known to be important in hyperacute rejection and may play a role in acute rejection, the most important mechanisms mediating rejection are probably cellular in nature.

OVERVIEW OF TRANSPLANTATION REJECTION

Transplant rejection involves both antigen independent and antigen dependent mechanisms. Early in the rejection process, adhesion molecules cause antigen independent adhesion of the lymphocytes to the foreign tissue (2,3). Within minutes of stimulation by ischemia, tissue manipulation, or other insults, activated vascular endothelium in the transplant begin to express a group of adhesion molecules termed selectins, primarily P-, and then E-selectin (4-6). These selectins cause increased adhesion from leukocytes perfusing the transplant. The increased leukocyte adhesion causes the leukocytes to increase their expression of selectin L which in cascade-like fashion increases the adhesion of the leukocytes. The binding of the leukocytes to the endothelial wall occurs particularly in areas of high cytokine concentrations (7) which induces an increase in expression of another class of adhesion molecules called integrins. This upregulation in integrin expression is critical for leukocyte extravasation into allogeneic or inflammatory sites. Once the lymphocytes are adhered to the endothelial cells and diapedesis occurs into the graft, antigen recognition and T cell activation can occur. Adhesion molecules belonging to the immunoglobulin gene superfamily, such as intracellular adhesion molecule 1 (ICAM-1), are involved in T cell activation and proliferation. Table 1 lists a number of the adhesion molecules involved in transplantation rejection and T cell activation. ICAM-1 interactions have been best studied with regard to transplantation rejection. ICAM-1 is expressed constitutively on a wide variety of cells, including endothelial cells and leukocytes, and is dramatically upregulated on endothelial cells during either inflammation or early antigen recognition. Rose et al (8) demonstrated that the appearance of rejection in human heart allografts corresponded with the expression of the HLA class I antigen on the normally negative myocardial plasma membrane and ICAM-1 on the intercalating discs. Moolenaar et al (9) and Faull and Russ (10) demonstrated that the appearance of rejection in renal transplants was associated with the de novo presence of ICAM-1 on tubular epithelial cells which closely paralleled increased MHC class II expression on endothelial cells and detection of T cell receptor expression on infiltrating host lymphocytes. Through adhesion molecule interactions, such

Table 1. Adhesion Molecules

Selectins:	
E-Selectin (ELAM-1)	
P-Selectin (GMP-140, PADGEM, CD62)	
L-Selectin (LECAM-1, MEL 14, LAM 1, Leu 8, TQ1, DREG-56)	
Integrins:	
Family:	Ligand:
ß1	
VLA-1	Laminin, Collagen
VLA-2	Collagen
VLA-3	Fibronectin, Laminin
VLA-4	Fibronectin, VCAM-1
VLA-5	Fibronectin
VLA-6	Laminin
VLA-7	Vibronectin RC-ß1
ß2	
LFA-1, Leu	ICAM-1, ICAM-2
CAMa	ICAM-3
MAC-1, CR3, Leu, CAMb	ICAM-1, iC3b
p150, 95, Leu, CAMc	iC3b
Immunoglobulin superfamily:	
Member:	Ligand:
CD2	LFA-3
CD3, TCR	MHC
CD4	MHC-II
CD8	MHC-I
ICAM-1, ICAM-2	LFA-1
LFA-3	CD2
MHC-I	CD8
MHC-II	CD4
VCAM-1	VLA-4

Heeman UW et al. Ann. Surg. 1994, 219:4-12.

as LFA-1/ICAM-1 (11), signal transduction to T cells is facilitated, leading to antigen recognition and cellular activation.

REJECTION MECHANISMS

T lymphocyte-mediated rejection is primarily directed against the major histocompatibility complex antigen, HLA, in humans. The immune response to foreign HLA has been demonstrated to be both strong and rapid. Precursor frequencies for T cells capable of recognizing a foreign HLA molecule have been demonstrated to be from ten to one hundred-fold higher than for T cells capable of recognizing a particular peptide plus HLA combination (12,13). In fact, it has been estimated that as many as 2 per cent of an individual's T cells are capable of recognizing and responding to a single foreign MHC molecule (1). Thus, recognition of foreign HLA molecules is a cross-reaction of a normal T cell receptor which also recognizes self HLA plus foreign peptide. Explanations for the high number of cross-reactive T cells are 1) foreign HLA molecules differ from self HLA molecules at multiple amino acid residues, each of which individually or in combination may produce a determinant recognized by a different cross-reactive T cell clone; 2) different bound self peptides, in combination with one foreign HLA molecule, may produce determinants recognized by different cross-reactive T cell clones (1); and 3) thymocytes, which have a strong affinity for self HLA, are deleted (negative selection), whereas T cells with the "proper" affinity for self HLA are selected for differentiation and proceed from the thymus (positive selection). Therefore, in the developing T cell repertoire, there exist T cells capable of high affinity interactions with "non-self" HLA types. Under non-transplant circumstances, such potential "high affinity" T cell interactions with foreign HLA would not exist; however, through organ transplantation, mature T cells "artificially" encounter non-self HLA to which some T cells will respond with high affinity (13).

The early T cell response to an alloantigen is primarily by the CD4+ helper cells that detect the foreign HLA class II antigens (14). In humans, vascular endothelial cells along with dendritic cells, B lymphocytes, and mononuclear phagocytes constitutively express class II MHC molecules and provide the initial stimulation of alloreactive CD4+ cells. CD8+ cytotoxic lymphocytes are also important in allograft rejection, however, in most situations are dependent on CD4+ lymphocytes for differentiation. Activation of the CD8+ cytotoxic T lymphocytes causes these T cells to lyse foreign cells through direct contact. The functional subdivision of CD4+ and CD8+ alloreactive T cells into helper cells and cytotoxic cells in humans, however, is not absolute. CD4+ class II specific cytotoxic cells can be detected in the mixed lymphocyte reaction in humans. Moreover, CD8+ T cells with cytokine production profiles similar to CD4+ cells have also been detected in human allograft rejection (1). B lymphocytes are also able to participate in antibody-dependent cell-mediated cytotoxicity through production of graft specific antibodies which may be involved in graft rejection.

Another mechanism of graft destruction is through the release of mediators that directly injure cells by activation of nonspecific effector mechanisms. These nonspecific effector mechanisms include: 1) activation of macrophages leading to release of cytokines, eicosanoids, and reactive oxygen intermediates, 2) recruitment of polymorphonuclear lymphocytes through release of cytokines 3) secondary effects of platelet and coagulation activation leading to graft ischemia 4) INF-gamma activation of cytotoxic T lymphocytes into antigen nonspecific natural killer cells and 5) cytokines released within the graft which have direct nonspecific cellular necrosis capability (14).

DETECTION OF TRANSPLANT REJECTION

Detection of early rejection is of great interest and allows intervention in the rejection process prior to complete loss of the graft. In the early years of transplantation, rejection was often assessed by biopsy. Now rejection severity is mainly assessed, with the exception of cardiac transplants which are still biopsied, through function of the grafted organ. For example, renal transplants are assessed through measurement of plasma creatinine levels and liver allografts may be assessed through measuring bile excretion. Table 2 illustrates some methods currently utilized to assess graft rejection. Several non-specific markers which indicate immunologic activation such as soluble IL-2 receptors, neopterin, adhesion molecule expression, cytokine production, and detection of the up-regulation of MHC molecules have been investigated. However, the use of the non-specific markers has not yielded much promise in assessing early transplant rejection. Assessment of the activation state and precursor frequencies of alloreactive T cells would directly measure the effectors of the rejection process and hopefully identify early graft rejection. Measurement of the alloreactive T cells has in the past been accomplished through the use of the mixed leukocyte reaction (MLR) and limiting dilution analysis (LDA) assays. The LDA has been utilized to estimate the precursor frequencies of the alloreactive T cells in an individual. The MLR is an in vitro model of T cell recognition of foreign MHC gene products. MLRs and LDAs are often used

Table 2. Detection of Rejection

Biopsy	e.g. Cardiac
Organ Function	e.g.: Renal transplants-plasma creatinine levels Liver transplants-bile excretion Pancreatic transplants-insulin requirements, C-peptide
Immune Markers	
Non-specific	Il-2R, neopterin, adhesion molecules cytokine production, MHC molecule expression
Specific (T-cells)	Limiting dilution analysis Mixed leukocyte reaction Mixed lymphocyte islet coculture Antigen-specific T cell assays

to assess the response of recipient lymphocytes to alloantigens expressed on donor or third party lymphocytes (15, 16). The MLR and LDA assay systems are developed using peripheral blood lymphocytes (PBLs) requiring that lymphocytes from the organ donor be prepared at the time of transplantation and then stored long-term in liquid nitrogen. The preparation of donor lymphocytes is not always possible, particularly when the donor is not living or is not local to the transplant center, and not all centers have the facilities to store large numbers of cells in this way. Therefore, the establishment of other T cell assays that would allow rejection to be identified early enough to intervene, has been an area of important research over the past number of years.

INSULIN-DEPENDENT DIABETES MELLITUS (IDDM)

In a normally functioning immune system, breakdowns sometimes occur in the self and non-self recognition mechanism and occasionally autoimmune diseases occur. Insulin Dependent Diabetes (IDDM) is an organ-specific autoimmune disease characterized by immune-mediated destruction of beta cells within the islets of Langerhans. The destructive process leading to clinical disease is believed to occur over a number of years. Clinical IDDM is manifested when the majority of the beta cells become severely impaired or have been destroyed. Preceding clinical disease, the pancreas is infiltrated with immune cells (insulitis). The insulitis has been demonstrated to consist predominantly of T lymphocytes and macrophages (16). The role of the macrophage is speculated to be in antigen presentation and the production of cytokines while the T lymphocytes are hypothesized to be the effector cells of beta cell destruction.

At diagnosis of IDDM, autoantibodies to a number of islet cell antigens are present. Islet cell antibodies (ICA) are found in 70-90% of newly diagnosed Caucasian IDDM patients (17), insulin autoantibodies (IAA) are present in 40-60% (18) prior to insulin treatment and antibodies to glutamatic acid decarboxylase (GAD) in 60-90% of patients (19). These antibodies, however, appear to primarily reflect beta cell damage, rather than mediate the disease process. In recent years, the use of these antibodies in prediction of individuals susceptible to IDDM has been of great interest. High titer ICA are associated with increased risk of developing diabetes (17), whereas the presence of IAA alone demonstrates only a slight risk as compared to controls (20, 21). It is believed that the presence of increasing types of autoantibodies is associated with an increased risk of developing IDDM.

LYMPHOCYTES IN IDDM

The islet cell antigen(s) that initiate the IDDM disease process is unknown. During the past few years, researchers have identified a number of islet cell proteins stimulatory for lymphocytes (23). Table 3 illustrates a few of the islet cell antigens that have been identified in recent years. However, many of the islet cell antigens capable of stimulating T cells in IDDM patients were first investigated due to their reactivity with antibodies. Since B and T lymphocytes are often specific for different protein epitopes (24), some or many of the T cell stimulating antigens may be overlooked. Moreover, most studies to date investigating cellular reactivity in the context of IDDM use either T cell lines or clones. The use of T cell lines and clones is limited to the detection of the antigen recognized by the particular line or clone. Analysis of the bulk population of stimulated lymphocytes allows for the majority of the stimulating antigens to be identified. To investigate the specificity of bulk populations of T cells in diabetic NO D(non-obese diabetic) mice to the islet cell proteins, Bieg et al (25) utilized normal rat beta cell extracts and various subcellular fractions of a transplantable parental rat insulinoma tumor (RIN) to stimulate unfractionated populations of purified splenic T lymphocytes. These investigators demonstrated that a large array of proteins from both the rat islet cell and RIN fractions stimulated proliferation of T cells from NOD mice (Figure 1). Gelber et al (26) also demonstrated, using peripheral T cells from diabetic and pre-diabetic NOD mice and extracts of pancreatic beta cell lines, that the murine T cells responded to multiple beta cell proteins in the absence of priming and before the manifestation of histologically detectable insulitis. These investigators also observed that at a very early stage in the disease process, the T cells responded not to the already identified putative autoantigens (GAD-65, GAD-67, Hsp 65, insulin, ICA 69, carboxypeptidase-H, and peripherin), but were specific for unidentified beta cell autoantigens. Also, these investigators observed that the NOD T cells responded to an extract of human islets, suggesting potentially shared antigenic determinants between human and mouse beta cells.

In our laboratory, we have established cellular immunoblotting to investigate responses of peripheral blood mononuclear (PBM) cells from IDDM patients to separated islet cell proteins. Cellular immunoblotting is a technique whereby human islet cell proteins are separated using SDS-PAGE and then electroblotted onto nitrocellulose. The nitrocellulose containing the islet cell proteins is solubilized using DMSO to produce antigen-bearing particles. The particles are then utilized to stimulate the PBM cells from IDDM patients in vitro. We have observed that newly diagnosed IDDM patients (within one year of diagnosis) respond to multiple islet cell proteins with positive proliferation (2 Stimulation Index). Whereas, PBM cells from normal controls do not respond to similar antigen doses. Figure

Table 3. Islet Autoantigens Identified in IDDM Patients

Insulin, Proinsulin
Glycolipids, Ganglioside GT3
64 kD antigen, Glutamic acid decarboxylase
Carboxypeptidase H, PM-1, Polar antigen
38 kD Secretory granule membrane component
Peripherin
Heat shock protein 65
Insulin receptor
Endocrine cell antigens
Cytoskeleton proteins (tubulin, actin), Reticulin
Nuclear antigens (ssDNA, ssRNA)

Boitard C. Diabetologia 1992, 35: 1101-1112.

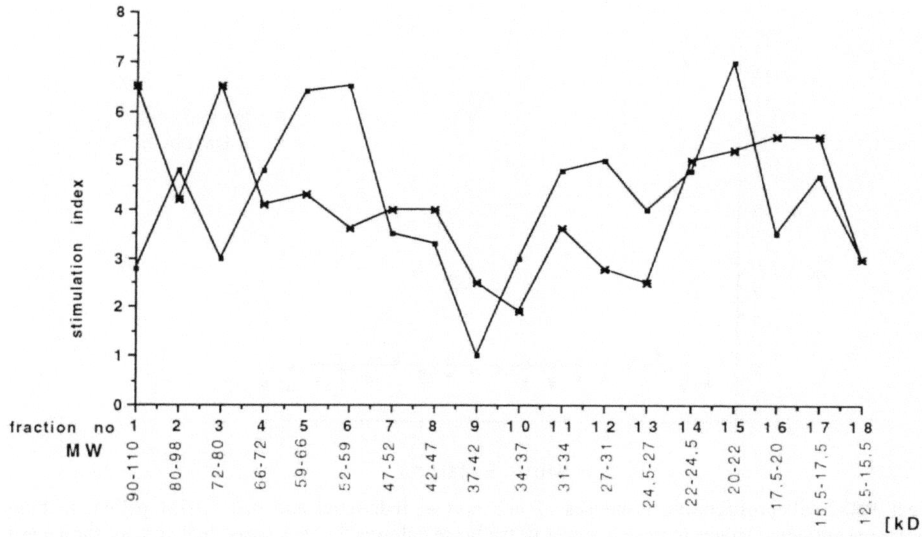

Figure 1. Proliferation of splenic NOD T cell with fractionated proteins derived from RIN insulinoma cytoplasmic (—x—) and microsomal membrane (—) fractions after stimulation with 18 different subfractions. The fractions were electroeluted from SDS polyacrylamide gel strips of different molecular weights in the range from 12.5-120 kDa. Three different concentrations of each of these fractions were tested and the highest stimulation index (SI) values obtained at one of these concentrations was plotted. Bieg et al. Diabetologia 1993, 36: 385-390.

2 illustrates a typical proliferative response of PBM cells from a normal control and IDDM patient to islet cell proteins. Moreover, normal controls and IDDM patients responded similarly to tetanus toxoid-bearing nitrocellulose, phytohema-gglutinin (PHA), and anti-CD3 (data not shown). Normal human spleen cells, and proteins from a human osteosarcoma cell line prepared in a similar manner as the islet cell proteins did not stimulate IDDM patients or normal controls. Figure 3 illustrates a typical proliferative response of PBM cells from a

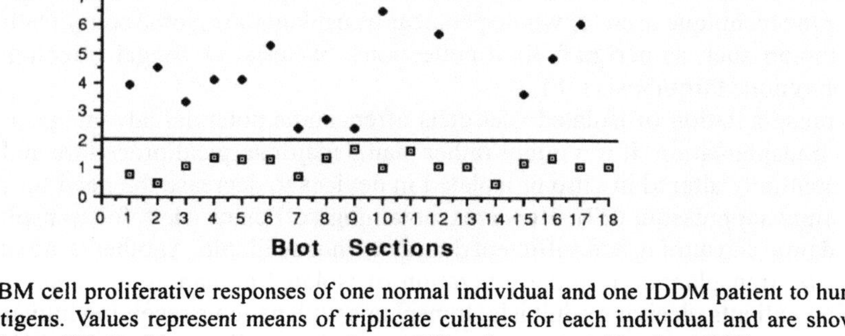

Figure 2. PBM cell proliferative responses of one normal individual and one IDDM patient to human adult islet cell antigens. Values represent means of triplicate cultures for each individual and are shown as the stimulation index (SI). Positive responses are taken as 2SI as demonstrated by the solid line.

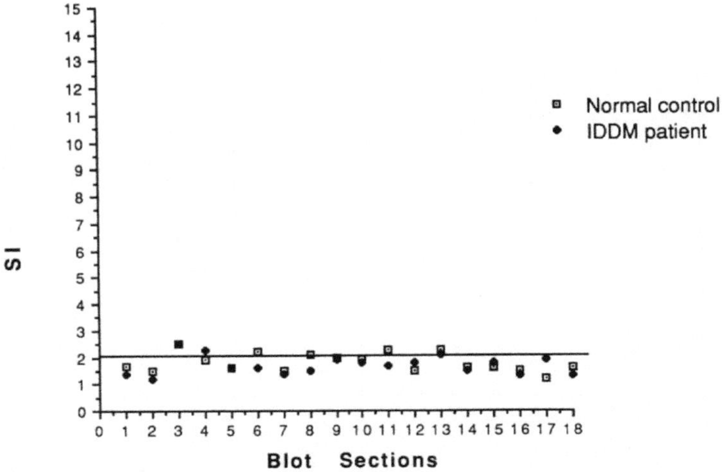

Figure 3. PBM cell proliferative responses of one normal individual and one IDDM patient to human osteosarcoma antigens. Values represent means of triplicate cultures for each individual and are shown as the stimulation index (SI). Positive responses are taken as 2SI as demonstrated by the solid line.

normal control and IDDM patient to the human osteosarcoma cells. These studies demonstrate that at the time of disease onset, PBM cells from IDDM patients respond to multiple islet cell proteins.

PANCREAS TRANSPLANTATION

Presently, treatment for IDDM consists of subcutaneous insulin injections, insulin pumps, and pancreatic or islet cell transplantation. Replacement of a patient's islets of Langerhans either by pancreas transplantation or by isolated islet transplantation is the only treatment of IDDM that results in a constant normoglycemic state (27). However, there are the associated concerns involved in the acceptance of the pancreatic or islet cell allograft in the recipient along with the added concern of autoimmune destruction of the transplant. Treatment of IDDM through transplantation has used whole pancreatic transplants, or human adult or fetal isolated islet cells with or without encapsulation. The advantage of whole pancreas over isolated islet transplantation is that the transplant is intact, unprocessed tissue with normal architecture and good vascularization. However, in these conditions, islets are surrounded by exocrine parenchyma whose secretion has to be diverted or blocked (28). Whatever the technique used for whole pancreas transplantation, some complications appear to be common such as perigraft fluid collections, bacterial or fungal infection, or acute arterial or venous thrombosis (28).

Transplantation of isolated islet cells offers some potential advantages over whole pancreas transplantation. It is a minor rather than a major surgical procedure and islet cells can be potentially altered in vitro or isolated in devices to decrease the need for post-transplant immunosuppression (27). However, obtaining sufficient islets for transplantation is costly and time consuming and sufficient donors are not available. Another issue surrounding isolated islet transplantation is the utilization of isolated human adult versus fetal islets. Comparing patients receiving adult islet transplants with patients receiving human fetal islet tissue, Hering et al (29) reported that a reduction in the insulin requirements in both sets of patients occurred some time during the first year post-transplant. However, in contrast to patients with adult islet transplants, the patients receiving human fetal transplants had no clear increases of C-peptide levels. Warren et al (30) and Hao et al (31) demonstrated in a mouse model of fetal versus adult islet transplants that rejection of the islet graft differs in cellular activation requirements. In the adult islet rejection is a CD8+ T cell dependent process, whereby the islet is damaged by a cytotoxic process and cytokine production by the T cells increases antigen density on the target surface. In the case of purified adult islets, CD4+ cells are essential to the activation of the CD8+ cells. However, when the islet tissue is fetal pancreas, CD8+ T cells alone can initiate and consummate the destructive process (32). Therefore, when considering all facets of rejection, it is yet unknown as to whether adult or fetal islet transplants or whole islet transplants will be better tolerated by the recipients.

METABOLIC ASSESSMENT OF PANCREAS REJECTION

Completely successful pancreatic or islet cell transplantation results in cessation of exogenous insulin requirements with normalization of plasma glucose and glycosylated hemoglobin A_{1c} (HbA_{1c}) levels. Increased insulin requirements are often present after transplantation due to insulin resistance induced by the immunosuppressive therapy. Since glucose homeostasis is dependent not only on beta-cell function but also on insulin sensitivity, both peripheral insulin (OGTT and IVGTT) and C-peptide concentrations have been used often in the estimation of beta cell function following transplantation. Other metabolic parameters commonly followed are fasting blood glucose, and HbA_{1c} levels (31, 32). There are, however, several limitations of using insulin and C-peptide concentrations as an index of insulin secretion after pancreas transplantation (33). The peripheral hyperinsulinemia observed in both the fasting and poststimulatory states in transplant patients may not indicate augmented insulin secretion when compared to peripheral insulin levels in normal subjects. Also, in most insulin assays there exists cross-reactivity between proinsulin and proinsulin conversion intermediates. Recipients of kidney/pancreas transplants have been demonstrated to have increased levels of proinsulin and proinsulin conversion intermediates (33). An alternative is to measure C-peptide levels following pancreas allografts. However, it has been demonstrated recently that pancreas transplant recipients have a reduced clearance of C-peptide and consequently elevated levels may not necessarily mean increased secretion.

T LYMPHOCYTES IN PANCREATIC TRANSPLANTATION

Assessment of T cell reactivity in IDDM patients receiving islet or pancreas transplants must address both T cell alloreactivity induced by the transplant and autoreactivity intrinsic to the underlying IDDM disease process. Kuttler et al (34) using the diabetic BB rat transplanted with Lewis rat islets, isolated viable graft lymphocytes and characterized these cells morphologically and functionally. They observed that in the graft there was a marked accumulation of both CD4+ and CD8+ T cells although the BB/OK rats are characterized by a drastic peripheral T cell lymphopenia. Also, when peripheral blood lymphocytes from the transplant recipient were incubated with the donor islets, a significant increase of cell-mediated cytotoxicity against the islets was observed in normoglycemic BB/OK rats 9 days before allograft rejection was completed and the animals had developed hyperglycemia. An adaption of the mixed lymphocyte response (MLR) called the mixed lymphocyte islet coculture (MLIC) has been used to investigate human islet immunogenicity in human islet transplants (35). Using intact exocrine-free human islets as stimulators and

Table 4. Summary of T Cell Assays on PBM Cells from IDDM Patients Receiving Human Fetal Islet Transplants

Patient	Antigen (Pre-transplant)	Antigen (Post-transplant)
1.	Adult Islet	Adult/Fetal/Tumor
		Adult/Fetal/Tumor
2.	Adult Islet	Adult/Fetal Islet
3.	Adult/Fetal Islet	Adult/Fetal/Spleen/Tumor
4,5.	Adult/Fetal/Spleen	Adult/Fetal/Spleen
6,7.	Adult/Fetal/Spleen	

HLA-mismatched peripheral blood lymphocytes as responders a strong proliferative response was observed. In contrast, HLA matching of the islets and lymphocytes resulted in very little proliferative responses. These results suggest that assays capable of detecting the autoreactive or alloreactive T cells would be of great value.

In collaboration with Dr. Lois Jovanovic-Peterson, Kieran Healy, and Dr. Karen Braun at Sansum Medical Research Foundation, Santa Barbara, CA, we have been assaying the T cell responses of IDDM patients undergoing islet cell transplants using cellular immunoblotting. We have been applying this technique to investigate the islet cell specific PBM responses of IDDM patients receiving human fetal islet cell transplants. Adult human islet cell proteins, human fetal islet cell proteins, normal human spleen proteins, and proteins from a human osteosarcoma cell line have been used as antigens. Patients are assessed before transplant and at intervals after transplant. Table 4 lists the patients and antigens utilized for the individual assays to date. Preliminary data suggest that two patterns of T cell responses using cellular immunoblotting have been identified. After transplant with normal fetal islets, 2 patients had PBM cells that responded with an increased proliferative response to adult human islets, human fetal islets, normal spleen and/or tumor. The T cell responses to adult human islets before and after transplant of one of these two patients is shown in Figure 4. Figure 5 illustrates the same patient's T cell responses to human fetal islets and human osteosarcoma antigens post-transplant. In the other patients there is no increased T cell

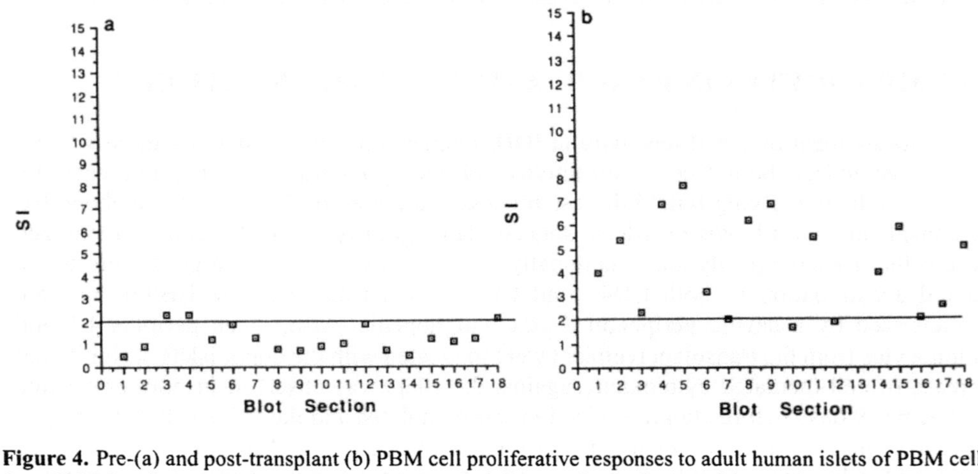

Figure 4. Pre-(a) and post-transplant (b) PBM cell proliferative responses to adult human islets of PBM cells from IDDM patient #1. Values represent means of triplicate cultures for each blot section and are shown as the stimulation index (SI). Positive responses are taken as 2SI as demonstrated by the solid line.

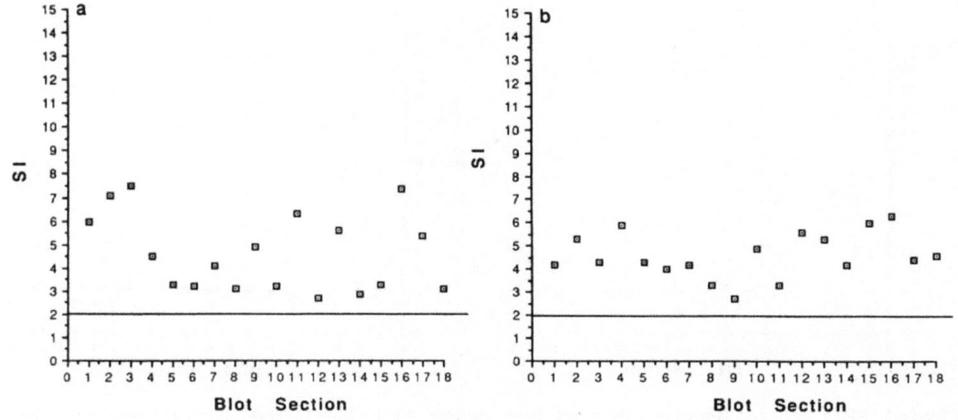

Figure 5. PBM cell proliferative responses from patient #1 to human fetal islet antigens (a) and human osteosarcoma cell antigens (b) post-transplant. Values represent means of triplicate cultures for each blot section and are shown as the stimulation index (SI). Positive responses are taken as 2SI as demonstrated by the solid line.

response either before or after transplantation to any of the antigens tested. T cell responses to human adult islet cells (Figure 6), and human fetal islets (Figure 7) from one of these patients pre- and post-transplant are illustrated. The T cell responses of the same patient post-transplant to human osteosarcoma antigens are shown in Figure 8.

The preliminary T cell data from the transplant recipients suggests that it may be possible to follow the reactivation of the autoimmune destructive process occurring in the islet transplant recipients by observing the T cell responses from the patients to the adult and fetal islet antigen preparations. The use of the normal human spleen and/or human osteosarcoma antigens may allow for us to identify an alloreactive response occurring in the patients that are rejecting their transplants. More patients need to be followed for longer periods of time in order to determine if this hypothesis is valid. Also, the amount of transplanted tissue and the number of donors which may influence the T cell response must be taken into

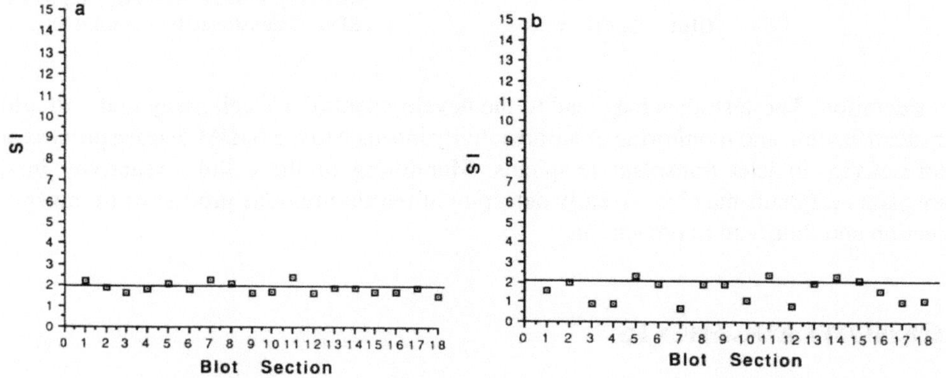

Figure 6. PBM cell proliferative responses from IDDM patient #3 to human adult islet antigens pre- (a) and post-transplant (b). Values represent means of triplicate cultures for each blot section and are shown as the stimulation index (SI). Positive responses are taken as 2SI as demonstrated by the solid line.

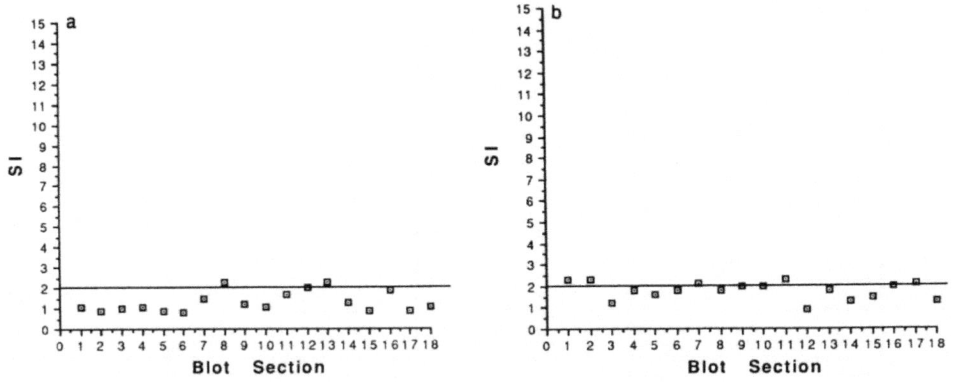

Figure 7. PBM cell proliferative responses from patient #3 to human fetal islet antigens pre- (a) and post-transplant (b). Values represent means of triplicate cultures for each blot section and are shown as the stimulation index (SI). Positive responses are taken as 2SI as demonstrated by the solid line.

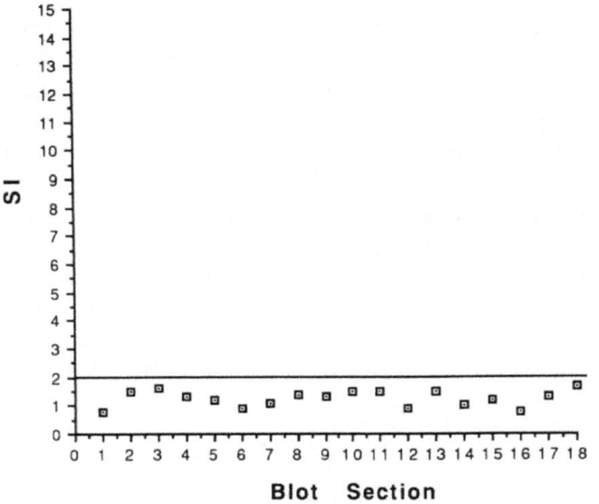

Figure 8. PBM cell proliferative responses from patient #3 to human osteosarcoma antigens post-transplant. Values represent means of triplicate cultures for each blot section and are shown as the stimulation index (SI). Positive responses are taken as 2SI as demonstrated by the solid line.

consideration. These studies may lead to the development of a T cell assay that will allow for identification and monitoring of autoreactivity intrinsic to the IDDM disease process and alloreactivity in islet transplant recipients. Monitoring of the cellular reactivity in the transplant recipients may lead to early detection of the autoimmune process or of transplant rejection and thus lead to prevention.

ACKNOWLEDGMENTS

This work was supported in part by a grant from the Medical Research Service of the Department of Veterans Affairs through a VA Merit Review grant and by National Institutes of Health (NIH) grants DK17047 and DK02456.

REFERENCES

1. Abbas AK, Lichtman AH, Pober JS. Immunity to tissue transplants, In: Cellular and Molecular Immunology. WB Saunders Co, Philadelpha AP 1991, 317-334.
2. Patarroyo M., Makgoba MW. Leucocyte adhesion to cells in immune and inflammatory responses. Lancet 1989, ii: 1139-41.
3. Heemann UW, Tullius SG, Azuma H., Kuprec-Weglinsky J., Tilney NL. Adhesion molecules and transplantation. Annals of Surgery 1994, 219: 4-12.
4. Lawrence MB, Springer TA. Leukocytes roll on a selectin at physiologyic flow rates: distinction from and prerequisite for adhesion through integrins. Cell 1991, 114: 181-217.
5. Bevilaequa MP, Stengelin S. Gimbrone MA Jr., Seed B. Endothelial leucocyte adhesion molecule 1: an inducible receptor for neutrophils related to complement regulatory proteins and lectins. Science 1989, 243: 1160-1165.
6. Smith CW, Kishimoto TK, Abbassi O, et al. Chemotactic factors regulate lectin adhesion molecule 1 (LECAM-1)-dependent neutrophil adhesion to cytokine-stimulated endothelial cells in vitro. J Clin Invest 1991, 87: 609-618.
7. Shimizu Y., Shaw S, Graber N. et al. Activation-independent binding of human memory T cells to adhesion molecule ELAM-1. Nature 1991, 349: 799-802.
8. Rose M., Page C, Hengstenberg C, Yacoub M. Immunocytochemical markers of activation in cardiac transplant rejection. Eur Heart J 1991, 12 (Suppl D): 147-150.
9. Moolenaar W, Bruijn JA, Schrama E, et al. T cell receptors and ICAM-1 expression in renal allografts during rejection. Transpl Int 1991, 4: 140-145.
10. Faull RJ, Russ GR. Tubular expression of intracellular adhesion molecule-1 during renal allograft rejection. Transplantation 1989, 48: 226-230.
11. David V, Leca G, Corvaia N, et al. Proliferation of resting lymphocytes is induced by triggering T cells through an epitope common to the three CD18/CD11 leucocyte adhesion molecules. Cell Immunol 1991, 136: 519-524.
12. Krensky AM. T cells in autoimmunity and allograft rejection. Kidney International 1994, 45(Suppl. 44): S50-56.
13. Krensky AM, Weiss A, Crabtree G, Davis MM, Parham P. T-lymphocyte-antigen interactions in transplantation rejection. N Eng J Med 1990, 322: 510-517.
14. Chandler C, Passaro E. Jr. Transplant rejection: Mechanisms and treatment. Arch Surg 1993, 128: 279-283
15. Barber WH, Mankin JA, Laskow DA, Drierhoi MH, Julian BA, Curtis JJ, Diethelm AG. Longterm results of a controlled prospective study with transfusion of donor-specific bone marrow in 57 cadaveric renal allograft recipients. Transplantation 1991; 51: 70-75.
16. Bottazzo GF, Dean BM, McNally JM, MacKay EH, Gamble RD. In situ characterizaton of autoimmune phenomena and expression of HLA molecules in pancreas in diabetic insulitis. N Eng J Med 1985, 313: 353-360.
17. Palmer JP. Predicting IDDM. Use of humoral immune markers. Diabetes Reviews 1993, 1: 104-115.
18. Hegewald MJ, Schoenfeld SL, McCulloch DK, Greenbaum DJ, Klaff LJ, Palmer JP. Increased specificity and sensitivity of insulin autoantibody measurements in autoimmune thyroid disease and type 1 diabetes. J Immunol Method 1992, 1154: 61-68.
19. Greenbaum DJ, Brooks-Worrell BM, Palmer JP, Lernmark A. Autoimmuntiy and prediction of insulin dependent diabetes mellitus. In: Diabetes Annual 8, Marshall SM, Home PD, eds., Elsevier Science BV 1994, in press.
20. Neifing JL, Greenbaum CJ, Kahn SK, McCulloch DK, Barmeier H, Lernmark A, Palmer JP. Prospective evaluation of beta cell function in insulin autoantibody-positive relatives of insulin-dependent diabetic patients. Metabolism 1993, 42: 482-486.
21. Ziegler A, Aiegler R, Vardi P, Jackson R, Soeldner R, Soeldner J, Eisenbarth G. Lifetable analysis of progression to diabetes of anti-insulin autoantibody-positive relatives of individuals with type 1 diabetes. Diabetes 1989, 38: 1320-1325.
22. Nepom GT. MHC Class II molecules and autoimmunity. Ann Rev Immunol 1991, 9: 493-525.
23. Dallmann MJ, Shiho O., Page TH, Wood KJ, Morris PJ. Peripheral tolerance to alloantigen results from altered regulation of the interleukin-2 pathway. J Exp Med 1991, 173: 79-87.
24. Anasetti C, Tan P, Hansen JA, Martin PJ. Induction of specific unresponsiveness in unprimed human T cells by anti-CD3 antibody and alloantigen. J Exp Med 1990, 172: 1691-1700.
25. Bieg S., Tailyes EM, Yassin N., Amann J, Herberg L, McGregor AM, Scherbaum WA, Banga JP. A multiplicity of protein antigens in subcellular fractions of rat insulinoma tissue are able to stimulate T cells obtained from non-obese diabetic mice. Diabetologia 1993, 36: 385-390.

26. Gelber C, Paborsky L, Singer S, McAteer D, Tisch R, Jolicoeur C, Buelow R, McDivitt H, Garrison Fathman C. Isolation of nonobese diabetic mouse T-cells that recognize novel autoantigens involved in the early events of diabetes. Diabetes 1994, 43: 33-39.
27. Bretzel RG, Alejandro R, Hering BJ, Van Suylichem PTR, Ricordi C. Clinical islet transplantation: guidelines for islet quality control. Transplant Proceed 1994, 26: 388-392.
28. Dubernard JM, Martin X, Lefrancois N, Cloix P, Brunet M. Technical aspects of pancreas transplantation. Transplant Proceed 1994, 26: 384-385.
29. Hering BJ, Browtzki CC, Schultz AO, Bretzel RG, Federlin K. Islet transplant registry report on adult and fetal islet allografts. Transplant Proceed 1994, 26(2): 565-568.
30. Warren HS, Simeonovic CJ, Dixon JE et al. Transplant Proceed 1986, 18: 310.
31. Hao L, WangY, Gill RG. et al. Transplant Proceed 1989, 21: 2697.
32. Lafferty KJ, Hao L. Approaches to the prevention of immune destruction of transplanted pancreatic islets. Transplant Proceed 1994, 26: 399-400.
33. Christiansen E, Tibell A, Groth CG, Rasmussen K, Pedersen O, Burcharth F, Christensen NJ, Volund A, Madsbad S, and the Danish-Swedish study group of metabolic effect of pancreas transplantation. Limitations in the use of insulin or C-peptide alone in the assessment of beta-cell function in pancreas transplant recipients. Transplant Proceed 1994, 26: 467-468.
34. Kuttler B, Wanka H, Hahn HJ. Cell-mediated cytotoxicity of peripheral lymphocytes as a new approach to early diagnosis of ongoing allograft rejection. Transplant Proceed 1994, 26: 731-731.
35. Swift SM, Rose Sh, London NJM, James RFL. Standardization of the human mixed lymphocytes islet coculture. Transplant Proceed 1994, 26: 732.

14

NETWORKING FOR THE COLLECTION OF FETAL ISLET TISSUES

Leatrice Ducat and Jane S. Schultz

The National Disease Research Interchange
Philadelphia, Pennsylvania 19103

INTRODUCTION

Growing social pressure to reduce the dependency on animal models in research and the increased difficulty in obtaining tissues locally has prompted scientists to look vigorously for a reliable source of experimental materials. The Human Tissue and Organ Resource for Research (HTOR) program of the National Disease Research Interchange (NDRI) is positioned to meet the demand for alternative resources.

HISTORY OF NDRI

In 1984, NDRI was a fledgling prototype known as the National Diabetes Research Interchange, established with a grant from the Pew Charitable Trusts of Philadelphia and operated as a program of the Juvenile Diabetes Foundation. Scientists recognized the importance of this resource to provide the basic human materials they would need to transition their research on diabetes and related disorders from the laboratory to the clinic. Their interest and support prompted NDRI to establish the first national clinical trials on human islet cell transplantation. Since 1984 more than 78 islet cell researchers have received more than 2300 adult pancreata.

NDRI has distributed nearly 80,000 samples of human cells, tissues and organs to nearly 2000 investigators since its inception, impacting researchers on both a national and international scale. In 1993 alone, NDRI collected and distributed nearly 11,000 tissues and organs of many varieties, in addition to 715 cell lines and 2757 aliquots of DNA distributed through its Human Biological Data Interchange (HBDI) program. Since 1989, NDRI has received funding from NIH's National Center for Research Resources (NCRR).

For diseases related to the aging process and other neurological and degenerative disorders where no animal models exist, the NDRI is often the only resource available to researchers. New technologies have helped make human tissues and cells increasingly viable tools for understanding the molecular basis of disease and for performing various types of genetic, biochemical and immunological analyses, thereby increasing the need for a reproducible and economic source of human biomaterials.

Fetal Islet Transplantation
Edited by C. M. Peterson, L. Jovanovic-Peterson, and B. Formby, Plenum Press, New York, 1995

The importance of using human tissue to understand human disease has been underscored through the growing and increasingly widespread use of the HTOR resource. NDRI has successfully recruited researchers at the rate of approximately 20% per year. Researchers in 41 states, Canada, Puerto Rico and Europe have received usable tissues and organs from the HTOR/NDRI program. Tissues in great demand include lung, liver, heart, and kidney from potential organ donors which cannot be used for transplantation. Tissues from diseased donors have included those with diabetes, glaucoma, atherosclerosis, sickle cell anemia, cerebral palsy, and schizophrenia.

Eye and tissue banks, hospitals and organ procurement organizations in 40 states now provide specimens from surgery, autopsy, and heart beating cadavers to NDRI. Preservation methods available include a variety of fixation techniques, such as fresh, frozen, snap frozen and ornithine carbamyl transferase cryomolds.

In 1984 NDRI began a program of fetal pancreas procurement in order to supply a source of these organs for fetal islet isolation, preparation and experimental transplantation for the treatment of type I diabetes. The program began in February of 1984 and rose to a high of 140 pancreata in the month of May, 1985. In 1984, 447 fetal pancreata were collected followed by 1155 in 1985, 1663 in 1886 and 1457 in 1987 for a four year total of 4722 tissues collected for 15 research groups.

Late in 1987 a moratorium on the use of fetal tissue obtained by induced abortion for therapeutic purposes was declared by the executive branch of the federal government. Collection of fetal tissue from induced abortuses by many reputable agencies ceased after the moratorium was declared because research utilizing fetal tissue obtained in this manner could no longer be funded by a federal government agency. But, since prior studies had demonstrated that research using fetal tissue was extremely important in the development of treatments for a number of serious diseases including diabetes, a presidential decision was made to support a network of centers to serve as human fetal tissue resources using tissue obtained from spontaneous abortions and ectopic pregnancies. The current administration was committed to developing these centers for scientific studies. The NDRI submitted a proposal the long term objective of which was to enhance the ability of the NDRI to serve as a primary participant in a national network of human fetal tissue banks depending entirely on tissue from the sources described above. These tissues were to be retrieved in a viable fashion and subsequently preserved, and stored, in a second phase, distributed throughout the Untied States as high quality, well characterized tissue for use in research and human transplantation therapy. The first phase granting period ran from September 1992 to September 1993.

With the expert assistance of Dr. Michael McCormack, coinvestigator on its grant application, NDRI began working with hospitals in the greater Philadelphia area, (Hospital of the University or Pennsylvania and Thomas Jefferson Hospital) and affiliates of the University of Medicine and Dentistry of New Jersey (Kennedy Memorial Hospitals: Stratford Division and Washington Township Division). Other institutions were later added to the network. Collected tissue was restricted to fetuses from 5 to 16 weeks gestation. Anticipated difficulties in collection of suitable tissues included the fact that many spontaneous abortions occur outside of the hospital and those tissues are frequently autolyzed or necrotic. Tissues may also be rendered unusable because of infection or improper handling. Ectopic pregnancies are often treated medically rather then surgically so that, in many cases, no tissue is available from this source.

The results of the studies supported the veracity of the anticipated difficulties. A total of 357 events were tracked by the NDRI staff, 285 spontaneous abortions and 72 ectopic pregnancies. Products of conception (333, POCs) were retrieved but only 13 potential usable fetuses were among them (one ectopic pregnancy and 12 spontaneous abortions). All specimens were examined to determine gestational age and to identify structural abnormalities and obvious necrosis. Histologic examination and cytogenetic testing were also carried out. However, the major research question to be answered by this study was the viability for transplantation of pancreatic cells which were obtained from these specimens. Dr. Alberto Hayek (University of California, San Diego) evaluated the tissue viability and found that only one specimen was viable pancreatic cells which could possibly be used for transplantation. There was also one viable central nervous system tissue. However, non-sterile procurement, as well as lack of serological testing and donor consent for transplantation obviated any transplant experimentation. Of 86 total tissues retrieved, six were cytogenically tested and two were abnormal. Most of the 231 rejected specimens contained no discernible fetal tissues. It was clear from this study that spontaneous abortuses and ectopic pregnancies would not serve as alternatives to tissue from induced abortuses for either research or therapeutic purposes. The second phase of the study was canceled because of lack of funding.

PRESENT CONSTRAINTS ON USE OF FETAL TISSUE

In January 1993 President Clinton lifted the funding moratorium imposed by previous administrations on "research involving the transplantation of fetal tissue from induced abortions"(1). Although this event would, on the surface, seem to have completely removed the barriers to use of fetal tissue from induced abortions for transplantation research, this is not entirely true. There is still a series of regulations written into the Public Law which govern the use of this tissue for the stated purpose.

The rules which were included in Public Law are as follows:

1. The research being conducted must serve a therapeutic purpose. (What is the definition of therapeutic? Is experimental transplantation to determine the fate of cells, for example, to be considered therapeutic per se?)
2. The mother must agree to the tissue's transplantation research use but must not know the identity of the recipient.
3. The physician must state that consent for abortion was obtained before the consent to donate tissue and that the timing, method or procedure for terminating the pregnancy have not been altered for the purpose of obtaining suitable research tissue. He/She must also state that the abortion has been carried out in accordance with state law, that the mother has been informed of medical risks, risks to privacy and any interest the physician has in the research.
4. The recipient researcher must state that he/she is aware that the tissue is human fetal tissue, was donated for research purposes and may have been obtained following abortion or stillbirth and must supply this information to anyone else involved in the research. The researcher must further guarantee that he or she has had no part in the decision to terminate the pregnancy.
5. If the fetal tissue is to be used for transplantation, the transplant recipient must state that he/she has been informed of the source of the tissue and how the fetus died.
6. All pertinent state laws must be observed.

PRESENT POSITION OF NDRI WITH RESPECT TO FETAL TISSUE

Since NDRI's activities relative to fetal tissue collection have been centered around the states of New Jersey and Pennsylvania, the laws of these states with respect to fetal tissue were reviewed. New Jersey has no laws which specifically address human fetal tissue research, nor did 24 other states as of May, 1990. Pennsylvania's law (2) permits the use of fetal tissue for therapeutic research with certain caveats: appropriate donor consent is obtained after the decision to have an abortion has been made, sale of tissue is prohibited, and the donor may not designate the recipient of the tissue. In 1990 ten other states had laws similar to Pennsylvania's. At that time six states, including California, permitted research using fetal tissue with some restrictions and eight states had outright prohibitions against the use of fetal tissue for research.

Additional complications are presented by the issuance of the report of a Presidential panel which has been meeting since February of 1994 (released September 1994) which contains new policy for the use of *embryonic* tissue for research. It is expected that the latter policy will become national policy. Moreover, what is permissible in the use of embryonic tissue for research, while substantively similar to what is permissible for the use of fetal tissue, differs in one important aspect: the age until which the organism may be used. Since the major differences between fetal tissue and embryonic tissue is implantation status, the nature of the legal distinction in unclear as are the reasons for the different regulations which apply to each. For this reason, the rationale for the regulatory distinction might well be questioned in the future.

The September 27, 1994 policy recommendation of the Human Embryo Panel applies to policies governing preimplantation embryos i.e. ova fertilized in vitro that have never been transferred or implanted in a uterus. The sense of this report is that it is acceptable public policy to provide federal funding for research involving human embryos if the research follows stringent guidelines. In general these guidelines state that the researcher must be scientifically qualified, that clear scientific of clinical benefit could be attributed to the research, that the research design be valid, that there be adequate preliminary studies and a minimal sample number, that informed consent and IRB approval be obtained, that there be no sale or purchase of tissue, that there be "equality of samples and benefits among population subgroups"(3) and that research not be permitted beyond 14 days gestation. The discussion among the meeting participants raised several additional points, among them the advisability that a special review committee, similar to the Recombinant DNA Advisory Committee, be formed which would review research protocols, that the permissible embryo age for research be extended to the time of onset of closure of the neural tube (18 days) and that research involving the development of embryotic stem cells from embryos fertilized especially for this purpose be permitted. In spite of the latter recommendation, President Clinton has instructed government agencies not to fund research on embryos which are solely created for research purposes but to limit funding to research using embryos "left over" from in vitro fertilization.

In would seem that placing an age limit of 18 days beyond which human embryos resulting from in vitro fertilization could not be used for research is inconsistent with permitting research on induced abortuses up to approximately 16 weeks gestation or at least until the tissues in question have differentiated.

These grey legal areas have caused NDRI to very carefully review the ethical/legal question involving networking the collection and distribution of human fetal islet cells and other human fetal tissues. Our legal advisors feel that proceeding with this effort is consistent with current regulations. The NDRI steering committee has also strongly urged NDRI to resume fetal tissue collection and distribution. However, no funding for the specific and specialized collection necessary for a fetal tissue initiative appears to be forthcoming from federal agencies. NDRI, therefore, needs the continuing advice of the research community, to insure that collection of these valuable research materials proceeds in a manner consistent with the standards of NDRI.

REFERENCES

1. Public Law 42 u.s.c. 289 g-2
2. Pa. C.S.A. 3216
3. Major Conclusions and Recommendations from the Final Report of the NIH Embryo Research Panel, September 27, 1994. Prepared by the Washington Fax.

15

CONSENSUS SESSION SUMMARY: SECOND INTERNATIONAL SYMPOSIUM ON FETAL ISLET TRANSPLANTATION

Paul E. Lacy, Moderator
Stellan Sandler, Alberto Hayek, Jerry Palmer, Section Chairs
Charles M. Peterson, Recording Secretary

The study of fetal pancreatic tissue is being pursued at a number of centers throughout the world. These studies are important not only because these tissues provide a potential source of insulin secreting cells for transplantation into persons with diabetes, but also because improved understanding of the growth, development, and immunology of fetal tissues will be of immense benefit to all who are trying to restore insulin secretory capacity for persons with diabetes mellitus. Because of the importance of the work, an attempt was made to achieve consensus in three areas. While consensus was not always achieved, there was agreement in a number of areas. The following summarizes the areas of agreement as well as identifies those areas where further work and definition were felt to be required.

CRITERIA FOR SCREENING OF FETAL TISSUE PRIOR TO TRANSPLANTATION

There was agreement that maternal blood needs to be analyzed and screened prior to transplantation of fetal pancreatic tissue. The tests that were recommended to be performed on maternal serum included screening for antibodies against human immunodeficiency virus (HIV), hepatitis A, B, and C and an IgM antibody test against cytomegalovirus (CMV). The consent process for such testing as well as the communication of test results vary among centers. Further consensus development in these areas would be helpful. An elevated maternal IgG but low IgM level against CMV was not felt to be a contraindication to use of the tissue. The desirable goal of developing polymerase chain reaction assays for these diseases was emphasized. Such testing could replace the above methods if sensitivity, specificity and comparisons with a standard method can be shown.

Testing for syphilis, herpes simplex II, rubella and toxoplasmosis has been performed at some centers. The general feeling was that in view of the low yield and/or threat from these pathogens, these forms of testing should not be mandatory.

Donor exclusion based on the presence of underlying disease was also felt not to be necessary. Specifically maternal insulin-dependent diabetes (IDDM), non-insulin-dependent

Fetal Islet Transplantation
Edited by C. M. Peterson, L. Jovanovic-Peterson, and B. Formby, Plenum Press, New York, 1995

diabetes (NIDDM), and gestational diabetes (GDM) were not felt to be contraindications to the use of fetal tissue from these gestations. Likewise the use of fetal tissue known to contain genetic abnormalities such as trisomy or hemoglobinopathies was not felt to be contraindicated. The one indication for historical source screening would be to avoid the use of tissue from a maternal source who had received pituitary hormones of cadaver origin such as growth hormone, follicular stimulating hormone, or luteinizing hormone. These latter maternal sources should be avoided. Tissue obtained from spontaneous abortions has been found to be rarely, if ever, suitable for transplantation studies.

The tissue itself needs to be screened for bacterial and fungal contamination prior to transplantation. Such screening should include testing for mycoplasma as well as for routine pathogenic bacteria and fungi.

The development of tissue banks for fetal pancreatic tissue is important. These resources will not only provide for the potentially advantageous HLA and blood group matching of tissue to recipient, but also will allow more time for extensive testing for potential pathogens. Even with cryopreservation, complete matching would be difficult especially as multiple donors will probably be necessary.

Determination of viability of tissue prior to transplantation was recommended. The most useful form of viability testing was felt to be a validation of insulin secretory capacity. These tests are usually performed as static batch incubations. In the case of cryopreserved tissue, the optimum time for secretory testing was felt to be after 24 hours following thawing. Most centers reported best results with cryopreservation of explants and development of islet like cell clusters or tissue fragments for transplantation after thawing. Thus it was felt that secretory screening prior to freezing as a predictor of tissue viability for transplantation would be less meaningful.

CRITERIA FOR EFFICACY OF A FETAL ISLET TRANSPLANT

Efficacy in islet transplantation was felt to comprise two categories: 1. Success and 2. Partial Success. For either form of success to be documented, careful evaluation of the recipient prior to the procedure is critical. Recipients with insulin-dependent diabetes mellitus need to be characterized in terms of C-peptide levels in the fasting state as well as following a provocative challenge that can be repeated at intervals following the transplant procedure. Insulin requirements are best expressed as units per kilogram. Reporting of insulin requirements is most meaningful when determined in an individual who has already achieved reasonable glucose control with a hemoglobin A_{1c} value around or below 7% (mean plasma glucose around 150 mg%) on an intensive management program.

"Transplant success" could be viewed as having occurred in a well characterized individual as noted above who had achieved insulin independence with a rise in C-peptide to the normal range and maintenance of normoglycemia with normal hemoglobin A_{1c} levels for one year. "Clinical success" evaluations need to include an assessment of adverse effects of the procedure as well as an evaluation of lifestyle changes. It was felt that biopsy evaluation of the graft in such a situation would be desirable but might be contravened by ethical or humanistic constraints.

Documentation of partial transplant success requires more rigorous evaluation of the recipient. Partial success could be defined as a 50% or greater decrement in insulin requirement and an increase in C-peptide values exceeding 3 fold the standard deviation of the baseline assay result. In view of the importance of the C-peptide values, the development of a centralized C-peptide assay facility was encouraged. An alternative to centralized C-peptide assays is to characterize each assay by documenting the limit of sensitivity and intra- and inter-assay coefficients of variation of the assay in the range(s) of the published data. For documentation of partial success, the importance of a biopsy demonstrating insulin containing tissue at the implantation site increases.

Because documentation of partial success is more difficult than success as defined above, control groups were considered. Most participants felt that inclusion of a control group was difficult unless the procedure were completely benign. Furthermore, protocols resulting in "partial success" might be best viewed as feasibility studies that indicate that further protocol development is needed. Thus the priority was felt to be to improve protocols that provide partial success with an eye toward achieving success in increasing numbers rather than to design extensive controlled trials at the stage of partial success. The need for immunosuppressive therapy was raised. Many felt that this was necessary, but no consensus was reached.

The availability of the Diabetes Control and Complications Trial (DCCT), while not providing a true control group, was felt to be helpful (1). Trials of transplantation leading to improved glycemia could use the DCCT results to evaluate potential toxicity with respect to hypoglycemia and weight gain. In addition, trials that may incorporate factors designed to facilitate tissue growth or vascularization or immunomodulation may find the cumulative incidence data of eye, kidney, and neural pathology from the DCCT useful as a benchmark.

IMMUNOLOGIC SURVEILLANCE OF RECIPIENTS

The development of assays for the evaluation of the autoimmune as well as allograft response to implanted fetal tissue was felt to be an important area. Development of benign means of retrieving tissue during the hyperacute rejection period or first month following implantation is also important to define the immunolgic response of the recipient.

At the present time, antibody studies of the recipient are most feasible. Whether and to what extent recipients develop antibodies to major histocompatibility antigens, blood group proteins (A,B,O or Rh), or islet cell antibodies remains to be determined in clinical trials to date.

Studies of T cell responses are in a stage of development. Development and evaluation of T cell assays such as limiting dilution assays, mixed lymphocyte islet co-culture systems, or cellular immunoblotting for specific or nonspecific immune responses are needed. These approaches will be important to correlate immune response with graft survival or rejection.

FUTURE DIRECTIONS

There was a general appreciation of the remarkable progress being made in studies of the fetal pancreas. The field is moving rapidly on a number of fronts ranging from genetics, cell biology, immunology, and embryology to transplantation. Such explosive growth makes it especially important that investigators have a forum to share findings, achieve consensus, and identify areas that require further work.

REFERENCE

1. Diabetes Control and Complications Trial Research Group. The effect of intensive treatment of diabetes on the development and progression of long term complications in insulin dependent diabetes mellitus. New Eng J Med 329:977-986, 1993.

CONTRIBUTORS

Tausif Alam, Ph.D.
Department of Surgery
University of Wisconsin
H4/749 CSC
600 Highland Ave
Madison, WI 53792

Arne Andersson, M.D., Ph.D.
Department of Medical Cell Biology
Uppsala University
Biomedicum, P. O. Box 571
S-751 23 Uppsala, Sweden

Gillian M. Beattie
The Islet Research Laboratory at The Whittier Institute
Department of Pediatrics
The University of California, San Diego
School of Medicine, 9894 Genesee Avenue
La Jolla, CA 92037

Wendy Bevier, Ph.D.
Sansum Medical Research Foundation
2219 Bath Street
Santa Barbara, California 93105

Barbara Brooks-Worrell, Ph.D.
Veterans Affairs Medical Center and
University of Washington, Seattle, Washington
Veterans Affairs Medical Center
Endocrinology (111)
1660 S. Columbian Way
Seattle WA 98108

Hui Min Chen, Ph.D.
Sansum Medical Research Foundation
2219 Bath Street
Santa Barbara, California 93105

Wei-Ping Dong
Diabetes Research Laboratory
Shanghai First People's Hospital
Shanghai Medical University
190 North Suzhou Road
Shanghai 200085
The People's Republic of China

Leatrice Ducat
National Disease Research Interchange
1880 John F. Kennedy Boulevard 6th Floor
Philadelphia, PA 19103

Jean Falzone
Sansum Medical Research Foundation
2219 Bath Street
Santa Barbara, California 93105

Gyula Farkas, M.D., Ph.D.
Department of Surgery
Albert Szent-Györgyi Medical University
Szeged
P. O. Box 464, H-6701
Hungary

Bent Formby, Ph.D., D.Sc.
Sansum Medical Research Foundation
2219 Bath Street
Santa Barbara, California, USA

Alberto Hayek, M.D.
The Islet Research Laboratory at The Whittier Institute
Department of Pediatrics
The University of California, San Diego
School of Medicine
9894 Genesee Avenue
La Jolla, CA 92037

Claes Hellerström, M.D., Ph.D.
Department of Medical Cell Biology, Uppsala University
Biomedicum, P. O. Box 571
S-751 23 Uppsala, Sweden

Yuan-Feng Hu, M.D.
Diabetes Research Laboratory
Shanghai First People's Hospital
Shanghai Medical University
190 North Suzhou Road
Shanghai 200085
The People's Republic of China

Debra A. Hullett, Ph.D.
Department of Surgery
University of Wisconsin
H4/749 CSC
600 Highland Ave
Madison, WI 53792

Leif Jansson, M.D., Ph.D.
Department of Medical Cell Biology
Uppsala University
Biomedicum, P. O. Box 571
S-751 23 Uppsala, Sweden

Lois Jovanovic-Peterson, M.D.
Sansum Medical Research Foundation
2219 Bath Street
Santa Barbara, California 93105

Barbara E.K. Klein, M.D., MPH
Department of Ophthalmology and Visual Sciences
University of Wisconsin Medical School
Madison, Wisconsin 53792-3220

Ronald Klein, M.D., M.P.H.
Department of Ophthalmology and Visual Sciences
University of Wisconsin Medical School
Madison, Wisconsin 53792-3220

Paul E. Lacy, M.D., M. Sc., Ph.D.
Department of Pathology
Washington University School of Medicine
Euclid Ave and Kingshighway Department of Pathology
St Louis, MO 63110-1093

Yu Li
Diabetes Research Laboratory
Shanghai First People's Hospital
Shanghai Medical University
190 North Suzhou Road
Shanghai 200085
The People's Republic of China

Sheng Loh
Sansum Medical Research Foundation
2219 Bath Street
Santa Barbara, California 93105

Debra A. MacKenzie, Ph.D.
Department of Surgery
University of Wisconsin
H4/749 CSC
600 Highland Ave
Madison, WI 53792

Scot E. Moss, M.A.
Department of Ophthalmology and Visual Sciences
University of Wisconsin Medical School
Madison, Wisconsin 53792-3220

Yoko Mullen, M.D., Ph.D.
Department of Surgery
University of California at Los Angeles
and VA Medical Center, West Los Angeles
Diabetes Research Center
675 Cirle Drive South
Los Angeles, CA 90024-7036

Jerry Palmer, M.D.
Veterans Affairs Medical Center and
University of Washington, Seattle, Washington
Veterans Affairs Medical Center
Endocrinology (111)
1660 S. Columbian Way
Seattle, WA 98108

Charles M. Peterson, M.D.
Sansum Medical Research Foundation
2219 Bath Street
Santa Barbara, California 93105

Richard B. Pearce, Ph.D.
Sansum Medical Research Foundation
2219 Bath Street
Santa Barbara, California 93105

Margaret Rose, Ph.D.
Department of Surgery
Prince Henry Hosptial
Sydney, New South Wales 2036
Australia

Navid Salari-Lak, M.Sc. Pharm.
Department of Medical Cell Biology
Uppsala University
Biomedicum, P. O. Box 571
S-751 23 Uppsala, Sweden

Jan-Olov Sandberg, M.Sc. Pharm.
Department of Medical Cell Biology
Uppsala University
Biomedicum, P. O. Box 571
S-751 23 Uppsala, Sweden

Stellan Sandler, M.D., Ph.D.
Department of Medical Cell Biology
Uppsala University
Biomedicum, P. O. Box 571
S-751 23 Uppsala, Sweden

Jane S. Schulz, Ph.D.
National Disease Research Interchange
1880 John F. Kennedy Boulevard 6th Floor
Philadelphia, PA 19103

Ann M. Simpson, Ph.D.
Department of Endocrinolgy
Prince of Wales Hospital
Randwick, Sydney
New South Wales 2031
Australia

Murray S.R. Smith, Ph.D., M.H.P. Ed.
School of Anatomy
The University of New South Wales
Sydney, New South Wales 2052
Australia

Hans W. Sollinger M.D., Ph.D.
Department of Surgery
University of Wisconsin
H4/749 CSC
600 Highland Ave
Madison, WI 53792

Patrick Soon-Shiong, M.D.
Islet Transplant Center
St. Vincents Medical Center
Los Angeles, CA 90404

Jian Tu, M.D.
Department of Endocrinolgy
Prince of Wales Hospital
Randwick, Sydney
New South Wales 2031
Australia

Bernard E. Tuch, F.R.A.C.P., Ph.D.
Department of Endocrinolgy
Prince of Wales Hospital
Randwick, Sydney
New South Wales 2031
Australia

Liberty Walker, B.A., M.A.
Sansum Medical Research Foundation
2219 Bath Street
Santa Barbara, California 93105

Yu-Fei Wang, Ph.B.
Diabetes Research Laboratory
Shanghai First People's Hospital
Shanghai Medical University
190 North Suzhou Road, Shanghai 200085
The People's Republic of China

Patrick Waugh, B.Sc.
School of Anatomy
The University of New South Wales
Sydney, New South Wales 2052
Australia

Anthony J. Weinhaus, B.Sc.
Department of Endocrinolgy
Prince of Wales Hospital
Randwick
New South Wales 2031
Australia

Alison Okada Wollitzer, Ph.D.
Sansum Medical Research Foundation
2219 Bath Street
Santa Barbara, California 93105

Jing-Juan Xu, Ph.D.
Diabetes Research Laboratory
Shanghai First People's Hospital
Shanghai Medical University
190 North Suzhou Road, Shanghai 200085
The People's Republic of China

Hong-De Zhang, M.D.
Diabetes Research Laboratory
Shanghai First People's Hospital
Shanghai Medical University
190 North Suzhou Road, Shanghai 200085
The People's Republic of China

Sheng-Rong Zhong, Ph.B.
Diabetes Research Laboratory
Shanghai First People's Hospital
Shanghai Medical University
190 North Suzhou Road
Shanghai 200085
The People's Republic of China

INDEX

MIX
Papier aus verantwortungsvollen Quellen
Paper from responsible sources
FSC® C105338

If you have any concerns about our products,
you can contact us on
ProductSafety@springernature.com

In case Publisher is established outside the EU,
the EU authorized representative is:
Springer Nature Customer Service Center GmbH
Europaplatz 3, 69115 Heidelberg, Germany

Printed by Libri Plureos GmbH
in Hamburg, Germany